# CONTENTS

| | | |
|---|---|---|
| **GUIDELINE DEVELOPMENT GROUP MEMBERS** | | **5** |
| **ACKNOWLEDGEMENTS** | | **7** |
| **1** | **PREFACE** | **8** |
| | 1.1 National clinical guidelines | 8 |
| | 1.2 The national common mental health disorders guideline | 11 |
| **2** | **COMMON MENTAL HEALTH DISORDERS** | **13** |
| | 2.1 Introduction | 13 |
| | 2.2 The disorders | 14 |
| | 2.3 Treatment | 31 |
| | 2.4 Identification, assessment and pathways to care | 34 |
| **3** | **METHODS USED TO DEVELOP THIS GUIDELINE** | **41** |
| | 3.1 Overview | 41 |
| | 3.2 The scope | 41 |
| | 3.3 The guideline development group | 42 |
| | 3.4 Review questions | 43 |
| | 3.5 Systematic clinical literature review | 44 |
| | 3.6 Health economic methods | 51 |
| | 3.7 From evidence to recommendations | 55 |
| | 3.8 Stakeholder contributions | 56 |
| | 3.9 Validation of the guideline | 57 |
| **4** | **ACCESS TO HEALTHCARE** | **58** |
| | 4.1 Introduction | 58 |
| | 4.2 Factors affecting access | 60 |
| | 4.3 Adapting models of service delivery and therapeutic interventions | 69 |
| | 4.4 Service developments and interventions specifically designed to promote access | 76 |
| | 4.5 Recommendations | 89 |
| **5** | **CASE IDENTIFICATION AND FORMAL ASSESSMENT** | **91** |
| | 5.1 Introduction | 91 |
| | 5.2 Case identification | 92 |
| | 5.3 Formal assessment of the nature and severity of common mental health disorders | 119 |
| | 5.4 Recommendations | 133 |

*Contents*

**6 FURTHER ASSESSMENT OF RISK AND NEED FOR TREATMENT, AND ROUTINE OUTCOME MONITORING**    **136**
6.1   Introduction   136
6.2   Risk assessment   136
6.3   Factors that predict treatment response   143
6.4   Routine outcome monitoring   180

**7 SYSTEMS FOR ORGANISING AND DEVELOPING LOCAL CARE PATHWAYS**    **188**
7.1   Introduction   188
7.2   Clinical evidence review   190
7.3   Health economic evidence   211
7.4   From evidence to recommendations   212
7.5   Recommendations   213

**8 SUMMARY OF RECOMMENDATIONS**    **215**
8.1   Improving access to services   215
8.2   Stepped care   217
8.3   Step 1: identification and assessment   217
8.4   Steps 2 and 3: treatment and referral for treatment   222
8.5   Developing local care pathways   227

**9 APPENDICES**    **230**

**10 REFERENCES**    **277**

**11 GLOSSARY**    **303**

**12 ABBREVIATIONS**    **308**

# COMMON MENTAL HEALTH DISORDERS

## IDENTIFICATION AND PATHWAYS TO CARE

**National Clinical Guideline Number 123**

**National Colla**borative Centre for Mental **Health**

*commissioned by the*

**National Insti**tute for **Clinical Excel**lence

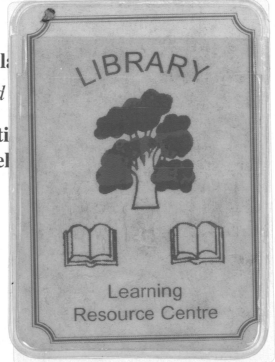

*published by*
**The British Psychological Society and The Royal College of Psychiatrists**

**British Library Cataloguing-in-Publication Data**

A catalogue record for this book is available from the British Library.

ISBN-: 978-1-908020-31-4

Printed in Great Britain by Stanley L. Hunt (Printers) Ltd.

Additional material: data CD-Rom created by Pix18 (www.pix18.co.uk)

| | |
|---|---|
| *developed by* | National Collaborating Centre for Mental Health<br>The Royal College of Psychiatrists<br>4th Floor, Standon House<br>21 Mansell Street<br>London<br>E1 8AA<br>www.nccmh.org.uk |
| *commissioned by* | National Institute for Health and Clinical Excellence<br>MidCity Place, 71 High Holborn<br>London<br>WC1V 6NA<br>www.nice.org.uk |
| *published by* | The British Psychological Society<br>St Andrews House<br>48 Princess Road East<br>Leicester<br>LE1 7DR<br>www.bps.org.uk |

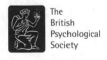

*and*

The Royal College of Psychiatrists
17 Belgrave Square
London
SW1X 8PG
www.rcpsych.ac.uk

# GUIDELINE DEVELOPMENT GROUP MEMBERS

**Professor Tony Kendrick (Chair)**
Professor of Primary Care and Dean, Hull York Medical School; General
Practitioner, Hull Primary Care Trust

**Professor Stephen Pilling (Facilitator)**
Director, National Collaborating Centre for Mental Health (NCCMH); Director,
Centre for Outcomes Research and Effectiveness, University College London

**Mr Mike Bessant**
Mental Health Nurse, Regional Mental Health Lead, NHS Direct, Bristol

**Ms Mary Burd**
Head of Psychology and Counselling (until December 2009), Tower Hamlets
Primary Care Trust

**Dr Alan Cohen**
Director of Primary Care, West London Mental Health Trust; National Primary Care
Advisor, Improving Access to Psychological Therapies, Department of Health

**Dr Barbara Compitus**
General Practitioner, Southville, Bristol

**Ms Lillian Dimas**
Service user and carer member

**Ms Beth Dumonteil**
Project Manager (2009 to 2010), NCCMH

**Mr David Ekers**
Nurse Consultant, Primary Care Mental Health, Tees Esk and Wear Valleys NHS
Foundation Trust; Honorary Clinical Lecturer, Centre for Mental Health Research,
Durham University

**Professor Linda Gask**
Professor of Primary Care Psychiatry, University of Manchester, and Honorary
Consultant Psychiatrist, Salford Primary Care Trust

**Ms Laura Gibbon**
Project Manager (from 2010), NCCMH

*Guideline development group members*

**Professor Simon Gilbody**
Professor of Psychological Medicine and Health Services, Hull York Medical School

**Ms Flora Kaminski**
Research Assistant (from 2010), NCCMH

**Dr Dimitra Lambrelli**
Health Economist, NCCMH

**Mr Terence Lewis**
Service user and carer member

**Mr Francesco Palma**
Service user and carer member

**Dr Matthew Ridd**
General Practitioner, Portishead; Clinical Lecturer, National Institute for Health Research, Bristol

**Ms Caroline Salter**
Research Assistant (2009 to 2010), NCCMH

**Ms Christine Sealey**
Centre Manager, NCCMH

**Professor Roz Shafran**
Professor of Psychology, School of Psychology and Clinical Language Sciences, University of Reading

**Ms Melinda Smith**
Research Assistant (from 2010), NCCMH

**Ms Sarah Stockton**
Senior Information Scientist, NCCMH

**Mr Rupert Suckling**
Deputy Director of Public Health; Consultant in Public Health Medicine, Doncaster Primary Care Trust

**Dr Clare Taylor**
Senior Editor, NCCMH

**Dr Amina Yesufu-Udechuku**
Systematic Reviewer, NCCMH

**Dr Craig Whittington**
Senior Systematic Reviewer, NCCMH

6

# ACKNOWLEDGEMENTS

**Editorial assistance**
Ms Nuala Ernest, Assistant Editor, NCCMH

# 1    PREFACE

This guideline has been developed to advise on common mental health disorders. The guideline recommendations have been developed by a multidisciplinary team of healthcare professionals, people with a common mental health disorder, a carer and guideline methodologists after careful consideration of the best available evidence. It is intended that the guideline will be useful to clinicians and service commissioners in providing and planning high-quality care for people with a common mental health disorder, while also emphasising the importance of the experience of care for them and their families and carers (see Appendix 1 for more details on the scope of the guideline).

Although the evidence base is rapidly expanding there are a number of major gaps, and future revisions of this guideline will incorporate new scientific evidence as it develops. The guideline makes a number of research recommendations specifically to address gaps in the evidence. In the meantime, it is hoped that the guideline will assist clinicians, and people with a common mental health disorder and their families and carers, by identifying the merits of particular approaches where the evidence from research and clinical experience exists.

## 1.1    NATIONAL CLINICAL GUIDELINES

### 1.1.1    What are clinical guidelines?

Clinical practice guidelines are 'systematically developed statements that assist clinicians and patients in making decisions about appropriate treatment for specific conditions' (Mann, 1996). They are derived from the best available research evidence, using predetermined and systematic methods to identify and evaluate the evidence relating to the specific condition in question. Where evidence is lacking, the guidelines incorporate statements and recommendations based upon the consensus statements developed by the Guideline Development Group (GDG).

Clinical guidelines are intended to improve the process and outcomes of healthcare in a number of different ways. They can:

- provide up-to-date evidence-based recommendations for the management of conditions and disorders by healthcare professionals
- be used as the basis to set standards to assess the practice of healthcare professionals
- form the basis for education and training of healthcare professionals
- assist patients and carers in making informed decisions about their treatment and care
- improve communication between healthcare professionals, patients and carers
- help to identify priority areas for further research.

### 1.1.2 Uses and limitation of clinical guidelines

Guidelines are not a substitute for professional knowledge and clinical judgement. They can be limited in their usefulness and applicability by a number of different factors: the availability of high-quality research evidence, the quality of the methodology used in the development of the guideline, the generalisability of research findings and the uniqueness of individuals with a common mental health disorder.

Although the quality of research in this field is variable, the methodology used here reflects current international understanding on the appropriate practice for guideline development (Appraisal of Guidelines for Research and Evaluation Instrument [AGREE]; www.agreecollaboration.org; AGREE Collaboration, 2003), ensuring the collection and selection of the best research evidence available and the systematic generation of treatment recommendations applicable to the majority of people with a common mental health disorder. However, there will always be some people for whom and situations in which clinical guideline recommendations are not readily applicable. This guideline does not, therefore, override the individual responsibility of healthcare professionals to make appropriate decisions in the circumstances of the individual, in consultation with the person with a common mental health disorder and their family or carer.

In addition to the clinical evidence, cost-effectiveness information, where available, is taken into account in the generation of statements and recommendations of the clinical guidelines. While national guidelines are concerned with clinical and cost effectiveness, issues of affordability and implementation costs are to be determined by the National Health Service (NHS).

In using guidelines, it is important to remember that the absence of empirical evidence for the effectiveness of a particular intervention is not the same as evidence for ineffectiveness. In addition and of particular relevance in mental health, evidence-based treatments are often delivered within the context of an overall treatment programme, including a range of activities the purpose of which may be to help engage the person and provide an appropriate context for the delivery of specific interventions. It is important to maintain and enhance the service context in which these interventions are delivered otherwise the specific benefits of effective interventions will be lost. Indeed, the importance of organising care in order to support and encourage a good therapeutic relationship is at times as important as the specific treatments offered.

### 1.1.3 Why develop national guidelines?

The National Institute for Health and Clinical Excellence (NICE) was established as a Special Health Authority for England and Wales in 1999, with a remit to provide a single source of authoritative and reliable guidance for service users, professionals and the public. NICE guidance aims to improve standards of care, diminish unacceptable variations in the provision and quality of care across the NHS and ensure that the health service is patient-centred. All guidance is developed in a transparent and collaborative manner using the best available evidence and involving all relevant stakeholders.

NICE generates guidance in a number of different ways, three of which are relevant here. First, national guidance is produced by the Technology Appraisal Committee to give robust advice about a particular treatment, intervention, procedure or other health technology. Second, NICE commissions public health intervention guidance focused on types of activity (interventions) that help to reduce people's risk of developing a disease or condition, or help to promote or maintain a healthy lifestyle. Third, NICE commissions the production of national clinical practice guidelines focused upon the overall treatment and management of a specific condition. To enable this latter development, NICE has established four National Collaborating Centres in conjunction with a range of professional organisations involved in healthcare.

### 1.1.4    The National Collaborating Centre for Mental Health

This guideline has been commissioned by NICE and developed within the National Collaborating Centre for Mental Health (NCCMH). The NCCMH is a collaboration of the professional organisations involved in the field of mental health, national service user and carer organisations, a number of academic institutions and NICE. The NCCMH is funded by NICE and is led by a partnership between the Royal College of Psychiatrists and the British Psychological Society's Centre for Outcomes Research and Effectiveness, based at University College London.

### 1.1.5    From national clinical guidelines to local protocols

Once a national guideline has been published and disseminated, local healthcare groups will be expected to produce a plan and identify resources for implementation along with appropriate timetables. Subsequently, a multidisciplinary group involving commissioners of healthcare, primary care and specialist mental health professionals, and service users and their carers should undertake the translation of the implementation plan locally, taking into account both the recommendations set out in this guideline and the priorities set in the National Service Framework for Mental Health (Department of Health, 1999) and related documentation. The nature and pace of the local plan will reflect local healthcare needs and the nature of existing services; full implementation may take considerable time, especially where substantial training needs are identified.

### 1.1.6    Auditing the implementation of clinical guidelines

This guideline identifies key areas of clinical practice and service delivery for local and national audit. Although the generation of audit standards is an important and necessary step in the implementation of this guidance, a more broadly-based imple-mentation strategy will be developed. Nevertheless, it should be noted that the Care Quality Commission will monitor the extent to which Primary Care Trusts, trusts responsible for mental health and social care, and Health Authorities have imple-mented these guidelines.

## 1.2 THE NATIONAL COMMON MENTAL HEALTH DISORDERS GUIDELINE

### 1.2.1 Who has developed this guideline?

The GDG was convened by the NCCMH and supported by funding from NICE. The GDG included two people with a common mental health disorder, a carer and profes-sionals from psychiatry, clinical psychology, general practice and nursing.

Staff from the NCCMH provided leadership and support throughout the process of guideline development, undertaking systematic searches, information retrieval, appraisal and systematic review of the evidence. Members of the GDG received training in the process of guideline development from NCCMH staff, and the service users and carer received training and support from the NICE Patient and Public Involvement Programme. The NICE Guidelines Technical Adviser provided advice and assistance regarding aspects of the guideline development process.

All GDG members made formal declarations of interests at the outset, which were updated at every GDG meeting. The GDG met a total of nine times throughout the process of guideline development. It met as a whole, but key topics were led by a national expert in the relevant topic. The GDG was supported by the NCCMH tech-nical team, with additional expert advice from special advisers where needed. The group oversaw the production and synthesis of research evidence before presentation. All statements and recommendations in this guideline have been generated and agreed by the whole GDG.

### 1.2.2 For whom is this guideline intended?

This guideline will be relevant for adults with common mental health disorders including depression and anxiety disorders. It covers the care provided by primary, community and secondary care, and other healthcare professionals who have direct contact with and make decisions concerning the care of adults with common mental health disorders.

The guideline will also be relevant to the work, but will not cover the practice, of those in:
- occupational health services
- social services
- the independent sector.

The experience of people with a common mental health disorder can affect the whole family and often the community. The guideline recognises the role of both in the treatment and support of people with common mental health disorders.

### 1.2.3    Specific aims of this guideline

The guideline makes recommendations for identification and pathways to care for people with common mental health disorders. It aims to:

- review aspects of service delivery critical to the effective provision of clinical interventions for common mental health disorders
- review aspects of service delivery critical to effective implementation of existing NICE guidelines covering these disorders
- evaluate models of service delivery designed to promote access to services
- evaluate the role of methods for identification and assessment
- develop treatment and referral advice for common mental health disorders through adaptation and adoption of recommendations from existing NICE guidelines
- evaluate the role of systems for organising and developing local care pathways for these disorders
- consider the experience of care from the perspective of people with a common mental health disorder, and their families and carers
- promote the implementation of best clinical practice through the development of recommendations tailored to the requirements of the NHS in England and Wales.

### 1.2.4    The structure of this guideline

The guideline is divided into chapters, each covering a set of related topics. The first three chapters provide a summary of the clinical practice and research recommendations, a general introduction to guidelines and the topic, and to the methods used to develop this guideline. Chapter 4 to Chapter 7 provide the evidence that underpins the recommendations.

Each evidence chapter begins with a general introduction to the topic that sets the recommendations in context. Depending on the nature of the evidence, narrative reviews or meta-analyses were conducted, and the structure of the chapters varies accordingly. Where appropriate, details about current practice, the evidence base and any research limitations are provided. Clinical summaries are then used to summarise the evidence presented. Health economic evidence is then presented (where appropriate), followed by a section ('From evidence to recommendations') that draws together the clinical and health economic evidence, and provides a rationale for the recommendations. On the CD-ROM, Appendix 14 provides further details about clinical study characteristics.

# 2    COMMON MENTAL HEALTH DISORDERS

## 2.1    INTRODUCTION

This guideline is concerned with the care and treatment of people with a common mental health disorder, including depression, generalised anxiety disorder (GAD), panic disorder, phobias, social anxiety disorder, obsessive-compulsive disorder (OCD) and post-traumatic stress disorder (PTSD). It makes recommendations about the delivery of effective identification, assessment and referral for treatment in primary care. The guideline will also be applicable to secondary care, and relevant (but does not make specific recommendations) for the prison service and non-NHS services such as social services, and the voluntary and independent sectors. A particular purpose of this guideline is to integrate existing NICE guidance on the identification and assessment of common mental health disorders and to provide recommendations to support the development of local care pathways for these disorders.

The purpose of this introductory chapter is to provide an overview of the epidemiology and treatment of the common mental health disorders, and to highlight important issues related to identification and assessment of the disorders and the relevant local care pathways within the NHS.

This guideline does not cover interventions to treat the disorders and should be used in conjunction with other relevant NICE guidelines, which give evidence of the effectiveness of interventions for the specific disorders, including drug treatments and psychological therapies:

- *Self-harm: the Short-term Physical and Psychological Management and Secondary Prevention of Self-harm in Primary and Secondary Care* (NICE, 2004c; NCCMH, 2004b).
- *Obsessive-compulsive Disorder* (NICE, 2005a; NCCMH, 2006).
- *Post-traumatic Stress Disorder (PTSD)* (NICE, 2005b; NCCMH, 2005).
- *Antenatal and Postnatal Mental Health* (NICE, 2007a; NCCMH, 2007).
- *Depression* (NICE, 2009a; NCCMH, 2010b).
- *Depression in Adults with a Chronic Physical Health Problem* (NICE, 2009b; NCCMH, 2010a).
- *Generalised Anxiety Disorder and Panic Disorder (with or without Agoraphobia) in Adults* (NICE, 2011a; NCCMH, 2011a).
- *Self-harm: Longer-Term Management* (NICE, 2011c; NCCMH, forthcoming).
  A NICE guideline on social anxiety disorder is expected in 2013.

## 2.2 THE DISORDERS

This guideline covers the following common mental health disorders in adults (18 years and older):

- depression (including subthreshold disorders)
- anxiety disorders (including GAD, panic disorder, phobias, social anxiety disorder, OCD and PTSD).

The guideline will also cover, where relevant, issues relating to comorbidity; however, as no separate NICE guideline addresses comorbid presentations of common mental health disorders, this will not be a key topic of the guideline. Groups not covered include adults with subthreshold mixed anxiety and depression, adults with psychotic and related disorders (including schizophrenia and bipolar disorder), people for whom drug and alcohol misuse are the primary problem, people with eating disorders, and children and people younger than 18 years old.

### 2.2.1 Symptoms and presentation

*Depression*
Depression refers to a wide range of mental health problems characterised by the absence of a positive affect (a loss of interest and enjoyment in ordinary things and experiences), low mood and a range of associated emotional, cognitive, physical and behavioural symptoms. Distinguishing the mood changes between clinically significant degrees of depression (for example, major depression) and those occurring 'normally' remains problematic and it is best to consider the symptoms of depression as occurring on a continuum of severity (Lewinsohn *et al.*, 2000).

Commonly, mood and affect in a major depressive illness are unreactive to circumstance remaining low throughout the course of each day, although for some people mood varies diurnally, with gradual improvement throughout the day only to return to a low mood on waking. In other cases a person's mood may be reactive to positive experiences and events, although these elevations in mood are not sustained with depressive feelings often quickly re-emerging (Andrews & Jenkins, 1999).

Behavioural and physical symptoms typically include tearfulness, irritability, social withdrawal, an exacerbation of pre-existing pains, and pains secondary to increased muscle tension (Gerber *et al.*, 1992). A lack of libido, fatigue and diminished activity are also common, although agitation and marked anxiety can frequently occur. Typically there is reduced sleep and lowered appetite (sometimes leading to significant weight loss), but some people sleep more than usual and have an increase in appetite. A loss of interest and enjoyment in everyday life, and feelings of guilt, worthlessness and deserved punishment are common, as are lowered self-esteem, loss of confidence, feelings of helplessness, suicidal ideation and attempts at self-harm or suicide. Cognitive changes include poor concentration and reduced attention, pessimistic and recurrently negative thoughts about oneself, one's past and the future, mental slowing and rumination (Cassano & Fava, 2002).

*Generalised anxiety disorder*

The essential feature of GAD is excessive anxiety and worry (apprehensive expectation), occurring on more days than not for a period of at least 6 months, about a number of events or activities. The person with GAD finds it difficult to control the anxiety and worry, which is often accompanied by restlessness, being easily fatigued, having difficulty concentrating, irritability, muscle tension and disturbed sleep (Brown *et al.*, 2001).

The focus of the anxiety and worry in GAD is not confined to features of another disorder, for example having panic attacks (as in panic disorder) or being embarrassed in public (as in social anxiety disorder). Some people with GAD may become excessively apprehensive about the outcome of routine activities, in particular those associated with the health of or separation from loved ones. Some people often anticipate a catastrophic outcome from a mild physical symptom or a side effect of medication. Demoralisation is said to be a common consequence, with many individuals becoming discouraged, ashamed and unhappy about the difficulties of carrying out their normal routines. GAD is often comorbid with depression and this can make accurate diagnosis problematic (Wittchen *et al.*, 2002).

*Panic disorder*

People with panic disorder report intermittent apprehension, and panic attacks (attacks of sudden short-lived anxiety) in relation to particular situations or spontaneous panic attacks, with no apparent cause. They often take action to avoid being in particular situations in order to prevent those feelings, which may develop into agoraphobia (Breier *et al.*, 1986).

The frequency and severity of panic attacks varies widely. Situational triggers for panic attacks can be external (for example, a phobic object or situation) or internal (physiological arousal). A panic attack may be unexpected (spontaneous or uncued), that is, one that an individual does not immediately associate with a situational trigger.

The essential feature of agoraphobia is anxiety about being in places or situations from which escape might be difficult, embarrassing or in which help may not be available in the event of having a panic attack. This anxiety is said to typically lead to a pervasive avoidance of a variety of situations that may include: being alone outside the home or being home alone; being in a crowd of people; travelling by car or bus; being in a particular place, such as on a bridge or in a lift.

*Obsessive-compulsive disorder*

OCD is characterised by the presence of either obsessions or compulsions, but commonly both. An obsession is defined as an unwanted intrusive thought, image or urge that repeatedly enters the person's mind. Obsessions are distressing, but are acknowledged as originating in the person's mind and not imposed by an external agency. They are usually regarded by the individual as unreasonable or excessive. Common obsessions in OCD include contamination from dirt, germs, viruses, body fluids and so on, fear of harm (for example, that door locks are not safe), excessive concern with order or symmetry, obsessions with the body or physical symptoms, religious, sacrilegious or blasphemous thoughts, sexual thoughts (for example, of being a paedophile or a homosexual), an urge to hoard useless or worn out possessions, or thoughts of violence or aggression (for example, stabbing one's baby) (Lochner & Stein, 2003).

Compulsions are repetitive behaviours or mental acts that the person feels driven to perform. A compulsion can either be overt and observable by others, or a covert mental act that cannot be observed. Covert compulsions are generally more difficult to resist or monitor than overt ones because they can be performed anywhere without others knowing and are easier to perform. Common compulsions include checking (for example, gas taps), cleaning, washing, repeating acts, mental compulsions (for example, repeating special words or prayers in a set manner), ordering, symmetry or exactness, hoarding/collecting and counting (Foa *et al.*, 1995). The most frequent presentations are checking and cleaning, and these are the most easily recognised because they are on a continuum with everyday behaviour. A compulsion is not in itself pleasurable, which differentiates it from impulsive acts such as shopping or gambling, which are associated with immediate gratification.

### Post-traumatic stress disorder

PTSD often develops in response to one or more traumatic events such as deliberate acts of interpersonal violence, severe accidents, disasters or military action. Those at risk of PTSD include survivors of war and torture, of accidents and disasters, and of violent crime (for example, physical and sexual assaults, sexual abuse, bombings and riots), refugees, women who have experienced traumatic childbirth, people diagnosed with a life-threatening illness, and members of the armed forces, police and other emergency personnel (Foa *et al.*, 2008).

The most characteristic symptoms of PTSD are re-experiencing symptoms. People with PTSD involuntarily re-experience aspects of the traumatic event in a vivid and distressing way. Symptoms include flashbacks in which the person acts or feels as if the event is recurring; nightmares; and repetitive and distressing intrusive images or other sensory impressions from the event. Reminders of the traumatic event arouse intense distress and/or physiological reactions. As a result, hypervigilance for threat, exaggerated startle responses, irritability, difficulty in concentrating, sleep problems and avoidance of trauma reminders are other core symptoms. However, people with PTSD also describe symptoms of emotional numbing. These include inability to have any feelings, feeling detached from other people, giving up previously significant activities and amnesia for significant parts of the event.

Two further common mental health disorders, social anxiety disorder and specific phobias, are briefly described below. However, because no NICE guidelines currently exist for these disorders they will not be discussed in detail in the remainder of this chapter.

### Social anxiety disorder

Social anxiety disorder, also referred to as social phobia, is characterised by an intense fear in social situations that results in considerable distress and in turn impacts on a person's ability to function effectively in aspects of their daily life. Central to the disorder is a fear of being judged by others and of being embarrassed or humiliated. This leads to the avoidance of a number of social situations and often impacts significantly on educational and vocational performance. The fears can be triggered by the actual or imagined scrutiny from others. The disorder often begins in early adolescence, and although an individual may recognise the problem as outside of normal experience, many do not seek help (Liebowitz *et al.*, 1985).

Social anxiety disorder is characterised by a range of physical symptoms including excessive blushing, sweating, trembling, palpitations and nausea. Panic attacks are common, as is the development of depressive symptoms as the problem becomes chronic. Alcohol or drug misuse can develop because people use these substances in an attempt to cope with the disturbing and disabling symptoms. It is also often comorbid with other disorders such as depression (Kessler *et al.*, 1999).

*Specific phobias*
A specific phobia is an unwarranted, extreme and persistent fear of a specific object or situation that is out of proportion to the actual danger or threat (Humphris *et al.*, 1995). The fear and anxiety occur immediately upon encountering the feared object or situation and tend to lead to avoidance or extreme discomfort. The person with a specific phobia recognises that the fear is excessive, unwarranted or out of proportion to the actual risk. Specific phobias result in significant interference with the activities of daily life; they are usually grouped under a number of subtypes including animal, natural environment, blood-injection-injury and situational.

### 2.2.2    Incidence and prevalence

Estimates of the prevalence of common mental health disorders vary considerably depending on where and when surveys are carried out, and the period over which prevalence is measured.

The 2007 Office for National Statistics (ONS) household survey of adult psychiatric morbidity in England found that 16.2% of adults aged 16 to 64 years met the diagnostic criteria for at least one disorder in the week prior to interview (McManus *et al.*, 2009). In the three ONS surveys carried out so far, the proportion of adults meeting the criteria for at least one disorder increased between 1993 and 2000 but did not change between 2000 and 2007 (15.5% in 1993, 17.5% in 2000 and 17.6% in 2007). The largest increase in the rate of disorders found between 1993 and 2007 was in women aged 45 to 64 years, among whom the rate went up by about one fifth (McManus *et al.*, 2009).

More than half of the adults identified with a common mental health disorder in the ONS survey presented with a mixed anxiety and depressive disorder (9% in the past week). The 1-week prevalence for the other common mental health disorders were 4.4% for GAD, 2.3% for a depressive episode, 1.4% for phobia, 1.1% for OCD and 1.1% for panic disorder (McManus *et al.*, 2009).

In the US, Kessler and colleagues conducted the National Comorbidity Survey, a representative household interview survey of 9,282 adults aged 18 years and over, to estimate the lifetime (Kessler *et al.*, 2005a) and 12-month (Kessler *et al.*, 2005b) prevalence rates of mental disorders classified using the *Diagnostic and Statistical*

*Manual of Mental Disorders* (4th text-revision version; DSM-IV-TR) of the American Psychiatric Association (APA, 2000). A summary of their findings can be seen in Table 1. Of the 12-month cases in the US National Comorbidity Survey, 22.3% were classified as serious, 37.3% as moderate and 40.4% as mild. Fifty-five per cent carried only a single diagnosis, 22% two diagnoses and 23% three or more diagnoses. Latent class analysis identified three highly comorbid classes representing 7% of the population, and the authors concluded that, although mental disorders are widespread, serious cases are concentrated among a relatively small proportion of people with high comorbidity (Kessler *et al.*, 2005b).

In summary, at any given time common mental health disorders can be found in around one in six people in the community, and around half of these have significant

**Table 1: Summary of prevalence rates for common mental health disorders**

| Disorder | Prevalence estimates | Reference |
|---|---|---|
| Major depression | 4 to 10% (worldwide)<br>6.7% (12-month)<br>16.6% (lifetime) | Waraich and colleagues (2004)<br>Kessler and colleagues (2005b)<br>Kessler and colleagues (2005a) |
| Dysthymia | 2.5 to 5% (worldwide)<br>1.5% (12-month)<br>2.5% (lifetime) | Waraich and colleagues (2004)<br>Kessler and colleagues (2005b)<br>Kessler and colleagues (2005a) |
| GAD | 3.1% (12-month)<br>5.7% (lifetime) | Kessler and colleagues (2005b)<br>Kessler and colleagues (2005a) |
| Panic disorder | 2.7% (12-month)<br>4.7% (lifetime) | Kessler and colleagues (2005b)<br>Kessler and colleagues (2005a) |
| Agoraphobia without panic disorder | 0.8% (12-month)<br>1.4% (lifetime) | Kessler and colleagues (2005b)<br>Kessler and colleagues (2005a) |
| Phobia (specific) | 8.7% (12-month)<br>12.5% (lifetime) | Kessler and colleagues (2005b)<br>Kessler and colleagues (2005a) |
| Social anxiety disorder | 6.8% (12-month)<br>12.1% (lifetime) | Kessler and colleagues (2005b)<br>Kessler and colleagues (2005a) |
| OCD | 1.0% (12-month)<br>1.6% (lifetime) | Kessler and colleagues (2005b)<br>Kessler and colleagues (2005a) |
| PTSD | 1.5% to 1.8% (1-month)<br>1.3 to 3.6% (12-month)<br><br>6.8% (lifetime) | Andrews and colleagues (1999)<br>Creamer and colleagues (2001) and Narrow and colleagues (2002)<br>Kessler and colleagues (2005a) |

symptoms that would warrant intervention from healthcare professionals. Most have non-specific mixed anxiety and depressive symptoms, but a proportion have more specific depressive disorder or anxiety disorders including panic disorder, phobias, OCD or PTSD.

The location, time and duration of the survey are not the only factors to influence prevalence rates. A number of demographic and socioeconomic factors are associated with a higher risk of disorders, including gender, age, marital status, ethnicity and socioeconomic deprivation. These will be discussed below.

### Gender

Depression and anxiety disorders tend to have a higher prevalence in women. Prevalence rates of depression have consistently been found to be between 1.5 and 2.5 times higher in women than men (Waraich *et al.*, 2004). In the ONS survey (McManus *et al.*, 2009) women were more likely than men to have a disorder (19.7 and 12.5%, respectively), with rates significantly higher for women across all categories of disorder except for panic disorder and OCD. The greatest difference between genders was among South Asian adults where the age-standardised rate among women (34.3% of South Asian women) was three times that of men (10.3% of South Asian men). Reasons cited in the 2007 ONS survey (McManus *et al.*, 2009) include the impact of having children (Bebbington *et al.*, 1991), exposure to domestic or sexual violence (Patel *et al.*, 2006), adverse experiences in childhood and women's relative poverty (Patel *et al.*, 1999; Piccinelli & Wilkinson, 2000).

### Age

In the 2007 ONS survey (McManus *et al.*, 2009) rates varied by age, with those aged 75 years and over least likely to have a disorder (6.3% of men and 12.2% of women). In women, the rate peaked among 45- to 54-year-olds of whom 25% met the criteria for at least one disorder. Among men, the rate was highest in 25- to 54-year-olds (14.6% of 25- to 34-year-olds, 15.0% of 35- to 44-year-olds and 14.5% of 45- to 54-year-olds).

### Marital status

Women across all marital-status categories were more likely than their male counterparts to have disorders in the 2007 ONS survey (McManus *et al.*, 2009), except for divorced people in whom the prevalence for men and women was very similar (26.6% for women and 27.7% for men). Among men, those currently divorced had the greatest likelihood of having a disorder, but variation by other marital status categories was less pronounced. For women the rate of disorder was high for divorced women, but even higher for separated women (33.0%). Men and women who were married or widowed had the lowest observed rates of disorder (10.1% of married men and 16.3% of married women; 10.4% widowed men and 17.4% widowed women).

### Ethnicity

In the 2007 ONS survey (McManus *et al.*, 2009), after age-standardisation of the data, there was little variation between white, black and South Asian men in the rates of any disorder. However, among women rates of all disorders (except phobias) were higher in the South Asian group. The number of South Asian women in the sample was small, so while the differences were pronounced they were only significant for disorders as a whole for GAD and panic disorder.

*Socioeconomic factors*
In the 2007 ONS survey (McManus *et al.*, 2009), people living in households with the lowest levels of income were more likely to have a disorder than those living in the highest income households. A number of socioeconomic factors significantly affected prevalence rates in the 2000 ONS survey (Singleton *et al.*, 2001): those with a depressive episode were more likely than those without a disorder to be unemployed, to belong to social classes 4 and below, to have no formal educational qualifications, to live in Local Authority or Housing Association accommodation, to have moved three or more times in the last 2 years and to live in an urban environment.

An illustration of the social origins of depression can be found in a general practice survey in which 7.2% (ranging 2.4 to 13.7%, depending upon the practice) of consecutive attendees had a depressive disorder. Neighbourhood social deprivation accounted for 48.3% of the variance among practices. Other variables were the proportion of the population having no or only one car and neighbourhood unemployment (Ostler *et al.*, 2001). The evidence therefore overwhelmingly supports the view that the prevalence of common mental health disorders, however it is defined, varies according to gender and social and economic factors.

*Learning disabilities*
The rates of common mental health disorders in adults with learning disabilities are generally considered to be higher, but limited data and methodological problems (Smiley, 2005) mean that precise estimates are often not available and so uncertainty remains. In contrast, there is clearer evidence that other mental disorders such as problem behaviour have a higher rate of learning disabilities (Cooper *et al.*, 2007). Rates of mental disorders may vary with the severity of the learning disability, being higher in more severe disability (Whitaker & Read, 2006), and challenges in assessment and diagnosis are considerable especially for those with more severe learning disabilities (Smiley, 2005; Whitaker & Read, 2006). However, some indication of the possible differential incidence of common mental health disorders can be obtained from the following studies. Richards and colleagues (2001) report a four-fold increase in the rates of affective disorders for people with mild learning disability. Rates of problems may also vary with the disorder; for example, Collacott (1999) reports a higher rate of depression in adults with Down's syndrome than in adults with other causes of learning disability. With regard to anxiety disorders, Cooper (1997) reports a rate of 2.5% for OCD in adults with a learning disability, which is higher than in the general adult population.

## 2.2.3 Aetiology

The aetiology of common mental health disorders is multi-factorial and involves psychological, social and biological factors. Many of the common mental health disorders have similar aetiologies. For example, King and colleagues (2008) identi-fied five immutable risk factors for depression. These were younger age, female gender, lower educational achievement, previous history of depression and family history of depression. Brewin and colleagues (2000) and Ozer and colleagues (2003) identified similar risk factors for PTSD, including a previous personal or family history of anxiety disorders or affective disorders, neuroticism, lower intelligence, female gender and a history of previous trauma. The ONS survey (McManus *et al.*, 2009) identified factors that may be associated with increased duration of an episode of depression or anxiety. These can be broadly defined as biological factors, social stresses and life events. These risk factors will now be discussed in general. For infor-mation regarding factors for specific disorders, please refer to the relevant NICE guideline (see Section 2.1).

There is good evidence for biological factors in the development of many psycho-logical disorders. Biological factors can be biochemical, endocrine and neurophysio-logical (Goodwin, 2000; Malhi *et al.*, 2005) or genetic (Kendler & Prescott, 1999), and can interact with early trauma ultimately leading to psychological distress (Heim & Nemeroff, 2001).

Support for this claim often comes from family-history studies (Angst *et al.*, 2003). A family history of depressive illness has been linked with an increased chance of developing depression (Kendler *et al.*, 2001). Similarly, the risk of GAD in first-degree relatives of patients with GAD was five times that of controls (Noyes *et al.*, 1987). Although specific genes conferring vulnerability to GAD have not yet been reliably identified, the genes involved in the transmission of GAD appear to increase susceptibility to other anxiety disorders such as panic disorder and agoraphobia as well as major depression (Hettema *et al.*, 2001 and 2005; Kendler, 1996). There is some evidence to suggest that personality traits such as neuroticism may have a role in the development of common mental health disorders. Personality traits such as neuroticism have been identified as risk factors for both depression (Fava & Kendler, 2000) and GAD (Hettema *et al.*, 2004). However, the specific role of neurotransmit-ters and other chemical mediators in the aetiology of common mental health disorders is currently unclear.

According to a stress-vulnerability model (Nuechterlein & Dawson, 1984), it is not only biological factors that can trigger the development of a common mental health disorder. Social triggers may also play an important role (Harris, 2000). The ONS survey (McManus *et al.*, 2009) identified perceived financial strain (Weich & Lewis, 1998a), work stress (Stansfeld *et al.*, 1999), poor housing (Weich & Lewis, 1998b) and social isolation (Bruce & Hoff, 1994) as key factors that can influence the development of common mental health disorders. In the UK, an influential study found that social vulnerability factors for depression in women in Camberwell, south-east London, included: having three or more children under the age of 14 years living at home; having no paid employment outside the home; and not having a confiding relationship with another person (Brown & Harris, 1978). The importance of a confiding relationship has been further reiterated by Patten (1991) who found that a lack of such a relationship was a strong risk factor for depression.

Negative life events, particularly those relating to health, can also impact on the development of depression and anxiety, although vulnerabilities will vary between individuals (Harris, 2000). The ONS survey identified poor physical health and problems with alcohol use as predictors of anxiety and depression (Salokangas & Poutanen, 1998), while King and colleagues (2008) found that current poorer physical and mental health functional status, based on the 12-Item Short Form Health Survey (SF-12) questionnaire, was linked to the development of depression. However, it is also important to note that depression may lead to secondary disability that compounds, and is difficult to distinguish from, the depression itself.

Early life experiences as well as current social stressors must also be considered. A poor parent–child relationship, marital discord and divorce, neglect, and physical and sexual abuse almost certainly increase a person's vulnerability to depression in later life (Fava & Kendler, 2000) and can play a vital role in the development of GAD. Barlow (2000) reported that good parenting experiences are important in providing children with a secure base from which to explore the world. Problems in child–parent attachment have been linked to feelings of diminished personal control of potentially threatening events (Barlow, 2000), which can in turn increase susceptibility to psychological illness.

However, when considering the importance of life events it is important to remember that events may not have a causal impact on the development of symptoms. Instead, they may act as a trigger among people who are biologically or psychologically predisposed to a disorder, for example OCD (Gothelf *et al.*, 2004; Khanna *et al.*, 1988). The authors of the ONS survey make the point that although these risk factors are associated with disorders and tend to increase the duration of episodes it is not clear whether or not they cause the onset of an episode.

### 2.2.4 Development, course and prognosis

For many people the onset of common mental health disorders occurs in adolescence or early adult life, but the disorders can affect people at any point. Earlier onset is generally associated with poorer outcomes. Kessler and colleagues (2005a) reported an estimated median age of onset for anxiety disorders of 11 years and for mood disorders of 30 years in their US National Comorbidity sample. Half of all lifetime cases had started by 14 years and three quarters by 24 years. Many anxiety disorders also have a chronic course. This chronic course may be associated with a considerable delay in presenting to services, with consequent significant personal and social impairment. Therefore, Kessler and colleagues (2005a) concluded that interventions aimed at prevention or early treatment needed to focus on young people.

*Depression*
The average age of the first episode of major depression is the mid-20s and although the first episode may occur at any time, from early childhood through to old age, a substantial proportion of people have their first depressive episode in childhood or adolescence (Fava & Kendler, 2000).

Although depression has been understood to be a time-limited disorder lasting on average 4 to 6 months with complete recovery afterwards, it is now clear that incomplete recovery and relapse are common. The World Health Organization (WHO) study of mental disorders in 14 centres across the world found that 50% still had a diagnosis of depression 1 year later (Simon *et al.*, 2002) and at least 10% of patients have persistent or chronic depression (Kessler *et al.*, 2003). At least 50% of people following their first episode of major depression will go on to have at least one more episode (Kupfer, 1991), and after the second and third episodes the risk of further relapse rises to 70 and 90%, respectively (Kupfer, 1991). Early-onset depression (at or before 20 years of age) and depression occurring in old age have a significantly increased vulnerability to relapse (Giles *et al.*, 1989; Mitchell & Subramaniam, 2005). Thus while the outlook for a first episode is good, the outlook for recurrent episodes over the long term can be poor with many patients experiencing symptoms of depression over many years (Akiskal, 1986).

*Generalised anxiety disorder*
Most clinical studies suggest that GAD is typically a chronic condition with low rates of remission over the short and medium term. Evaluation of prognosis is complicated by the frequent comorbidity with other anxiety disorders and depression, which worsen the long-term outcome and accompanying burden of disability (Tyrer & Baldwin, 2006). In the Harvard-Brown Anxiety Research Program, which recruited patients from Boston hospitals, the mean age of onset of GAD was 21 years, although many patients had been unwell since their teens. The average duration of illness in this group was about 20 years and despite treatment the outcome over the next 3 years was relatively poor, with only one in four patients showing symptomatic remission from GAD (Yonkers *et al.*, 1996). The proportion of patients who became free from all psychiatric symptomatology was even smaller, at about one in six. In patients who remitted from GAD, the risk of relapse over the next year was about 15% increasing to about 30% in those who achieved only partial symptomatic remission (Yonkers *et al.*, 1996).

The participants in the above study were recruited from hospital services and may not be representative of GAD in general. In a naturalistic study in the UK, Tyrer and colleagues (2004) followed up patients with anxiety and depression identified in psychiatric clinics in primary care and found that 12 years later 40% of those initially diagnosed with GAD had recovered, in the sense of no longer meeting criteria for any DSM-III psychiatric disorder. The remaining participants remained symptomatic, but only 3% still had GAD as the principal diagnosis; in the vast majority of patients, conditions such as dysthymia, major depression and agoraphobia were now more prominent. This study confirms the chronic and fluctuating symptomatic course of GAD in clinically-identified patients. It should be noted, however, that the majority of people with GAD in the community do not seek medical help for their symptoms (Wittchen & Jacobi, 2005) and the course of the illness in these circumstances is not established.

*Panic disorder*
Panic disorder comprises two main subtypes; panic disorder without agoraphobia and panic disorder with agoraphobia, with different presentations and often different

23

courses. Panic disorder with agoraphobia (about one third of all presentations of panic disorder) is characterised by an avoidance of situations from which escape may not be possible or help not available in the event of a panic attack. Panic disorder with agoraphobia is also more common in women by a factor of approximately two to one. In contrast, panic disorder without agoraphobia is not situation-specific and symptoms may develop with no obvious or apparent cause (Weissman & Merikangas, 1986).

The most common age of onset is from the mid-teens to the mid-20s; however, onset may occur at any time. Panic disorder often begins with occasional panic attacks that increase in frequency and which in time lead to a pattern of a generalised avoidance. The course of this disorder often follows a chronic pathway for many people with panic disorder, with agoraphobia likely to have an even more chronic course (Francis *et al.*, 2007).

Panic attacks commonly occur in many other disorders including specific phobias and social anxiety disorder, but they can also occur in GAD, drug or alcohol misuse, personality disorders and a number of physical disorders.

*Obsessive-compulsive disorder*

The mean age of onset of OCD is in late adolescence for men and early 20s for women, although age of onset covers a wide range of ages. However, it may take individuals between 10 and 15 years or longer to seek professional help. There is often comorbidity with a range of disorders, especially depression (for example, Abramowitz, 2004; Abramowitz *et al.*, 2003; Apter *et al.*, 2003), and other anxiety disorders (for example, Biederman *et al.*, 2004; LaSalle *et al.*, 2004; Nestadt *et al.*, 2003; Welkowitz *et al.*, 2000).

OCD may follow an acute, episodic or chronic course. In one of the largest follow-up studies, Skoog and Skoog (1999) conducted a 40-year prospective study and reported that approximately 60% of people with OCD displayed signs of general improvement within 10 years of illness, increasing to 80% by the end of the study. However, only 20% achieved full remission even after almost 50 years of illness; 60% continue to experience significant symptoms; 10% displayed no improvement; and 10% had deteriorated. A fifth of those who had displayed an early sustained improvement subsequently relapsed, even after 20 years without symptoms. This suggests that early recovery does not eliminate the possibility of very late relapse. Intermittent, episodic disorder was more common during the early stage of illness and predicted a more favourable outcome, whereas chronic illness predominated in later years. Worse outcome was predicted by early age of onset (particularly in males), experiencing obsessions and compulsions or magical thinking, poor social adjustment and early chronic course.

*Post-traumatic stress disorder*

The onset of symptoms in PTSD is usually in the first month after the traumatic event, but in a minority (less than 15%; McNally, 2003) there may be a delay of months or years before symptoms start to appear. PTSD also shows substantial natural recovery in the initial months and years after a traumatic event. Whereas a high proportion of trauma survivors will initially develop symptoms of PTSD, a substantial proportion of these individuals recover without treatment in the following years, with a steep decline in PTSD rates occurring in the first year (for example, Breslau *et al.*, 1991; Kessler *et al.*, 1995). On the other hand, at least one third of people who initially develop PTSD remain symptomatic for 3 years or longer and are at risk of secondary problems such as substance misuse (for example, Kessler *et al.*, 1995). In the 2007 ONS (McManus *et al.*, 2009) survey, screening positive for current PTSD declined with age, from 4.7% of 16- to 24-year-olds to 0.6% of adults aged 75 years or over.

## 2.2.5 Impairment, disability, secondary problems

*Depression*
Apart from the subjective suffering experienced by people who are depressed, the impact on social and occupational functioning, physical health and mortality is substantial. In fact, depressive illness causes a greater decrement in health state than major chronic physical illnesses such as angina, arthritis, asthma and diabetes (Moussavi *et al.*, 2007).

Depression is a major cause of disability across the world. In 1990 it was the fourth most common cause of loss of disability-adjusted life years (DALYs) in the world and by 2020 it is projected to become the second most common cause (World Bank, 1993). In 1994 it was estimated that about 1.5 million DALYs were lost each year in the West as a result of depression (Murray *et al.*, 1994). Depressive disorders account for 4.4% of the global disease burden or the equivalent of 65 million DALYs (Murray & Lopez, 1997; WHO, 2002).

Emotional, motivational and cognitive effects substantially reduce a person's ability to work effectively, with losses in personal and family income as well as lost contribution to society in tax revenues and employment skills. Wider social effects include: greater dependence upon welfare and benefits with loss of self-esteem and self-confidence; social impairments, including reduced ability to communicate and sustain relationships during the illness with knock-on effects after an episode; and longer-term impairment in social functioning, especially for those who have chronic or recurrent disorders. Some of the features of depression (such as lethargy) may impede access to appropriate healthcare.

Depression can also exacerbate the pain, distress and disability associated with physical health problems, and can adversely affect outcomes. Depression combined with chronic physical health problems incrementally worsens health compared with a physical health problem alone or even combinations of physical health problems (Moussavi *et al.*, 2007). In addition, for a range of physical health problems findings suggest an increased risk of death when comorbid depression is present (Cassano & Fava, 2002). In coronary heart disease, for example, depressive disorders are associated with an 80% increased risk both for its development and of subsequent mortality in people with established disease, at least partly because of common contributory factors (Nicholson *et al.*, 2006).

Suicide accounts for nearly 1% of all deaths and nearly two thirds are people with depression (Sartorius, 2001); putting it in another way, having depression leads to over a four-times higher risk of suicide compared with the general population, which rises to nearly 20 times in the most severely ill (Bostwick & Pankratz, 2000). Sometimes depression may also lead to acts of violence against others, and may even include homicide. Marital and family relationships are frequently negatively affected, and parental depression may lead to neglect of children and significant disturbances in children (Ramachandani & Stein, 2003).

*Generalised anxiety disorder*

Like major depression GAD is associated with a substantial burden of disability, equivalent to that of other chronic physical health problems such as arthritis and diabetes (Wittchen *et al.*, 2002). There is evidence that comorbid depression and anxiety has a worse prognosis and more persistent symptoms than either depression or anxiety disorders alone (Kroenke *et al.*, 2007). There is also evidence that, in the community, anxiety disorders are independently associated with several physical health problems and that this comorbidity is significantly associated with poor quality of life and disability (Sareen *et al.*, 2006), and high associated health and social costs (Simon *et al.*, 1995).

Studies have shown that the presence of GAD is also associated with significant impairments in occupational and social functioning. For example, over 30% of patients with GAD showed an annual reduction of work productivity of 10% or more compared with 8% of people with major depression. The figure for people with comorbid GAD and depression was over 45% (Wittchen *et al.*, 2000). A large part of the economic cost of anxiety disorders is attributable to the costs of non-medical psychiatric treatment. Patients with GAD have increased numbers of visits not only to primary care doctors but also to hospital specialists, particularly gastroenterologists (Kennedy & Schwab, 1997; Wittchen *et al.*, 2002). This may be a consequence of the distressing somatic symptoms that many people with GAD experience.

GAD also carries a considerable cost in personal suffering and difficulties. In the Harvard-Brown Program, one third of patients had never married and unemployment was higher than average (Yonkers *et al.*, 1996). Suicidal ideation and suicide attempts are significantly increased in GAD, particularly in women, and this increase is still greater in the presence of comorbid major depression (Cougle *et al.*, 2009).

*Panic disorder*

Panic disorder has considerable impact on the NHS, such as general practitioners (GPs), society as a whole (in terms of sickness and absence from work, labour turnover and reduced productivity), and individuals and families (Sherbourne *et al.*, 1996). The impact in any of these spheres is difficult to measure accurately and there may be an underestimation of the impact, but it is still substantial. A person with panic disorder may experience severe and enduring physical sensations, which may lead them to think that they have a physical illness; it can be difficult for healthcare professionals to provide adequate reassurance that this is not the case, which may lead to multiple consultations. Their economic wellbeing may also be affected (Edlund & Swann, 1987).

*Obsessive-compulsive disorder*

OCD is ranked by the WHO in the top ten of the most disabling illnesses by lost income and decreased quality of life (Bobes *et al.*, 2001). The severity of OCD differs markedly from one person to another. While some people may be able to hide their OCD from their own family, the disorder may have a major negative impact on social relationships leading to frequent family and marital discord or dissatisfaction, separation or divorce (Koran, 2000). It also interferes with leisure activities (Antony *et al.*, 1998) and with a person's ability to study or work, leading to diminished educational and/or occupational attainment and unemployment (Koran, 2000; Leon *et al.*, 1995). The social cost (that is the person's inability to fully function in society) has been estimated as US$5.9 billion in 1990, or 70.4% of the total economic cost of OCD (DuPont *et al.*, 1995).

*Post-traumatic stress disorder*

Symptoms of PTSD cause considerable distress and can significantly interfere with social, educational and occupational functioning. It is not uncommon for people with PTSD to lose their jobs either because re-experiencing symptoms, as well as sleep and concentration problems, make regular work difficult or because they are unable to cope with reminders of the traumatic event they encounter while at work (Zatzick *et al.*, 1997). The resulting financial problems are a common source of additional stress and may be a contributory factor leading to extreme hardship, such as homelessness. The disorder has adverse effects on the person's social relationships, leading to social withdrawal. Problems in the family and break-up of significant relationships are not uncommon.

People with PTSD may also develop further, secondary psychological disorders as complications of the disorder. The most common complications are:

- the use of alcohol, drugs, caffeine or nicotine to cope with their symptoms, which may eventually lead to dependence
- depression, including the risk of suicide
- other anxiety disorders, such as panic disorder, which may lead to additional restrictions in their life (for example, inability to use public transport).

Other possible complications of PTSD include somatisation, chronic pain and poor health (Schnurr & Green, 2003). People with PTSD are at greater risk of physical health problems, including circulatory and musculoskeletal disorders, and have a greater number of medical conditions than those without PTSD (Ouimette *et al.*, 2004).

The course and prognosis of all common mental disorders are affected by a range of social factors, a number of which have been already discussed above. However, a range of factors related to social exclusion have a specific effect on access to services. This means that a number of groups may have particular problems accessing services including: those involved with the criminal justice system; homeless or precariously housed people; travelling communities; some groups of younger people (including those who have been in care as children and adolescence); people who misuse drugs and alcohol; and those of uncertain immigration status.

### 2.2.6 Economic costs

The ONS report (McManus *et al.*, 2009) makes the point that although common mental health disorders are usually less disabling than major psychiatric disorders such as psychosis, their greater prevalence means that the cumulative cost to society is vast. Mixed anxiety and depression has been estimated to cause one fifth of days lost from work in Britain (Das-Munshi *et al.*, 2008). Even before the recent expansion of the European Union, it was estimated that work-related stress affected at least 40 million workers in its then 15 member states and that it cost at least €20 billion annually. In the UK, it has been suggested that over 40 million working days are lost each year due to stress-related disorders (European Agency for Safety and Health at Work, 2000).

*Costs of depression*

Depression is associated with high prevalence and treatment costs, and as stated above is considered one of the most important risk factors for suicide (Knapp & Illson, 2002). Furthermore, depression has a large impact on workplace productivity. As a result, depression places an enormous burden on both the healthcare system and the broader society.

Depression has a major financial impact on health and social services and the wider economy. A review was conducted by the King's Fund in 2006 to estimate mental health expenditure including depression in England for the next 20 years, to 2026 (McCrone *et al.*, 2008). The study estimated the total cost of services for depression in England in 2007 to be £1.7 billion, while lost employment increased this total to £7.5 billion. Based on the estimate that 1.45 million people would have depression in 2026, the authors estimated that the total service cost would be £12.2 billion when accounting for prescribed drugs, inpatient care, other NHS services, supported accommodation, social services and lost employment in terms of workplace absenteeism.

One of the key findings from the cost-of-illness literature is that the indirect costs of depression far outweigh the health service costs. A study by Thomas and Morris (2003) suggested that the effect on lost employment and productivity was 23 times larger than the costs falling to the health service. Other studies have also supported these findings. Based on UK labour-market survey data, Almond and Healey (2003) estimated that respondents with self-reported depression/anxiety were three times more likely to be absent from work (equivalent to 15 days per year) than workers without depression/anxiety. Furthermore, a US-based study suggests that depression is a major cause of reduced productivity at work, in terms of 'work cut-back days' (Kessler *et al.*, 2001). This reduced workplace productivity is unlikely to be adequately measured by absenteeism rates and further emphasises the 'hidden costs' of depression (Knapp, 2003). A recent study conducted by the the Centre for Economic Performance's Mental Health Policy Group estimated that the total loss of output (in terms of lost productivity, absenteeism from work or benefits received) due to depression and chronic anxiety is some £12 billion per year (Layard, 2006).

Other intangible costs of illness include the impact on the quality of life of people with depression and their families and carers. Certainly, the cost-of-illness calculations presented here and in Table 2 show that depression imposes a significant burden on individuals and their families and carers, the healthcare system and the broader economy through lost productivity and workplace absenteeism. Furthermore, it is anticipated that these costs will continue to rise significantly in future years. Therefore, it is important that the efficient use of available healthcare resources is used to maximise health benefits for people with depression.

*Costs of anxiety disorders*

Anxiety disorders place a significant burden on individuals as well as on the healthcare system. Although direct comparisons between studies are difficult to make due to variations in country, health services and year of interest, economic cost has been estimated at over US$40 billion (Andlin-Sobocki *et al.*, 2005; see Table 2 for further information). Estimated costs are incurred by healthcare resource utilisation such as mental health services, medication, hospitalisation, nursing homes and outpatient visits, productivity losses and, to a lesser extent, by provision of other services such as criminal justice services, social welfare administration and incarceration, as well as family care-giving (0.8%) (Andlin-Sobocki *et al.*, 2005).

Total healthcare cost is not the only important outcome to consider when investigating cost. Marciniak and colleagues (2005) found that the total medical cost per person with any anxiety disorder was estimated at US$6,475 in 1999. More specifically, when looking at GAD alone, the figure increased to US$2,138 when controlling for demographics and other disease states. This increased cost may be due to factors such as increased outpatient mental health service use or medical specialist service use. Furthermore, people with anxiety tend to miss more days of work or have a short-term disability than controls (Marciniak *et al.*, 2004).

Anxiety disorders are associated with a wide range of comorbidities, which result in a substantial increase in the total healthcare costs. Souêtre and colleagues (1994) estimated the total direct and indirect costs incurred by people with GAD with and without comorbidities using data on 999 people participating in a French cross-sectional study. Controlling for confounding variables, the prevalence of healthcare utilisation in terms of hospitalisation, laboratory tests and medications, and the respective medical costs were found to be significantly higher in people with GAD and other comorbidities than those without comorbidities. Moreover, comorbidities were associated with increased absenteeism from work. In particular, comorbid depression (Marciniak *et al.*, 2005; Wetherell *et al.*, 2007; Zhu *et al.*, 2009) and physical pain (Olfson & Gameroff, 2007; Zhu *et al.*, 2009) have been found to have a significant impact on treatment costs incurred by people with GAD.

*Costs of post-traumatic stress disorder*

In 2003 to 2004, social and welfare costs of claims for incapacitation and severe disablement from severe stress and PTSD amounted to £103 million, which is

**Table 2: Summary of cost of illness data for depression and anxiety**

| | Measurement of cost | Cost | Reference | Country |
|---|---|---|---|---|
| Depression | Estimated total service cost (2007 to 2026) | £1.7 to 3 billion | McCrone and colleagues (2008) | UK |
| | Estimated total service cost, accounting for lost employment (2007) | £7.5 to 12.2 billion | McCrone and colleagues (2008) | UK |
| Anxiety | Estimated total service cost (1990) | US$46.6 billion | DuPont and colleagues (1998) | US |
| | Estimated total service cost (1998) | US$63.1 billion | Greenberg and colleagues (1999) | US |
| | Estimated total service cost (2004) | €41 billion | Andlin-Sobocki and colleagues (2005) | Europe |
| | Average annual excess service cost (2004) | €1628 | Andlin-Sobocki and colleagues (2005) | Europe |
| | Estimated total annual cost of routine treatment for GAD (1997) | AU$112.3 million | Andrews and colleagues (2004) | Australia |
| | Estimated total annual cost of optimal, increased treatment for GAD (1997) | AU$205.1 million | Andrews and colleagues (2004) | Australia |
| | Total medical cost per person with any anxiety disorder (1999) | US$6475 | Marciniak and colleagues (2005) | US |
| | Increase in total medical cost per person, controlling for demographics and other disease states (1999) | US$2138 | Marciniak and colleagues (2005) | US |

£55 million more than was claimed 5 years previously (Hansard, 2004). Therefore, PTSD presents an enormous economic burden on families, the national health services and society as a whole.

## 2.3    TREATMENT

A number of treatments exist for common mental health disorders. However, because this guideline is predominantly interested in the identification and assessment of these conditions, the treatments will only be discussed briefly. For more information, please see the relevant guideline (see Section 2.1).

### 2.3.1    Pharmacological treatments

*Depression*
There is a wide range of antidepressant drugs available for people with depression. These can be grouped into tricyclic antidepressants, selective serotonin reuptake inhibitors (SSRIs), monoamine oxidase inhibitors and a range of other chemically unrelated antidepressants (*British National Formulary* [BNF] *59;* British Medical Association & the Royal Pharmaceutical Society of Great Britain, 2010).

*Generalised anxiety disorder*
Placebo-controlled trials indicate that a wide range of drugs with differing pharmacological properties can be effective in the treatment of GAD (Baldwin *et al.*, 2005). In recent years, antidepressant medications such as SSRIs have been increasingly used to treat GAD (Baldwin *et al.*, 2005).

Conventional antipsychotic drugs and the newer 'atypical' antipsychotic agents have also been used in the treatment in GAD, both as a sole therapy and as an 'add-on' to SSRI therapy when the latter has proved ineffective (Pies, 2009). However, the greater side-effect burden of antipsychotic drugs means that presently their use is restricted to people with refractory conditions, with prescribing being guided by secondary care physicians.

*Panic disorder*
There is evidence to support the use of pharmacological intervention in the treatment of panic disorder, in particular with SSRIs. When a person has not responded to an SSRI, other related antidepressants may be of benefit. There is little good evidence to support the use of benzodiazepines. In contrast to a number of other depressive and anxiety disorders, there is little evidence to support the use of pharmacological and psychological interventions in combination.

*Obsessive-compulsive disorder*
Pharmacological investigations have demonstrated effectiveness in OCD, in particular with SSRIs and related antidepressants (Montgomery *et al.*, 2001; Zohar & Judge,

1996) for moderate to severe presentations, especially if the problem has a chronic course; this may be in combination with psychological interventions.

*Post-traumatic stress disorder*
At present there is no conclusive evidence that any drug treatment helps as an early intervention for the treatment of PTSD-specific symptoms (NCCMH, 2005). However, for people who are acutely distressed and may be experiencing severe sleep problems, consideration may be given to the use of medication. Drug treatments for PTSD should not be used as a routine first-line treatment for adults (in general use or by specialist mental health professionals) in preference to a trauma-focused psychological therapy. Drug treatments should be considered for the treatment of PTSD in adults when a person with the disorder expresses a preference not to engage in a trauma-focused psychological treatment. The SSRI paroxetine is the only drug with a current UK product licence for PTSD.

### 2.3.2    Psychological treatments

*Depression*
Effective psychological treatments for depression identified in the NICE *Depression* guideline (NICE, 2009a) include: cognitive behavioural therapy (CBT), behavioural activation, interpersonal therapy (IPT), behavioural couples therapy and mindfulness-based cognitive therapy. For moderate to severe disorders these are often provided in conjunction with antidepressants. For subthreshold and milder disorders, structured group physical activity programmes, facilitated self-help and CCBT are effective interventions.

*Generalised anxiety disorder*
Cognitive and behavioural approaches are the treatments of choice for GAD. People who have moderate to severe disorder, particularly if the problem is long-standing, should be offered CBT or applied relaxation. For those with milder and more recent onset disorders, two options are available: facilitated or non-facilitated self-help based on CBT principles and psychoeducational groups also based on CBT principles.

*Panic disorder*
Cognitive and behavioural approaches are again the treatments of choice for panic disorder. People who have a moderate to severe GAD, particularly if it is long-standing, should receive between 7 and 14 hours of therapist-provided treatment over a 4-month period. For those with milder and more recent onset GAD, facilitated or non-facilitated self-help based on CBT principle are efficacious treatments.

*Obsessive-compulsive disorder*
CBT is the most widely used psychological treatment for OCD in adults (Roth & Fonagy, 2004). The main CBT interventions that have been used in the treatment of OCD are exposure and response prevention (ERP) (for example, Foa & Kozak, 1996;

Marks, 1997), different variants of cognitive therapy (Clark, 2004; Freeston *et al.*, 1996; Frost & Steketee, 1999; Krochmalik *et al.*, 2001; Rachman, 1998, 2002 and 2004; Salkovskis *et al.*, 1999; van Oppen & Arntz, 1994; Wells, 2000), and a combination of ERP and cognitive therapy (see Kobak *et al.*, 1998; Roth & Fonagy, 2004) ERP and cognitive therapy have different theoretical underpinnings, but may be used together in a coherent package.

*Post-traumatic stress disorder*

General practical and social support and guidance about the immediate distress and likely course of symptoms should be given to anyone following a traumatic incident. Trauma-focused psychological treatments are effective for the treatment of PTSD, either trauma-focused CBT or eye movement desensitisation and reprocessing (EMDR). These treatments are normally provided on an individual outpatient basis and are effective even when considerable time has elapsed since the traumatic event(s).

### 2.3.3 Current levels of treatment of common mental health disorders

It is concerning that, according to the 2007 ONS survey (McManus *et al.*, 2009), only one quarter (24%) of people with a disorder were receiving any treatment for it in the week prior to interview. Treatment received by that 24% was mostly in the form of medication: 14% were taking psychoactive medication only, 5% were in receipt of counselling or therapy and 5% were receiving both medication and counselling/therapy.

*Use of healthcare services*

Of the people reporting a common mental health disorder in the ONS survey (McManus *et al.*, 2009), 39% had used some type of healthcare service for a mental or emotional problem within the last year, compared with 6% of men and women without a disorder.

*Primary care services*

General practice services were the most common healthcare service used in the ONS survey. A total of 38% of people with a common mental health disorder contacted their GP for help. Depression and phobias were associated with the highest use of healthcare services for a mental or emotional problem (both 67%), and mixed anxiety and depression was associated with the lowest use (30%) (McManus *et al.*, 2009).

*Community care services*

All respondents in the ONS survey (McManus *et al.*, 2009), were asked about community and day care services used in the past year. Community and day care services were used less than healthcare services. Those with phobias made most use of community or day care services (49%), while mixed anxiety and depressive disorder was associated with the lowest rate of community or day care service use (12%).

*Summary*

In summary, common mental health disorders are associated with a range of symptoms that can lead to significant impairment and disability, and high costs both for the individual with the disorder and for society as a whole.

Effective treatments are available that differ depending on the disorder. As a result, early detection, assessment and intervention are key priorities for any healthcare system. This guideline, which is focused on primary care, will provide recommendations on how to best identify and assess common mental health disorders and the key indicators for treatment in order to help improve and facilitate access to care, and the route through care.

## 2.4 IDENTIFICATION, ASSESSMENT AND PATHWAYS TO CARE

Goldberg and Huxley (1992) described a useful model within which to consider issues relating to the identification, assessment and pathway to psychiatric care for people with a common mental health disorder (see Figure 1). They identified five levels of care, with 'filters' between them relating to the behaviour of those with the disorders and the behaviours of the healthcare practitioners with whom they came into contact, emphasising that only a small proportion of people with a mental disorder receive specialist psychiatric care.

The prevalence rates given above are taken from the original model and relate to proportions found in epidemiological surveys conducted before 1980. The Level 1 figures refer to all psychiatric disorders in the population, including psychotic and organic disorders, so the prevalence rates are somewhat higher than those given for the common mental health disorders in Section 2.2.2 above.

**Figure 1: Levels and filters model of the pathway to psychiatric care (adapted from Goldberg & Huxley, 1992)**

| | |
|---|---|
| Level 1. The community | Annual prevalence 260 to 315 per 1000 |
| Filter 1. Decision to consult a primary care physician | |
| Level 2. Primary care (total) | Annual prevalence 230 per 1000 |
| Filter 2. Recognition by the primary care physician | |
| Level 3. Primary care (conspicuous) | Annual prevalence 101 per 1000 |
| Filter 3. Referral by GP to secondary care | |
| Level 4. Psychiatric outpatient care | Annual prevalence 23 per 1000 |
| Filter 4. Decision by psychiatrist to admit | |
| Level 5. Psychiatric inpatient care | Annual prevalence 6 per 1000 |

For Filter 1 (the decision to consult a primary care physician), the key individual is the patient themselves. Level 2 refers to all psychiatric disorders in general practice, even if the GP has not diagnosed the disorder. Filter 2 refers to the detection and diagnosis of psychiatric disorder; Level 3 is 'conspicuous' or diagnosed psychiatric disorder within primary care. The third filter is the process of referral to secondary care, and Level 4 and Level 5 refer to the small proportion of patients with illnesses severe enough to need specialist secondary care.

## 2.4.1    Increasing access to care

There are significant concerns about a number of barriers to access to care. These may include stigma (both cultural and self, and stigmatisation), misinformation or cultural beliefs about the nature of mental disorder, social policy or other approaches that limit access to services.

*Presentation of people with a common mental health disorder to primary care*
Of the 130 cases of depression (including mild cases) per 1000 population, only 80 will consult their GP. The stigma associated with mental health problems generally (Sartorius, 2002), and the public view that others might view a person with depression as unbalanced, neurotic and irritating (Priest *et al.*, 1996), may partly account for the reluctance of depressed people to seek help (Bridges & Goldberg, 1987). The most common reasons given for reluctance to contact the family doctor include: did not think anyone could help (28%); a problem one should be able to cope with (28%); did not think it was necessary to contact a doctor (17%); thought problem would get better by itself (15%); too embarrassed to discuss it with anyone (13%); and afraid of the consequences (for example treatment, tests, hospitalisation or being sectioned under the Mental Health Act; 10%) (Meltzer *et al.*, 2000).

Most anxiety disorders are found more frequently in primary care than in the community except for social anxiety disorder and agoraphobia, both of which involve avoidance of public places such as doctors' surgeries (Bushnell *et al.*, 2005; Oakley Browne *et al.*, 2006; see Table 3). However, even when people with anxiety and depression do consult their GP, their disorder often goes unrecognised, partly because many do not present their psychological symptoms overtly.

Dowrick and colleagues (2010) carried out systematic reviews to identify groups for whom there are particular problems accessing mental health services, and to identify systems for promoting access. Poorer access to care has been found to be associated with lower social class, geographical location, ethnic minority groups, the presence of sensory or other impairments, the presence of learning difficulties, and particular demographic factors including age and gender (for example, older people or younger men).

This guideline seeks to identify service developments or changes that may be specifically designed to promote access, both for the general population and for specific outreach groups (see Chapter 4). Particular areas include: community outreach; providing education and information concerning the nature of mental

**Table 3: Twelve-month prevalence of anxiety disorders in New Zealand**
**(Oakley Browne *et al.*, 2006)**

| Condition | Prevalence (%) in primary care (N = 908) | Prevalence (%) in the community (N = 12,992) |
|---|---|---|
| Any anxiety disorder | 20.7 | 14.8 |
| Specific phobia | 11.0 | 7.3 |
| GAD | 6.6 | 2.9 |
| Social phobia | 3.7 | 5.1 |
| PTSD | 3.4 | 3.0 |
| OCD | 2.9 | 0.6 |
| Panic disorder without agoraphobia | 2.0 | 1.7 |
| Agoraphobia | 0.2 | 0.6 |

disorder; and new and adapted models of service delivery, which focus on the needs of black and minority ethnic (BME) groups and older people.

### 2.4.2    Identification

*Recognition of depression*
Of the 80 people with depression per 1000 population who do consult their GP, 49 are not recognised as depressed, mainly because most such patients are consulting for a somatic symptom and do not consider themselves mentally unwell despite the presence of symptoms of depression (Kisely *et al.*, 1995). People who present with somatic symptoms are especially unlikely to be recognised (Kisely *et al.*, 1995). GPs tend to be better at recognising more severe forms of the disorder (Goldberg *et al.*, 1998; Thompson *et al.*, 2001). With 50% of people with depression never consulting a doctor, 95% never entering secondary mental health services, and many more having their depression going unrecognised and untreated, this is clearly a problem for primary care.

*Recognition of anxiety disorders*
Anxiety symptoms are also often not recognised by primary healthcare professionals because, once again, patients may not complain of them overtly (Tylee & Walters, 2007). Cases of anxiety are especially likely to be missed when people frequently attend with multiple symptoms, despite reassurance. Instead, these symptoms are often characterised as possible symptoms of cardiovascular, respiratory, gastrointestinal, neurological or musculoskeletal disease (Blashki *et al.*, 2007).

For many people with a common mental health disorder, stigma and avoidance may contribute to under-recognition of their condition. Pessimism about possible treatment outcomes may further contribute to this. However, GPs themselves can contribute to the under-recognition of these conditions.

*Consultation skills*

GPs are immensely variable in their ability to recognise depressive illnesses, with some recognising virtually all of the patients found to be depressed at independent research interview, and others recognising very few (Goldberg & Huxley, 1992; Üstün & Sartorius, 1995).

The communication skills of the GP make a vital contribution to determining their ability to detect emotional distress, and those with superior skills allow their patients to show more evidence of distress during their interviews thus facilitating detection (Goldberg & Bridges, 1988; Goldberg et al., 1993).

According to Goldberg and colleagues (1980a and 1980b), ten behaviours are associated with greater detection. These include factors such as making eye contact, having good interview skills, asking well-formulated questions and focusing on more than just a symptom count. Attempts to improve GP behaviour have been successful (Ostler et al., 2001; Tiemens et al., 1999), although results are mixed (Kendrick et al., 2001; Thompson et al., 2000) and interventions sometimes fail to impact on patient outcomes despite changes in clinician behaviour (Gask et al., 2004).

*Case identification*

The fact that common mental health disorders often go undiagnosed among primary care attenders has led to suggestions that clinicians should systematically screen for hidden disorders. However, general screening is not without its problems and is currently not recommended in most countries, including the UK. Instead, targeted case identification, which involves screening a smaller group of people known to be at higher risk based on the presence of particular risk factors, may be a more useful method of improving recognition of psychological disorders in primary care.

Whooley and colleagues (1997) found that two questions were particularly sensitive in identifying depression:

- During the last month, have you often been bothered by feeling down, depressed or hopeless?
- During the last month, have you often been bothered by having little interest or pleasure in doing things?

The current NICE *Depression* guideline (NICE, 2009a) recommends that GPs be alert to possible depression in at-risk patients and consider asking the above Whooley questions when depression is suspected. If the person screens positive, further follow-up assessments should then be considered. Currently, no equivalent Whooley questions have been recommended for anxiety.

The view of the GDG for this guideline was that the development of separate case identification questions for each type of anxiety disorder would very likely be impractical and have no utility for routine use in primary care. The preference was to explore the possibility of a small number of case identification questions with general applicability for a range of anxiety disorders. A potentially positive response would then prompt a further assessment. This is dealt with in Chapter 5.

### 2.4.3   Assessment

Since April 2006, the UK general practice contract *Quality and Outcomes Framework Guidance for GMS Contract* (QOF) has incentivised GPs for measuring the severity of depression at the outset of treatment in all diagnosed cases, using validated questionnaires (British Medical Association & NHS Employers, 2008). The aim is to improve the targeting of treatment of diagnosed cases, particularly antidepressant prescribing, to those with moderate to severe depression, in line with the NICE guidelines.

A number of assessment tools have been identified as potentially useful for the assessment. The NICE *Depression* guideline (NICE, 2009a), for example, recommends the use of the nine-item Patient Health Questionnaire (PHQ-9) (Spitzer *et al.*, 1999), the depression scale of the Hospital Anxiety and Depression Scale (HADS) (Zigmond & Snaith, 1983) and the Beck Depression Inventory, 2nd edition (BDI-II) (Beck, 1996; Arnau *et al.*, 2001). The rationale for using such instruments is that doctors' global assessments of severity do not agree well with valid and reliable self-report measures of severity in terms of cut-off levels for case identification (Dowrick, 1995; Kendrick *et al.*, 2005; Lowe *et al.*, 2004; Williams *et al.*, 2002), which can result in over-treatment of mild cases and under-treatment of moderate to severe cases (Kendrick *et al.*, 2001 and 2005).

However, the QOF guidance, again in line with NICE guidance, also recommends that clinicians consider the degree of associated disability, previous history and patient preference when assessing the need for treatment rather than relying completely on the questionnaire score (British Medical Association & NHS Employers, 2006). This is especially important given that people with mental illness vary in the pattern of symptoms they experience, their family history, personalities, pre-morbid difficulties (for example, sexual abuse), physical illness, psychological mindedness, current relational and social problems and comorbidities – all of which may affect the outcomes of any intervention (for example, Cassano & Fava, 2002; Ramachandani & Stein, 2003).

Currently, evidence exists that points practitioners in the direction of well-validated tools. As a result, this guideline will not attempt to recommend specific tools because preferences vary between practices. Instead, this guideline will focus on ways to improve the assessment process, specifically, how to assess the nature and severity of a common mental health disorder, factors that may influence referral for treatment, routine outcome monitoring (ROM) and risk assessment.

### 2.4.4    Pathways to care

Given the complexity of healthcare organisations and the variation in the way care is delivered (inpatient, outpatient, day hospital, community teams and so on), choosing the right service configuration for the delivery of care to specific groups of people has gained increasing interest with regard to both policy (for example, see Department of Health, 1999) and research (for example, evaluating day hospital treatment [Marshall *et al.*, 2001]). Research using randomised controlled trial (RCT) designs has a number of difficulties; for example, using comparators such as 'standard care' in the US makes the results difficult to generalise or apply to countries with very different types of 'standard care'.

*Stepped care*
Currently, much of the UK mental health system is organised around the principles of stepped care. Stepped care (Scogin *et al.*, 2003) is a framework that is increasingly being used in the UK to provide a structure for best-practice clinical pathways to care. It is designed to increase the efficiency of service provision with an overall benefit to patient populations. The basic principle is that patients presenting with a common mental health disorder will 'step through' progressive levels of treatment as necessary, with the expectation that many of these patients will recover during the less intensive phases. High-intensity treatments are reserved for patients who do not benefit from low-intensity treatments, or for those who can be accurately predicted not to benefit from such treatments. Thus, stepped care has the potential for deriving the greatest benefit from available therapeutic resources (Bower & Gilbody, 2005) and has been recommended in a number of NICE guidelines including *Depression* (NICE, 2009a) and *Generalised Anxiety Disorder and Panic Disorder (With or Without Agoraphobia) in Adults* (NICE, 2011a).

A potential disadvantage of a stepped-care approach is that patients who do not benefit from low-intensity treatments may still have to undergo such treatments before a successful outcome is achieved. To maximise the efficiency of care delivery, patients who can be predicted as unlikely to respond to less intensive treatments ideally should be referred straight to higher levels; that is, care should be 'stratified' to an extent (Bower *et al.*, 2006). However, prognostic evidence to support such decisions is currently lacking.

*Improving Access to Psychological Therapies programme*
In 2004 the economist Richard Layard made the case for a major expansion in the availability of psychological treatments, which he suggested could bring a significant reduction in the welfare benefits bill and increased tax contributions of those helped back to work. In 2006 the government established the Improving Access to Psychological Therapies (IAPT) programme, based heavily on the stepped-care approach. Clark and colleagues (2009) reported on the initial success of two demonstration sites in Newham and Doncaster, and the IAPT programme proposes a phased national roll-out by 2013 (to date, over 50% of Primary Care Trusts have an IAPT service). Self-referral to IAPT services is also actively encouraged, with emerging evidence to suggest that it increases access for vulnerable groups, such as BME groups to psychological interventions (Clark *et al.*, 2009). In addition, an analysis of the first full year of operation of the first wave of roll-out sites (October 2008 to September 2009) has recently been published (Glover *et al.*, 2010). Anonymous

patient-level data were collected from 32 sites with the aim of evaluating whether the 'commitments relating to accessibility, the provision of NICE-approved therapies and detailed outcome monitoring were progressing appropriately'. The authors concluded that the large amount of outcome data collected is a remarkable achievement, although there are some limitations and shortcomings that need to be addressed. For example, the analysis suggests that the diagnostic coding frame needs to be extended to include panic disorder and more research needs to be conducted to establish how reliable diagnoses can be obtained. Furthermore, in terms of equality of access, the authors state that 'older people and men appeared under-represented in relation to expectation based on the patterns of morbidity shown by the psychiatric morbidity survey. The position for people with disabilities is not recorded at all in most sites, making it difficult to see how commissioners and providers can discharge their responsibilities to promote access to services for disabled people under disability discrimination legislation.' Also, 'after allowing for all other relevant factors for which data were available, Black people were significantly less likely to receive any treatment or to recover on either the two-scale or the three-scale makers, Asians were less likely to receive high intensity treatment (CBT or counselling), and both were significantly less likely to receive CBT'. More generally, with regard to treatment received, there was evidence to suggest that more needs to be done to ensure that the treatment given for specific diagnoses is aligned to that recommended in NICE guidelines.

# 3 METHODS USED TO DEVELOP THIS GUIDELINE

## 3.1 OVERVIEW

The development of this guideline drew upon methods outlined by NICE (further information is available in *The Guidelines Manual* [NICE, 2009d]). A team of health professionals, lay representatives and technical experts known as the Guideline Development Group (GDG), with support from the NCCMH staff, undertook the development of a patient-centred, evidence-based guideline. There are six basic steps in the process of developing a guideline:

1. Define the scope, which sets the parameters of the guideline and provides a focus and steer for the development work.
2. Define review questions considered important for practitioners and people with a common mental health disorder.
3. Develop criteria for evidence searching and search for evidence.
4. Design validated protocols for systematic review and apply to evidence recovered by search.
5. Synthesise and (meta-) analyse data retrieved, guided by the review questions, and produce Grading of Recommendations: Assessment, Development and Evaluation (GRADE) evidence profiles and summaries.
6. Answer review questions with evidence-based recommendations for clinical practice.

The clinical practice recommendations made by the GDG are therefore derived from the most up-to-date and robust evidence base for the clinical and cost effectiveness of the treatments and services used in the treatment and management of common mental health disorders. In addition, to ensure a patient and carer focus, the concerns of people with common mental health disorders and carers (regarding health and social care) have been highlighted and addressed by recommendations agreed by the whole GDG.

## 3.2 THE SCOPE

Guideline topics are selected by the Department of Health and the Welsh Assembly Government, which identify the main areas to be covered by the guideline in a specific remit (see *The Guidelines Manual* [NICE, 2009d] for further information). The NCCMH developed a scope for the guideline based on the remit. The purpose of the scope is to:

● provide an overview of what the guideline will include and exclude
● identify the key aspects of care that must be included
● set the boundaries of the development work and provide a clear framework to enable work to stay within the priorities agreed by NICE and the National

Collaborating Centre and the remit from the Department of Health/Welsh Assembly Government
- inform the development of the review questions and search strategy
- inform professionals and the public about expected content of the guideline
- keep the guideline to a reasonable size to ensure that its development can be carried out within the allocated period.

An initial draft of the scope was sent to registered stakeholders who had agreed to attend a scoping workshop. The workshop was used to:
- obtain feedback on the selected key clinical issues
- identify which patient or population subgroups should be specified (if any)
- seek views on the composition of the GDG
- encourage applications for GDG membership.

The draft scope was subject to consultation with registered stakeholders over a 4-week period. During the consultation period, the scope was posted on the NICE website (www.nice.org.uk). Comments were invited from stakeholder organisations and the Guideline Review Panel. Further information about the Guideline Review Panel can also be found on the NICE website. The NCCMH and NICE reviewed the scope in light of comments received, and the revised scope was signed off by the Guideline Review Panel. The scope is reproduced in Appendix 1.

## 3.3    THE GUIDELINE DEVELOPMENT GROUP

The GDG consisted of: professionals in psychiatry, clinical psychology, nursing and general practice; academic experts in psychiatry and psychology; two people with a common mental health disorder and a carer. The guideline development process was supported by staff from the NCCMH, who undertook the clinical and health economics literature searches, reviewed and presented the evidence to the GDG, managed the process, and contributed to drafting the guideline.

### 3.3.1    Guideline Development Group meetings

Nine GDG meetings were held between December 2009 and January 2011. During each day-long GDG meeting review questions and clinical and economic evidence were reviewed and assessed, and recommendations formulated. At each meeting, all GDG members declared any potential conflicts of interest, and service user and carer concerns were routinely discussed as part of a standing agenda.

### 3.3.2    Topic groups

The GDG divided its workload along clinically relevant lines to simplify the guideline development process, and GDG members formed smaller topic groups to undertake guideline work in that area of clinical practice: Topic Group 1 covered questions relating to access to healthcare; Topic Group 2 covered case identification; Topic Group 3 covered assessment; and Topic Group 4 covered systems for organising and developing local care pathways. These groups were designed to efficiently manage the large volume of evidence appraisal prior to presenting it to the GDG as a whole. Each topic group was chaired by a GDG member with expert knowledge of the topic area (one of the healthcare professionals). Topic groups were responsible for refining the review questions relevant to the topic, and assisted with the review and synthesis of the evidence. All decisions concerning recommendations were made by the full GDG. Topic group leaders reported the status of the group's work as part of the standing agenda. They also introduced and led the GDG discussion of the evidence review for that topic and assisted the technical staff from the NCCMH in drafting the section of the guideline relevant to the work of each topic group.

### 3.3.3    Service users and carers

Individuals with direct experience of services gave an integral service-user focus to the GDG and the guideline. The GDG included two people with a common mental health disorder and a carer. They contributed as full GDG members to writing the review questions, helping to ensure that the evidence addressed their views and preferences, highlighting sensitive issues and terminology relevant to the guideline, and bringing service-user research to the attention of the GDG. In drafting the guideline, they contributed to developing the evidence chapters and identified recommendations from the service user and carer perspective.

### 3.4    REVIEW QUESTIONS

Review (clinical) questions were used to guide the identification and interrogation of the evidence base relevant to the topic of the guideline. Before the first GDG meeting an analytic framework (see Appendix 4) was prepared by NCCMH staff, based on the scope and an overview of existing guidelines, and discussed with the guideline Chair. The framework was used to provide a structure from which the review questions were drafted. Both the analytic framework and the draft review questions were then discussed by the GDG at the first few meetings and amended as necessary. Where appropriate, the framework and questions were refined once the evidence had been searched and, where necessary, subquestions were generated. Questions submitted by stakeholders were also discussed by the GDG and the rationale for not including any questions was recorded in the minutes. The final list of review questions can be found in Appendix 4.

For questions about interventions or service delivery models, the PICO (patient/population, intervention, comparison and outcome) framework was used (see Table 4).

In some situations, the prognosis of a particular condition is of fundamental importance, over and above its general significance in relation to specific interventions.

**Table 4:  Features of a well-formulated question on effectiveness intervention – the PICO guide**

| Patients/ population | Which patients or population of patients are we interested in? How can they be best described? Are there subgroups that need to be considered? |
|---|---|
| Intervention | Which intervention, treatment or approach should be used? |
| Comparison | What is/are the main alternative/s to compare with the intervention? |
| Outcome | What is really important for the patient? Which outcomes should be considered: intermediate or short-term measures; mortality; morbidity and treatment complications; rates of relapse; late morbidity and readmission; return to work, physical and social functioning and other measures such as quality of life; general health status; costs? |

Areas where this is particularly likely to occur relate to assessment of risk, for example in terms of behaviour modification or case identification and early intervention. In addition, review questions related to issues of service delivery are occasionally specified in the remit from the Department of Health/Welsh Assembly Government. In these cases, appropriate review questions were developed to be clear and concise.

To help facilitate the literature review, a note was made of the best study design type to answer each question. There are four main types of review question of relevance to NICE guidelines. These are listed in Table 5: Best study design to answer each type of question. For each type of question, the best primary study design varies, where 'best' is interpreted as 'least likely to give misleading answers to the question'.

However, in all cases, a well-conducted systematic review (of the appropriate type of study) is likely to always yield a better answer than a single study.

Deciding on the best design type to answer a specific review question does not mean that studies of different design types addressing the same question were discarded.

## 3.5    SYSTEMATIC CLINICAL LITERATURE REVIEW

The aim of the clinical literature review was to systematically identify and synthesise relevant evidence from the literature in order to answer the specific review questions developed by the GDG. Thus, clinical practice recommendations are evidence-based where possible and, if evidence is not available, informal consensus methods are used (see Section 7.2) and the need for future research is specified.

**Table 5: Best study design to answer each type of question**

| Type of question | Best primary study design |
|---|---|
| Effectiveness or other impact of in an intervention | RCT; other studies that may be considered the absence of RCTs are the following: internally/externally controlled before and after trial, interrupted time-series |
| Accuracy of information (for example, risk factor, test and prediction rule) | Comparing the information against a valid gold standard in a randomised trial or inception cohort study |
| Rates (of disease, patient experience and rare side effects) | Prospective cohort, registry, cross-sectional study |
| Costs | Naturalistic prospective cost study |

### 3.5.1 Methodology

A stepwise hierarchical approach was taken to locating and presenting evidence to the GDG. The NCCMH developed this process based on methods set out by NICE (*The Guidelines Manual*; NICE, 2009d), and after considering recommendations from a range of other sources. These included:

- Clinical Policy and Practice Program of the New South Wales Department of Health (Australia)
- BMJ Clinical Evidence
- GRADE Working Group
- New Zealand Guidelines Group
- NHS Centre for Reviews and Dissemination
- Oxford Centre for Evidence-Based Medicine
- Oxford Systematic Review Development Programme
- Scottish Intercollegiate Guidelines Network (SIGN)
- The Cochrane Collaboration
- United States Agency for Healthcare Research and Quality.

### 3.5.2 The review process

*Scoping searches*

A broad preliminary search of the literature was undertaken in October 2009 to obtain an overview of the issues likely to be covered by the scope and to help define key areas. Searches were restricted to clinical guidelines, health technology assessment (HTA) reports, key systematic reviews and RCTs, and conducted in the following databases and websites:

- BMJ Clinical Evidence
- Canadian Medical Association Infobase (Canadian guidelines)
- Clinical Policy and Practice Program of the New South Wales Department of Health (Australia)
- Clinical Practice Guidelines (Australian guidelines)
- Cochrane Central Register of Controlled Trials (CENTRAL)
- Cochrane Database of Abstracts of Reviews of Effects (DARE)
- Cochrane Database of Systematic Reviews (CDSR)
- Excerpta Medical Database (EMBASE)
- Guidelines International Network (G-I-N)
- Health Evidence Bulletin Wales
- Health Management Information Consortium
- HTA database (technology assessments)
- Medical Literature Analysis and Retrieval System Online (MEDLINE)/ MEDLINE in Process
- National Health and Medical Research Council
- National Library for Health Guidelines Finder
- New Zealand Guidelines Group
- NHS Centre for Reviews and Dissemination
- OmniMedicalSearch
- Scottish Intercollegiate Guidelines Network (SIGN)
- Turning Research Into Practice
- United States Agency for Healthcare Research and Quality
- Websites of NICE and the National Institute for Health Research HTA programme for guidelines and HTAs in development.

Existing NICE guidelines were updated where necessary. Other relevant guidelines were assessed for quality using the AGREE instrument (AGREE Collaboration, 2003). Where an individual review from another guideline was used (rather than the full guideline), the systematic review methodology checklist was used instead of the AGREE instrument. The evidence base underlying high-quality existing guidelines was utilised and updated as appropriate. Further information about this process can be found in *The Guidelines Manual* (NICE, 2009d).

*Systematic literature searches*

After the scope was finalised, a systematic search strategy was developed to locate all the relevant evidence. The balance between sensitivity (the power to identify all studies on a particular topic) and specificity (the ability to exclude irrelevant studies from the results) was carefully considered and a decision made to utilise a broad approach to searching, to identify as complete a set as possible of clinically relevant studies.

Searches were conducted in the following databases:

- CDSR
- CENTRAL
- Cumulative Index to Nursing and Allied Health Literature (CINAHL)
- DARE
- EMBASE

- MEDLINE/MEDLINE In-Process
- Psychological Information Database (PsycINFO).

The search strategies were initially developed for MEDLINE before being translated for use in other databases/interfaces. Strategies were built up from a number of trial searches, and from discussions of the results of the searches with the review team/GDG, to ensure that all possible relevant search terms were covered.

*Reference Manager*

Citations from each search were downloaded into Reference Manager (a software product for managing references and formatting bibliographies) and duplicates removed. Records were then screened against the inclusion criteria of the reviews before being quality appraised (see below). The unfiltered search results were saved and retained for future potential re-analysis to help keep the process both replicable and transparent.

*Search filters*

To aid retrieval of relevant and sound studies, filters were used to limit the searches to systematic reviews, RCTs and observational studies. The systematic review and RCT filters are adaptations of designs constructed by the NHS Centre for Reviews and Dissemination and the Health Information Research Unit of McMaster University, Ontario. The observational studies filter was developed in-house. Each filter comprises index terms relating to the study type(s) and associated text words for the methodological description of the design(s).

*Date and language restrictions*

Systematic database searches were initially conducted in December 2009. The search for systematic reviews was restricted to the last 10 years because older reviews were considered to be less useful. Search updates were generated on a 6-monthly basis, with the final re-runs carried out in September 2010 ahead of the guideline consultation. After this point, studies were only included if they were judged to be exceptional by the GDG (for example, if the evidence was likely to change a recommendation).

Although no language restrictions were applied at the searching stage, foreign language papers were not requested or reviewed unless they were of particular importance to a clinical question. Date restrictions were applied for searches for systematic reviews and for updates of published reviews only (see Appendix 5). No date restrictions were imposed for the remainder of the searches.

*Post-guideline searching*

Following the draft guideline consultation, a search for systematic reviews on 'predictors of response' was undertaken for the period from 2003 up to January 2011.

*Other search methods*

Other search methods involved: (1) scanning the reference lists of all eligible publications (systematic reviews, stakeholder evidence and included studies) for more published reports and citations of unpublished research; (2) checking the tables of contents of key journals for studies that might have been missed by the database and reference list searches; (3) tracking key papers in the Science Citation Index (prospectively) over time for further useful references.

Full details of the MEDLINE search strategies/filters used for the systematic review of clinical evidence are provided in Appendix 6.

*Study selection and quality assessment*

All studies included after the first scan of citations were acquired in full and re-evaluated for eligibility at the time they were being entered into Review Manager 5 (Cochrane Collaboration, 2008) or evidence tables. More specific eligibility criteria were developed for each review question and are described in the relevant clinical evidence chapters. Eligible systematic reviews and primary-level studies were critically appraised for methodological quality (see Appendix 7 for methodology checklists). The eligibility of each study was confirmed by at least one member of the appropriate topic group.

For some review questions, it was necessary to prioritise the evidence with respect to the UK context (that is, external validity). To make this process explicit, the GDG took into account the following factors when assessing the evidence:
● participant factors (for example, gender, age and ethnicity)
● provider factors (for example, model fidelity, the conditions under which the intervention was performed and the availability of experienced staff to undertake the procedure)
● cultural factors (for example, differences in standard care and differences in the welfare system).

It was the responsibility of each topic group to decide which prioritisation factors were relevant to each review question in light of the UK context and then decide how they should modify their recommendations.

*Unpublished evidence*

The GDG used a number of criteria when deciding whether or not to accept unpublished data. First, the evidence must have been accompanied by a trial report containing sufficient detail to properly assess the quality of the data. Second, the evidence must have been submitted with the understanding that data from the study and a summary of the study's characteristics would be published in the full guideline. Therefore, the GDG did not accept evidence submitted as commercial in confidence. However, the GDG recognised that unpublished evidence submitted by investigators might later be retracted by those investigators if the inclusion of such data would jeopardise publication of their research.

### 3.5.3    Data extraction

Study characteristics and outcome data were extracted from all eligible studies, which met the minimum quality criteria, using Review Manager 5 (Cochrane Collaboration, 2008) or Microsoft Word-based evidence tables (Microsoft, 2007).

Consultation with another reviewer or members of the GDG was used to overcome difficulties with coding. Where possible, two independent reviewers extracted data from new studies. Where double data extraction was not possible, data extracted by one reviewer was checked by the second reviewer. Disagreements were resolved through discussion. Where consensus could not be reached, a third reviewer or GDG members resolved the disagreement. Masked assessment (that is, blind to the journal from which the article comes, the authors, the institution and the magnitude of the effect) was not used because it is unclear whether doing so reduces bias (Berlin, 1997; Jadad *et al.*, 1996).

### 3.5.4    Evidence synthesis and presentation

*Existing guidelines and systematic reviews*
Existing NICE guidelines (listed in Section 2.1) provided an important relevant source of evidence for the development of this guideline in terms of treatment and referral advice for common mental health disorders, and this was subject to narrative synthesis.

Methods for conducting narrative synthesis, based on the work of Popay and colleagues (2006), were used to synthesise existing NICE guidelines relevant to common mental health disorders and systematic reviews identified during the literature search. In most cases, a preliminary synthesis was made using tabulation. This was then used to write an evidence summary.

*Meta-analysis of diagnostic accuracy data*
Review Manager 5 was used to summarise diagnostic accuracy data from each study using forest plots and summary receiver operator characteristic (ROC) plots. Where more than two studies reported appropriate data, a bivariate diagnostic accuracy meta-analysis was conducted using Stata 10 (StataCorp, 2007) with the MIDAS (Module for Meta-analytical Integration of Diagnostic Test Accuracy Studies; Dwamena, 2007) command to obtain pooled estimates of sensitivity, specificity, likelihood ratios and diagnostic odds ratio (OR).

*Sensitivity and specificity*
The sensitivity of an instrument refers to the proportion of those with the condition who test positive. An instrument that detects a low percentage of cases will not be very helpful in determining the numbers of service users who should receive a known effective treatment because many individuals who should receive the treatment will not do so. This would lead to an under-estimation of the prevalence of the disorder, contribute to inadequate care and make for poor planning and costing of the need for treatment. As the sensitivity of an instrument increases, the number of false negatives it detects will decrease.

The specificity of an instrument refers to the proportion of those who do not have the condition and test negative. This is important so that healthy people are not offered treatments they do not need. As the specificity of an instrument increases, the number of false positives it detects will decrease.

To illustrate this: from a population in which the point prevalence rate of anxiety is 10% (that is, 10% of the population has anxiety at any one time), 1000 people are given a test that has 90% sensitivity and 85% specificity. It is known that 100 people in this population have anxiety, but the test detects only 90 (true positives) leaving ten undetected (false negatives). It is also known that 900 people do not have anxiety, and the test correctly identifies 765 of these (true negatives) but classifies 135 incorrectly as having anxiety (false positives). The positive predictive value of the test (the number correctly identified as having anxiety as a proportion of positive tests) is 40% (90/90 + 135), and the negative predictive value (the number correctly identified as not having anxiety as a proportion of negative tests) is 98% (765/765 + 10). Therefore, in this example, a positive test result is correct in only 40% of cases, while a negative result can be relied upon in 98% of cases.

The example above illustrates some of the main differences between positive predictive values and negative predictive values in comparison with sensitivity and specificity. For both positive and negative predictive values, prevalence explicitly forms part of their calculation (see Altman & Bland, 1994a). When the prevalence of a disorder is low in a population this is generally associated with a higher negative predictive value and a lower positive predictive value. Therefore, although these statistics are concerned with issues probably more directly applicable to clinical practice (for example, the probability that a person with a positive test result actually has anxiety), they are largely dependent on the characteristics of the population sampled and cannot be universally applied (Altman & Bland, 1994a).

On the other hand, sensitivity and specificity do not necessarily depend on prevalence of anxiety (Altman & Bland, 1994b). For example, sensitivity is concerned with the performance of an identification instrument conditional on a person having anxiety. Therefore the higher false positives often associated with samples of low prevalence will not affect such estimates. The advantage of this approach is that sensitivity and specificity can be applied across populations (Altman & Bland, 1994b). However, the main disadvantage is that clinicians tend to find such estimates more difficult to interpret.

When describing the sensitivity and specificity of the different instruments, the GDG defined values above 0.9 as 'excellent', 0.8 to 0.9 as 'good', 0.5 to 0.7 as 'moderate', 0.3 to 0.5 as 'low' and less than 0.3 as 'poor'.

*Receiver operator characteristic curves*
The qualities of a particular tool are summarised in a ROC curve, which plots sensitivity (expressed as a percentage) against (100-specificity) (see Figure 2).

A test with perfect discrimination would have an ROC curve that passed through the top left hand corner; that is, it would have 100% specificity and pick up all true positives with no false positives. While this is never achieved in practice, the area under the curve (AUC) measures how close the tool gets to the theoretical ideal. A perfect test would have an AUC of 1 and a test with AUC above 0.5 is better than chance. As discussed above, because these measures are based on sensitivity and 100-specificity, theoretically these estimates are not affected by prevalence.

**Figure 2: Receiver operator characteristic curve**

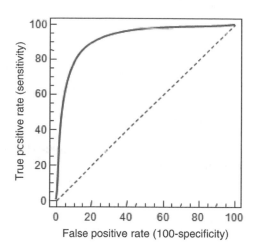

*Negative and positive likelihood ratios*

Negative and positive likelihood ratios (LR–/LR+) are considered not to be dependent on prevalence. LR– is calculated by sensitivity/1-specificity and LR+ is 1-sensitivity/specificity. A value of LR+ >5 and LR– <0.3 suggests the test is relatively accurate (Fischer *et al.*, 2003).

*Diagnostic odds ratio*

The diagnostic OR is LR+/LR–; a value of 20 or greater suggests a good level of accuracy (Fischer *et al.*, 2003).

*Publication bias*

Where there was sufficient data, the intention was to use funnel plots to explore the possibility of publication bias. Asymmetry of the plot would be taken to indicate possible publication bias and investigated further. However, due to a paucity of data, funnel plots could not be used.

## 3.6     HEALTH ECONOMIC METHODS

The aim of the health economics was to contribute to the guideline's development by providing evidence on the cost effectiveness of interventions for common mental health disorders covered in the guideline. This was achieved by:

● systematic literature review of existing economic evidence
● decision-analytic economic modelling.

Systematic reviews of economic literature were conducted in all areas covered in the guideline. Economic modelling was undertaken in areas with likely major resource implications, where available clinical evidence was sufficient to allow the development of an economic model that would provide fairly robust evidence on the cost effectiveness of interventions for the management of people with common mental health disorders. Prioritisation of areas for economic modelling was a joint decision between the health economist and the GDG. After considering areas with potentially significant resource implications and the availability of respective clinical data, the following economic question was selected as a key issue that was addressed by economic modelling:

● what is the cost effectiveness of case identification for people with common mental health disorders?

In addition, literature on the health-related quality of life (HRQoL) of people with common mental health disorders, especially anxiety and depression, was systematically searched to identify studies reporting appropriate utility scores that could be utilised in a cost-utility analysis.

The rest of this section describes the methods adopted in the systematic literature review of economic studies. Methods employed in economic modelling are described in the respective sections of the guideline.

### 3.6.1    Search strategy for economic evidence

*Scoping searches*

A broad preliminary search of the literature was undertaken in October 2009 to obtain an overview of the issues likely to be covered by the scope and help define key areas. Searches were restricted to economic studies and HTA reports, and conducted in the following databases:

● EMBASE
● HTA database (technology assessments)
● MEDLINE/MEDLINE In-Process
● NHS Economic Evaluation Database (NHS EED).

Any relevant economic evidence arising from the clinical scoping searches was also made available to the health economist during the same period.

*Systematic literature searches*

After the scope was finalised, a systematic search strategy was developed to locate all the relevant evidence. The balance between sensitivity (the power to identify all studies on a particular topic) and specificity (the ability to exclude irrelevant studies from the results) was carefully considered, and a decision made to utilise a broad approach to searching to maximise retrieval of evidence to all parts of the guideline. Searches were restricted to economic evidence (including full and partial economic evaluations) and HTA reports, and conducted in the following databases:

● EconLit
● EMBASE
● HTA database (technology assessments)

- MEDLINE/MEDLINE In-Process
- NHS EED
- PsycINFO.

Again, any relevant economic evidence arising from the clinical searches was also made available to the health economist during the same period.

The search strategies were initially developed for MEDLINE before being translated for use in other databases/interfaces. Strategies were built up through a number of trial searches, and through discussions of the results of the searches with the review team/GDG, to ensure that all possible relevant search terms were covered.

*Reference Manager*

Citations from each search were downloaded into Reference Manager and duplicates removed. Records were then screened against the inclusion criteria of the reviews before being quality appraised. The unfiltered search results were saved and retained for future potential re-analysis to help keep the process both replicable and transparent.

*Search filters*

The search filter for health economics is an adaptation of a pre-tested strategy designed by the NHS Centre for Reviews and Dissemination (2007). The search filter is designed to retrieve records of economic evidence (including full and partial economic evaluations) from the vast amount of literature indexed to major medical databases such as MEDLINE. The filter, which comprises a combination of controlled vocabulary and free-text retrieval methods, maximises sensitivity (or recall) to ensure that as many potentially relevant records as possible are retrieved from a search. Full details of the filter are provided in Appendix 8.

*Date and language restrictions*

Systematic database searches were initially conducted in January 2010 up to the most recent searchable date, with the final re-runs carried out in September 2010. After this point, studies were included only if they were judged by the GDG to be exceptional (for example, the evidence was likely to change a recommendation).

Although no language restrictions were applied at the searching stage, foreign language papers were not requested or reviewed unless they were of particular importance to an area under review. All the searches were restricted to research published from 1995 onwards in order to obtain data relevant to current healthcare settings and costs.

*Other search methods*

Other search methods involved scanning the reference lists of all eligible publications (systematic reviews, stakeholder evidence and included studies from the economic and clinical reviews) to identify further studies for consideration.

Full details of the search strategies and filters used for the systematic review of health economic evidence are provided in Appendix 8.

### 3.6.2 Inclusion criteria for economic studies

The following inclusion criteria were applied to select studies identified by the economic searches for further consideration:

- Only studies from the Organisation for Economic Co-operation and Development countries were included because the aim of the review was to identify economic information transferable to the UK context.
- Selection criteria based on types of clinical conditions and patients as well as interventions assessed were identical to the clinical literature review.
- Studies were included provided that sufficient details regarding methods and results were available to enable the methodological quality of the study to be assessed, and provided that the study's data and results were extractable. Poster presentations of abstracts were excluded.
- Full economic evaluations that compared two or more relevant options and considered both costs and consequences (that is, cost–consequence analysis, cost–effectiveness analysis, cost–utility analysis or cost–benefit analysis), as well as costing analyses that compared only costs between two or more interventions, were included in the review.
- Economic studies were included if they used clinical effectiveness data from an RCT, a prospective cohort study, or a systematic review and meta-analysis of clinical studies. Studies that had a mirror-image or other retrospective design were excluded from the review.
- Studies were included only if the examined interventions were clearly described. This involved the dosage and route of administration and the duration of treatment in the case of pharmacological therapies, and the types of health professionals involved, as well as the frequency and duration of treatment in the case of psychological interventions. Evaluations in which medications were treated as a class were excluded from further consideration.
- Studies that adopted a very narrow perspective, ignoring major categories of costs to the NHS, were excluded; for example, studies that estimated exclusively drug acquisition costs or hospitalisation costs were considered non-informative to the guideline development process.

### 3.6.3 Applicability and quality criteria for economic studies

All economic papers eligible for inclusion were appraised for their applicability and quality using the methodology checklist for economic evaluations recommended by NICE (2009d), which is shown in Appendix 9 of this guideline. The methodology checklist for economic evaluations was also applied to the economic models developed specifically for this guideline. All studies that fully or partially met the applicability and quality criteria described in the methodology checklist were considered during the guideline development process, along with the results of the economic modelling conducted specifically for this guideline. The completed methodology checklists for all economic evaluations considered in the guideline are provided in Appendix 12.

### 3.6.4    Presentation of economic evidence

The economic evidence considered in the guideline is provided in the respective evidence chapters, following presentation of the relevant clinical evidence. The references to included studies and the respective evidence tables with the study characteristics and results are provided in Appendix 10. Methods and results of economic modelling undertaken alongside the guideline development process are presented in the relevant evidence chapters.

### 3.6.5    Results of the systematic search of economic literature

The titles of all studies identified by the systematic search of the literature were screened for their relevance to the topic (that is, economic issues and information on HRQoL in people with common mental health disorders). References that were clearly not relevant were excluded first. The abstracts of all potentially relevant studies (235 references) were then assessed against the inclusion criteria for economic evaluations by the health economist. Full texts of the studies potentially meeting the inclusion criteria (including those for which eligibility was not clear from the abstract) were obtained. Studies that did not meet the inclusion criteria, were duplicates, were secondary publications of one study or had been updated in more recent publications were subsequently excluded. Economic evaluations eligible for inclusion (that is, one study on stepped care and one study on identification methods) were then appraised for their applicability and quality using the methodology checklist for economic evaluations. Of these, one economic study fully or partially met the applicability and quality criteria and was considered at formulation of the guideline recommendations.

### 3.7    FROM EVIDENCE TO RECOMMENDATIONS

Once the clinical and health economic evidence was summarised, the GDG drafted the recommendations. The GDG took account of the principles of stepped-care approaches when considering the evidence and formulating recommendations.

In making recommendations, the GDG took into account the trade-off between the benefits and downsides of the intervention/instrument, as well as other important factors such as economic considerations, values of the development group and society, the requirements to prevent discrimination and to promote equality[1] and the group's awareness of practical issues (Eccles *et al.*, 1998; NICE, 2009d).

Finally, to show clearly how the GDG moved from the evidence to the recommendations, each chapter has a section called 'From evidence to recommendations'. Underpinning this section is the concept of the 'strength' of a recommendation (Schünemann *et al.*, 2003). This takes into account the quality of the evidence, but is

---

[1]See NICE's equality scheme: www.nice.org.uk/aboutnice/howwework/NICEEquality Scheme.jsp

conceptually different. Some recommendations are 'strong' in that the GDG believes that the vast majority of healthcare professionals and patients would choose a particular intervention if they considered the evidence in the same way that the GDG has. This is generally the case if the benefits clearly outweigh the harms for most people and the intervention is likely to be cost effective. However, there is often a closer balance between benefits and harms and some patients would not choose an intervention whereas others would. This may happen, for example, if some service users are particularly averse to a side effect and others are not. In these circumstances the recommendation is generally weaker, although it may be possible to make stronger recommendations about specific groups of patients. The strength of each recommendation is reflected in the wording of the recommendation, rather than by using ratings, labels or symbols.

Where the GDG identified areas in which there are uncertainties or where robust evidence was lacking, they developed research recommendations. Those that were identified as 'high-priority' were included in the NICE version of the guideline, and in Appendix 11.

## 3.8    STAKEHOLDER CONTRIBUTIONS

Professionals, service users, and companies have contributed to and commented on the guideline at key stages in its development. Stakeholders for this guideline include:

- service user and carer stakeholders: the national service user and carer organisations that represent the interests of people with a common mental health disorder
- local service user and carer organisations: but only if there is no relevant national organisation
- professional stakeholders' national organisations: that represent the healthcare professionals who provide the services described in the guideline
- commercial stakeholders: companies that manufacture drugs or devices used in treatment of common mental health disorders and whose interests may be significantly affected by the guideline
- providers and commissioners of health services in England and Wales
- statutory organisations: including the Department of Health, the Welsh Assembly Government, NHS Quality Improvement Scotland, the Healthcare Commission and the National Patient Safety Agency
- research organisations: that have carried out nationally recognised research in the area.

Stakeholders have been involved in the guideline's development at the following points:

- commenting on the initial scope of the guideline and attending a briefing meeting held by NICE
- contributing possible review questions and lists of evidence to the GDG
- commenting on the draft of the guideline
- highlighting factual errors in the pre-publication check.

## 3.9    VALIDATION OF THE GUIDELINE

Registered stakeholders had an opportunity to comment on the draft guideline, which was posted on the NICE website during the consultation period. Following the consultation all comments from stakeholders and others were responded to and the guideline updated as appropriate. The Guideline Review Panel also reviewed the guideline and checked that stakeholders' comments had been addressed.

Following the consultation period, the GDG finalised the recommendations and the NCCMH produced the final documents. These were then submitted to NICE for the pre-publication check where stakeholders were given the opportunity to highlight factual errors. Any errors were corrected by the NCCMH, then the guideline was formally approved by NICE and issued as guidance to the NHS in England and Wales.

# 4. ACCESS TO HEALTHCARE

## 4.1 INTRODUCTION

### 4.1.1 Definition of access to healthcare

Many people with a range of mental disorders are disadvantaged because of poor access to care. This may either be because care is not available, or because their interaction with care givers deters or diverts their help seeking (Dowrick *et al.*, 2009a). Improving the quality of care requires addressing both effectiveness of *and* access to healthcare (Campbell *et al.*, 2000). Access to healthcare is a complex phenomenon that is notoriously difficult to define (Gulliford *et al.*, 2007). Considerations of access to mental healthcare for people with common mental health disorders have largely been restricted to concerns about recognition of mental health disorders by primary care 'gatekeepers' in the NHS and the difficulties of training professionals to improve recognition and referral. This deals only with a small part of a more complex experience of gaining access to healthcare for the individual, which has been recently characterised by Dixon-Woods and colleagues (2005) as consisting of several stages, outlined in the paragraph below.

*Candidacy* is defined as 'how people's eligibility for healthcare is a jointly negotiated interaction between individuals and healthcare services', and as a 'dynamic and contingent process, constantly being defined and redefined through interactions between individuals and professionals'. Following determination of candidacy, individuals undertake *navigation* to gain a point of entry to healthcare services. *Appearance* can involve a number of different approaches, including appearing before healthcare services through individual-initiated actions or through invitations (where people respond to healthcare services). *Adjudication* refers to professional judgements about the presentation of an individual for an intervention or service, influenced by categorisations made by professionals with reference to current services and relationships. Adjudication leads to an *offer* (or non-offer) of a healthcare service, which may be accepted or rejected. The concept of *recursivity* captures how the response of the system to individuals may reinforce or discourage future health behaviours (Rogers *et al.*, 1999).

### 4.1.2 Aim of the review

Access to healthcare is a large and diverse topic with a range of complex issues and considerations. For people experiencing mental health problems across a range of social and demographic groups, access to healthcare can be challenging. This chapter aims to identify factors that affect access for those who require mental healthcare. This chapter also aims to evaluate the effectiveness of adaptations to existing models and methods with the aim of improving access, as well as new service developments that are specifically designed to promote access.

Initial scoping reviews and advice from GDG members identified that, in addition to factors that affect access for all people, there are other factors that need to be considered for certain vulnerable groups. Previous research has evaluated inequalities in access to healthcare for a wide range of different groups, based on socioeconomic situation, ethnicity, age and gender (see, for example, Dixon-Woods *et al.*, 2005). The GDG therefore considered the evidence for all individuals requiring access to healthcare, as well as evidence (when available) for different vulnerable groups.

Although the literature search identified a number of groups whose access to services was disproportionately restricted, a great proportion of the evidence for vulnerable groups reviewed factors that affect access, and methods of improving access, for BME groups and older people in particular. There is considerable evidence that access to healthcare for BME groups is problematic in the UK (Department of Health, 2009). Similarly, a number of studies have identified older people has having poor access to healthcare and, in particular, mental healthcare services (Department of Health, 2001). The GDG therefore decided to focus this review on the general principles underpinning access to services for all members of the population (referred to in the rest of the chapter as the 'general population' and including people with a range of mental disorders and also some with physical health problems), and to also look at specific problems faced by two sub-populations: BME groups and older people. In view of the limitations of the data the GDG decided to undertake a narrative synthesis of the available evidence. See Chapter 3 for a rationale of the methods employed in this review.

*Black and minority ethnic groups*
Recent literature indicates that there are still disparities in access to mental healthcare for BME groups when compared with other ethnic groups. Although primary care utilisation appears to be high among BME groups (more for physical health problems than mental health disorders), the utilisation of secondary and tertiary services is not as high (Dixon-Woods *et al.*, 2005). Even after adjusting for variables such as region, place of residence and income, Van Voorhees and colleagues (2007) reported that people from BME groups were still less likely to receive treatment from mental healthcare services. Simpson and colleagues (2007) also found that there are racial disparities in the diagnosis and treatment of depression in the US, and that people from BME groups with depression are less likely to be identified, even when a screening tool is utilised, and less likely to receive medication or psychotherapy for the treatment of depression.

Similarly, in a review of UK specialist mental healthcare services, Bhui and colleagues (2003) reported that black Africans and black Caribbeans were less likely than south Asian and white people to be referred for specialist mental healthcare unless they presented to a GP who was already aware they had a mental health problem. Bhui and colleagues (2003) also identified that, as a consequence of this, black people were more likely to present in crisis, usually to an on-call emergency department psychiatrist. Moreover, black people (ethnicity not specified) are more likely to be admitted to psychiatric units compulsorily, held in locked wards and sectioned under the Mental Health Act in the UK (Dixon-Woods *et al.*, 2005). It also appears that people from BME groups may be less likely to maintain contact with specialist mental healthcare services compared with white people (although the evidence for this is inconsistent across studies) (Bhui *et al.*, 2003).

*Older people*
There are particular concerns about disadvantages in access to healthcare for older people (Department of Health, 2001). Studies consistently identify unmet needs and older people often lack family or similar support systems, which may contribute to under recognition and limited access to services. Consultation rates for psychiatric disorders in men in particular have been found to be low in older people (Shah *et al.*, 2001), and this may contribute further to poor access and consequent under treatment (see, for example, the work on depression in older people by Katona [2000]). Unsurprisingly, concerns have been raised about access to healthcare for older people from BME groups. For example, Lindesay and colleagues (1997) found that older Asian people had poorer uptake of services than white older people. However, it should be noted that research evaluating access to healthcare for older BME people is limited. It has also been suggested that sociodemographic factors also result in reduced access to healthcare for older people (Chaix *et al.*, 2005). Although Dixon-Woods and colleagues (2005) found no evidence for an urban-rural divide in access to healthcare for older people, they discerned that older individuals living in rural areas did not have equal access to domiciliary services or more centralised services.

## 4.2    FACTORS AFFECTING ACCESS

### 4.2.1    Introduction

Factors that affect access to healthcare exist at different points in the system and it is important to properly identify those factors that result from the behaviour of health-care professionals, and the performance of the wider health and social care system, and those that are related to individual or group behaviours, beliefs and attitudes towards mental health disorders and their care and treatment.

### 4.2.2    Clinical review protocol

The aim of this review is to provide a narrative synthesis of the evidence that assesses and identifies the possible factors that affect access to mental healthcare services for people with common mental health disorders. The review protocol, including the review question(s), information about databases searched and the eligibility criteria used in this section of the guideline can be found in Table 6. A search for systematic reviews published since 1995 was conducted. The GDG decided that systematic reviews conducted since 1995 would be most relevant, so the searches were therefore restricted. Furthermore, due to the large volume of literature retrieved from the

**Table 6: Clinical review protocol for the review of models of service delivery**

| Component | Description |
|---|---|
| Review question | In adults (18 years and older) at risk of depression or anxiety disorders* (in particular, BME groups and older people), what factors prevent people accessing mental healthcare services? |
| Objectives | To perform a narrative synthesis of the evidence that assesses and identifies potential factors affecting access to mental healthcare services |
| Subquestions | • What factors, or attributes of the individual who requires mental healthcare, can inhibit access to services?<br>• What practitioner-level factors or attributes can inhibit an individual from accessing healthcare?<br>• Do systems and processes utilised in mental healthcare services inhibit access to healthcare?<br>• What practical or resource-based factors inhibit access to mental healthcare services? |
| Population | Adults (18 years and older) identified as at risk of depression or anxiety disorders* |
| Intervention(s) | Not applicable |
| Comparison | Not applicable |
| Critical outcomes | Identified factors affecting access |
| Electronic databases | Systematic reviews: CDSR, CINAHL, DARE, EMBASE, MEDLINE, PsycINFO<br>RCTs: CENTRAL |
| Date searched | Systematic reviews: 1 January 1995 to 10 September 2010<br>RCTs: 1 January 2004 to 10 September 2010 |
| Study design | Systematic review and RCT |
| *Including GAD, OCD, panic disorder, PTSD, social anxiety disorder and specific phobias. | |

search, the GDG decided to only evaluate papers published in the previous 7 years. The GDG conducted an additional search for RCTs published between 2004 and 2010 with the aim of identifying studies that may not have been captured by the included systematic reviews (searching for RCTs published in the last 6 years would identify the studies included in the majority of systematic reviews). Further information about the rationale for the methods used here can be found in Chapter 3 and details of the search strategy can be found in Appendix 6.

### 4.2.3    Studies considered

The literature search for systematic reviews and RCTs yielded 7,534 papers. Of these, nine systematic reviews, COCHRANE2007 (Cochrane *et al.*, 2007*)*, DAS2006 (Das *et al.*, 2006), DENNIS2006 (Dennis & Chung-Lee, 2006), DIXONWOODS2005 (Dixon-Woods *et al.*, 2005*)*, JUNG2003 (Jung *et al.*, 2003*)*, PRINS2008 (Prins *et al.*, 2008), RODRIGUEZ2009 (Rodriguez *et al.*, 2009), SCHEPPERS2006 (Scheppers *et al.*, 2006) and VANVOORHES2007 (Van Voorhees *et al.*, 2007) met the eligibility criteria for inclusion in the narrative synthesis. Of the included reviews, five were focused on identifying factors that affect access to mental healthcare services (DAS2006, DENNIS2006, PRINS2008, RODRIGUEZ2009, VANVOORHES2007). DIXONWOODS2005 was the only UK-based systematic review. DENNIS2006, PRINS2008, SCHEPPERS2006, JUNG2003 and COCHRANE2007 did not limit the countries included in the review and included UK-based papers. DAS2006, VANVOORHES2007 and RODRIGUEZ2009 evaluated papers from the US alone. Of the nine systematic reviews included, five focused on improving access to mental healthcare services (DAS2006, DENNIS2006, PRINS2008, RODRIGUEZ2009, VANVOORHES2007) and one evaluated mental healthcare specifically (DIXON-WOODS2005). The other included studies evaluated factors that affect access to healthcare in general. The characteristics of the studies included in the narrative synthesis can be found in Table 7, with further information in Appendix 14.

### 4.2.4    Clinical evidence

On the basis of a systematic search of the literature, factors that affect access can be grouped around a number of themes, as identified in the clinical review protocol: individual-level factors (the attributes, beliefs, behaviours and characteristics of the individual) that may result in reduced access to healthcare; practitioner-level factors (the characteristics, beliefs, attitudes and behaviours of the healthcare professional) that may contribute to disparities in access to healthcare for the individual; system- and process-level factors (such as policy, service-organisational and structural factors) that may reduce access to healthcare for certain population groups; and resource-based or practical factors (such as transportation and childcare issues) that may reduce people's ability to access healthcare services. The initial scoping review suggested that there may be little evidence that relates to specific disorders or populations that were specific to common mental health disorders. As a result, the GDG took a view that they would first consider factors at the general level across all disorders, developing more specific recommendations only when the evidence supported doing so. Therefore, where possible, the identified factors are presented for all individuals, that is, the general population (all individuals who require mental healthcare, rather than specific demographic groups or people with particular mental health disorders, as well as for the identified vulnerable groups, that is, BME groups and older people).

**Table 7: Study information table for systematic reviews evaluating factors that affect access to healthcare**

| Study ID | COCHRANE 2007 | DAS2006[1] | DENNIS2006[1] | DIXON-WOODS2005 | JUNG2003 | PRINS2008[1] | RODRIGUEZ 2009[1] | SCHEPPERS 2006 | VANVOORHES 2007[1] |
|---|---|---|---|---|---|---|---|---|---|
| **Method used to synthesise evidence** | Qualitative thematic analysis | Narrative | Narrative | Meta-ethnography (critically interpretive synthesis) | Narrative | Narrative | Narrative | Narrative | Narrative |
| **Design of included studies** | Qualitative, surveys and mixed-model | Qualitative and quantitative | Qualitative | Qualitative | Not specified | Qualitative and quantitative | Qualitative, quantitative and reviews | Qualitative, quantitative and combined | Interventions studies |
| **Dates searched** | 1998 to 2007 | 1966 to 2004 | 1966 to 2005 | 1985 to 2005 | 1963 to 2001 | 1995 to 2006 | 1996 to 2008 | 1990 to 2003 | 1995 to 2006 |
| **No. of included studies** | 256 | 24 | 40 | 253 (general population); 103 (BME groups); 111 (older people) | 145 | 71 | 55 | 54 | 73 |
| **Participant characteristics** | General population | African–Americans | Postnatal depression only (does not include other perinatal mood disorders) | General population; BME groups; older people | Older patients | Patients with anxiety or depression | Women who have experienced domestic violence | General population | BME groups |

[1]Mental healthcare-specific.

63

*Individual-level factors*

**General population**

Individual attributes and beliefs may have an important impact on access to healthcare services, specifically mental healthcare services. Previous research has identified stigma, shame and fear of being diagnosed with a mental health disorder as possible factors affecting access to healthcare (COCHRANE2007, DAS2006, DENNIS2006, DIXONWOODS2005, PRINS2008, RODRIGUEZ2009, SCHEPPERS2006, VANVOORHES2007). Disparities in power have also been identified (DIXON-WOODS2005), with some individuals not seeking treatment to avoid feeling disempowered because they may view seeking help as the relinquishing of power and resignation of the self to one's symptoms. People have also been found to normalise symptoms of mental health disorders and view mental health disorders not as an illness but as a sign of weakness (DENNIS2006) or as not worthy of investigation (DIXON-WOODS2005). In the review by DENNIS2006, women from a variety of cultural and ethnic backgrounds viewed depression in the postnatal period as an inability to perform as a woman and a mother, and as an implied weakness or perceived failure. RODRIGUEZ2009 suggested that the word 'clinic', especially in reference to mental health services, can be frightening to individuals and can deter them from obtaining necessary help. Self-medicating (with illicit drugs and alcohol) and coexisting physical health problems may also mask depression and anxiety disorders (DAS2006).

Lack of knowledge about mental health disorders, services and available treatment options have also been identified as factors that affect access to treatment. Some individuals may not be aware they have symptoms of a mental health disorder (DENNIS2006, DIXONWOODS2005, PRINS2008, SCHEPPERS2006, VANVOORHES2007, COCHRANE2007). For mental healthcare services in particular, individual perceptions as to how much a service can help may also influence a person's decision to access healthcare services (DIXONWOODS2005). A fear of child protection becoming involved, and the concern that children will be taken away following diagnosis of a mental health disorder, may discourage individuals from accessing healthcare services (RODRIGUEZ2009, SCHEPPERS2006).

**Black and minority ethnic groups**

The combination of being from a BME group as well as having a mental health diagnosis may result in additional feelings of stigma (VANVOORHES2007). Furthermore, there is evidence to suggest that certain BME groups find treatment for mental health disorders (both medication and psychological therapies) less acceptable than other ethnic groups (DAS2006, VANVOORHES2007). In some BME groups there may also be a belief that health professionals are an inappropriate source of support and help for mental health disorders (COCHRANE2007, DENNIS2006, SCHEPPERS2006). BME groups may also believe in self-reliance for mental health problems (RODRIGUEZ2009, SCHEPPERS2006). All of this may contribute to individuals being unwilling to access healthcare services to discuss symptoms or treatment options, and preferring alternative sources of support. For example, BME groups may see religion as a way of coping with mental health disorders (RODRIGUEZ2009, SCHEPPERS2006, VANVOORHES2007).

Language barriers between the individual and practitioner can impair communication, resulting in the healthcare professional misunderstanding symptoms and the individual being unaware of treatment options and their care plan (DIXON-WOODS2005, RODRIGUEZ2009, SCHEPPERS2006). Access to healthcare may also be affected by cultural attitudes to mental disorders within their community and, therefore, they may be unfamiliar with or reject the treatments on offer and possibly prefer traditional methods of treatment (for example, traditional herbs and remedies) (RODRIGUEZ2009, SCHEPPERS2006). A lack of trust in state-run organisations, such as the healthcare system, and fear of immigration practices and laws can all act as factors that affect access to treatment (RODRIGUEZ2009, SCHEPPERS2006, VANVOORHES2007).

Although it has been reported (DAS2006) that black[2] people are just as likely as white people to discuss mental health disorders in primary care, previous research has also suggested that BME groups may exhibit somatic and neurovegetative symptoms of depression, rather than mood or cognitive symptoms, which could affect recognition by healthcare professionals and access to care pathways (DAS2006, VANVOORHES2007).

Due to the stigmatisation of mental health disorders that exists in some BME communities, friends and family can sometimes act as a factor that affects access to treatment by discouraging help seeking and being unwilling to discuss symptoms or problems outside the trusted family and community group (DENNIS2006, RODRIGUEZ2009, SCHEPPERS2006). Furthermore, peer and family social networks may have a strong influence on an individual's decision to seek treatment (DIXONWOODS2005) and may discourage it, preferring the community or religion-based support systems to healthcare services (VANVOORHES2007). There may also be community-based stigmatisation of those who leave the community to seek treatment outside (VANVOORHES2007).

**Older people**
In older people, 'acceptance' of problems or 'resignation' to symptoms and self-characterisation of symptoms such as low mood, anxiety and memory problems as inevitable and related to old age, may affect help-seeking behaviour (DIXON-WOODS2005). Evidence suggests that depression especially may be seen by some older people as not deserving of medical attention (DIXONWOODS2005). Older people may also see their identity as partly defined by good health, preferring not to be pitied or viewed as a burden on healthcare services (DIXONWOODS2005). Some older people may be more likely to believe in self-reliance for the treatment of mental health and other disorders (DIXONWOODS2005). Diagnosis of depression in older people has also been found to be difficult because they may present with somatic and anxiety symptoms as opposed to overt low mood or sadness, or symptoms are masked where there is physical comorbidity (DIXONWOODS2005).

---

[2]Both black-African and black-Caribbean people were included in this review.

JUNG2003 reviewed individual characteristics as predictors of individual preferences for treatment choice and care provision and found a significant association between older people and a preference for a 'traditional' practitioner (that is, an older, male and assertive practitioner). Older people also showed a preference for the GP coordinating hospital care, having the same practitioner on every visit, home visits when ill and the use of educational pamphlets. Older people also indicated that practitioners needed to spend more time explaining their health problems and symptoms as well as their care plan.

*Practitioner-level factors*
**General population**
Healthcare professionals can play a crucial role in either promoting help-seeking behaviour or in acting as a barrier to access (DIXONWOODS2005). This begins with the methods used by the practitioner in the detection of mental health disorders and has an effect on the consequent access and utilisation of mental healthcare services by individuals. For example, RODRIGUEZ2009 identified that few practitioners who are not mental healthcare specialists actively look for mental health disorders such as depression, which in turn acts as a factor that affects access to mental healthcare services.

Practitioners' communication style may also be a factor affecting diagnosis and consequently access to treatment (COCHRANE2007, DIXONWOODS2005, VANVOORHES2007). A practitioner displaying a disinterested and 'patronising' attitude to individuals may cause feelings of inadequacy in the service user, who is consequently less likely to seek treatment (DENNIS2006). Similarly, an overly formal, authoritative and confrontational practitioner can lead to shame and discomfort (COCHRANE2007, SCHEPPERS2006). In addition, conveying medical information to the individual in a formal manner using medical jargon can act as a factor that limits access (COCHRANE2007, SCHEPPERS2006). The personality and practice of the practitioner has also been found to affect access to healthcare through its influence on the management and organisation of the service (DIXONWOODS2005).

Inadequate assessment, insufficient time with the GP and poor referral practice to secondary specialist services have also been identified as factors that affect access to treatment (COCHRANE2007, DENNIS2006, SCHEPPERS2006). Inadequate referrals to mental healthcare services by the practitioner may arise from a lack of knowledge about available services, a desire to reduce or save costs, perceived or actual limited availability of mental healthcare services and long waiting times for specialist appointments (DENNIS2006).

The practitioner's opinion or attitudes about the nature of the presenting problem can also impact on an individual's access and consequent pathway to care (DIXONWOODS2005). For example, DIXONWOODS2005 suggests that how serious, interesting and deserving a problem is perceived to be by a practitioner, along with the practitioner's expertise and knowledge of resources and services, may all affect an individual's access to healthcare.

**Black and minority ethnic groups**
VANVOORHES2007 suggests that practitioners who are not mental healthcare specialists do not actively look for mental health symptoms and, as a consequence, there is under-recognition of mental health symptoms for BME groups in particular. Previous research also indicates that practitioners may be more likely to minimise or not identify symptoms of depression in people from BME groups (DAS2006) or post-natal depressive symptoms (DENNIS2006), and it has been suggested that this is especially apparent when there is not 'race-concordance'[3] between the individual and practitioner (DAS2006, VANVOORHES2007).

A lack of sensitivity about the cultural background and beliefs of an individual by the practitioner could also have a detrimental effect on that individual's access to healthcare (COCHRANE2007, DENNIS2006, SCHEPPERS2006). For example, race discrimination based on stereotypes about intelligence, education and social support can lead to poorer recognition of mental health disorders, and hence limit access to services for BME groups (DENNIS2006, SCHEPPERS2006).

*System- and process-level factors*
**General population**
There may be healthcare systems and processes in place that affect access to appropriate care. A lack of provision and capacity in mental healthcare services can be a factor that affects access to care for all individuals (DIXONWOODS2005). Long waiting-times for outpatient appointments were also found to influence help-seeking behaviour (DIXONWOODS2005). When services are available, allocation of resources as well as the quality of these services, especially in mental healthcare, may be unevenly distributed across different geographical areas and consequent inequalities in the provision of services may arise (DIXONWOODS2005). This can have particular ramifications for certain groups, for example people living in rural areas (DIXONWOODS2005).

Absence of clear policies and, where they exist, disruptions due to changes in the healthcare system and poor communication about referral procedures both between primary, secondary and tertiary healthcare, and across different service sectors (for example, health and social care), may also have an effect on access to healthcare for individuals, causing delays in being seen and miscommunication and may result in the individual feeling 'shuffled around' services (DIXONWOODS2005).

It has been suggested that the policies and procedures that govern access to healthcare can be implemented in a rigid, inflexible and bureaucratic manner, and this can in turn limit access because such implementation can impair the recognition of important cultural and religious dimensions. Communication difficulties about the nature of services, such as the lack of a 'common language', can lead to limited access (SCHEPPERS2006). The use of certain standard procedures and practices can also be experienced as alien, unfamiliar and frightening (COCHRANE2007,

---

[3]'Race' is used in this context by these studies to describe the biological heritage of the individual and not their 'ethnicity', which refers to learned cultural behaviours and practices through geographical location.

SCHEPPERS2006). For example, monitoring procedures associated with a referral system may make some individuals feel uncomfortable and can deter them from accessing healthcare services (SCHEPPERS2006). This is particularly problematic for mental health because some individuals may not be comfortable with the repeated discussion of the same issues with a number of different people before they obtain help. Lack of information and support has an impact on an individual's decision to seek help or take up treatment. In addition, difficulty in obtaining information about ways to manage the illness after diagnosis and about the support services available can be a factor that affects access (DIXONWOODS2005).

## Black and minority ethnic groups

It has been suggested that BME groups are more likely to have complex and prolonged pathways to specialist mental healthcare because they are less likely to be referred directly for specialist assessment and care (SCHEPPERS2006). Furthermore, general limitations in the availability of mental healthcare services may disproportionately affect BME groups when accessing mental healthcare services (VANVOORHES2007).

A lack of trained and available interpreters for people with limited English proficiency can also act as a factor that affects access to mental healthcare (RODRIGUEZ2009). In relation to this, the reliance on printed material as opposed to direct contact with BME groups, as well as the lack of materials and information translated into the individuals' language, have been proposed as factors that may also affect access to healthcare (SCHEPPERS2006).

## Older people

Older people in particular have been found to dislike having to seek referral to specialist services from GPs (DIXONWOODS2005). Although older people are often comfortable seeing their GP for minor physical ailments and prescriptions, they reported that having to access specialist services via their GP was a potential factor in their not seeking help.[4]

### *Resource-based or practical factors*

Practical factors that affect access, such as lack of time, were identified as influencing access to treatment for common mental health disorders (DIXONWOODS2005, PRINS2008). Transportation issues, for example irregular public transport, in both urban and rural areas can act as a factor that affects access for all individuals, but more substantially for older people and other vulnerable groups who may not have access to a private car (COCHRANE2007, DIXONWOODS2005, SCHEPPERS2006). Having to arrange childcare can also impact on ability to access healthcare (DIXONWOODS2005). Inflexible clinic hours may also be a factor that affects access for individuals such as those who work and need out-of-hours services (DIXONWOODS2005, SCHEPPERS2006). Furthermore, the length of processes

---

[4]The IAPT program has introduced a self-referral element. Initial reports suggest that this has improved access, in particular for BME groups (Clark *et al.*, 2009).

such as making and obtaining appointments, problems with scheduling and long waiting-times can also affect access to healthcare (DIXONWOODS2005). COCHRANE2007, DIXONWOODS2005, and SCHEPPERS2006 identified that for some groups (such as BME groups and older people) poverty can have an effect on the ability to attend appointments with a GP, due to physical access limitations such as lack of access to a car or funds for public transportation.

## 4.3 ADAPTING MODELS OF SERVICE DELIVERY AND THERAPEUTIC INTERVENTIONS

### 4.3.1 Introduction

One approach to improving access to services has been to focus on the systems for the organisation and delivery of interventions. These approaches have fallen into two broad categories; first, attempts to alter the configuration of services, for example by delivering a service in a community centre away from traditional healthcare settings (Powell, 2002), or by using novel methods of service delivery, for example computers (Gulliford *et al.*, 2007); second, to alter the nature of the intervention provided, for example by changing the structure and content of a psychological intervention in the light of information about the cultural beliefs or presentations of a disorder within a particular ethnic group (Bernal, 2006; Bernal & Domenech Rodriguez, 2009; Griner & Smith, 2006).

### 4.3.2 Clinical review protocol

The aim of this review was to perform a narrative synthesis of the evidence that assesses the effectiveness of adapting existing models, methods, services and interventions, with the aim of improving access to healthcare. The review protocol, including the review question, information about databases searched and the eligibility criteria used in this section of the guideline can be found in Table 8. A search for systematic reviews published since 1995 was conducted. The GDG decided that systematic reviews conducted before 1995 would not be useful in evaluating access to healthcare and so these were excluded. Furthermore, due to the large volume of literature retrieved from the search, the GDG decided to evaluate papers from the last 7 years alone. The GDG conducted an additional search for RCTs published between 2004 and 2010 with the aim of identifying studies that may not have been captured by the included systematic reviews (searching for RCTs published in the last 6 years would identify the studies included in the majority of systematic reviews). Further information about the rationale for the method employed here can be found in Chapter 3 and information about the search strategy can be found in Appendix 6. Where possible, the evidence was grouped and synthesised by the subquestions, that is, those that evaluated interventions for the general population, for mental healthcare services specifically and for identified hard-to-reach groups (for example, BME groups and older people).

**Table 8: Clinical review protocol for the review of models of service delivery**

| Component | Description |
|---|---|
| Review question | In adults (18 years and older) at risk of depression or anxiety disorders* (in particular, BME groups and older people), do changes to services and interventions (that is, community-based outreach clinics, clinics or services in non-health settings), increase the proportion of people from the target group who access treatment when compared with standard care? |
| Objectives | To perform a narrative synthesis of the evidence, which assesses the effectiveness of adapting or changing existing models, methods, services and interventions, with the aim of improving access to healthcare |
| Subquestions | • Do adaptations to existing services improve access to mental healthcare for all individuals?<br>• Do adaptations improve access to mental healthcare for vulnerable groups (for example, older people and people from BME groups)? |
| Population | Adults (18 years and older) identified as at risk of depression or anxiety disorders* (in particular, older people and people from BME groups) |
| Intervention(s) | • Service developments or changes that are specifically designed to promote access<br>• Specific models of service delivery (that is, community-based outreach clinics, clinics or services in non-health settings)<br>• Methods designed to remove barriers to access, including stigma (both cultural and self and stigmatisation), misinformation or cultural beliefs about the nature of mental disorder |
| Comparison | • Standard care |
| Critical outcomes | • Proportion of people from the target group who access treatment<br>• Uptake of treatment |
| Secondary outcomes | • Satisfaction, preference<br>• Anxiety about treatment |
| Electronic databases | Systematic reviews: CDSR, CINAHL, DARE, EMBASE, MEDLINE, PsycINFO<br>RCTs: CENTRAL |
| Date searched | Systematic reviews: 1 January 1995 to 10 September 2010<br>RCTs: 1 January 2004 to 10 September 2010 |
| Study design | Systematic review and RCT |
| *Including GAD, panic disorder, social anxiety disorder, OCD, specific phobias and PTSD. | |

### 4.3.3 Studies considered

The literature search for systematic reviews and RCTs yielded 7,534 papers. Of these, seven systematic reviews (BALAS1997 [Balas *et al.*, 1997], BEE2008 [Bee *et al.*, 2008], CHAPMAN2004 [Chapman *et al.*, 2004], GRILLI2002 [Grilli *et al.*, 2002], KAIRY2009 [Kairy *et al.*, 2009], KINNERSLEY2008 [Kinnersley *et al.*, 2008], PIGNONE2005 [Pignone *et al.*, 2005]) met the eligibility criteria for inclusion in the review. All included studies were published in peer-reviewed journals between 1997 and 2009, and included a total of 224 included studies identified from searches that ranged from database inception to 2007. The characteristics of the studies included in the narrative synthesis can be found in Table 9, with further information in Appendix 14.

In addition, nine reviews were excluded from the narrative synthesis. Of these, six were excluded because they were not relevant to the clinical question or did not have outcomes that evaluated access to healthcare (Akesson *et al.*, 2007; Azarmina & Wallace, 2005; Bower & Sibbald, 2000; Bunn *et al.*, 2005; O'Dwyer *et al.*, 2007; Harkness & Bower, 2009) and two were outside the scope (Anderson *et al.*, 2001; Beney *et al.*, 2000).

Of the seven systematic reviews included, one (BEE2008) was focused on improving access to mental healthcare services whereas the other six were not mental health-specific. Two reviews focused on improving access for vulnerable groups. CHAPMAN2004 evaluated recent UK innovations in service provision to improve access for BME groups and older people and PIGNONE2005 reviewed methods of improving access for those with poor literacy. Two systematic reviews performed formal meta-analyses of the included studies (BEE2008, KINNERSLEY2008) and the other included reviews were narrative summaries (BALAS1997, CHAPMAN2004, GRILLI2002, KAIRY2009, PIGNONE2005). BALAS1997 evaluated the effectiveness of various types of telephone or computer-based electronic communication versus control. BEE2008 evaluated the effectiveness of a psychological intervention delivered via remote communication versus control, conventional face-to-face therapy as well as different types of remote therapy. CHAPMAN2004 did not evaluate a specific intervention for improving access but described the effectiveness of various interventions aimed at improving access for vulnerable groups identified in the included literature. GRILLI2002 assessed the effectiveness of mass communication versus control in improving healthcare utilisation. KAIRY2009 evaluated the effectiveness of telerehabilitation compared with usual face-to-face care and the effects on attendance and adherence, satisfaction and healthcare utilisation. KINNERSLEY2008 reviewed information giving prior to consultation versus control (for example, usual care) and the effects on individuals' question asking, satisfaction and anxiety. PIGNONE2005 focused on literacy as a factor that affects access and hence evaluated interventions such as easy-to-read printed materials, the use of videotapes, CD-ROM, computer programs and interactive videodiscs, as well as practitioner-led instruction and the effects of these interventions on health behaviours, health outcomes and the use of health services.

**Table 9: Study information and results table for systematic reviews evaluating adapting models of service delivery and therapeutic interventions to improve access**

| Study ID | BALAS1997 | BEE2008[1] | CHAPMAN2004 | GRILLI2002 | KAIRY2009 | KINNERSLEY2008 | PIGNONE2005 |
|---|---|---|---|---|---|---|---|
| **Method used to synthesise evidence** | Narrative | Meta-analysis | Narrative | Narrative | Narrative | Meta-analysis | Narrative |
| **Design of included studies** | RCTs | RCTs | RCTs, systematic reviews, analytical intervention and observational studies | RCTs, controlled clinical trials, controlled before and after trials, and interrupted time series analyses | Experimental or observational intervention studies, including cross-over designs | RCTs | Controlled and uncontrolled trials |
| **Dates searched** | 1966 to 1996 | 1980 to 2006 | 1984 to 2004 | Database inception to 1999 | Database inception to 2007 | 1966 to 2006 | 1980 to 2003 |
| **No. of included studies** | 80 | 13 | 30 | 26 | 22 | 33 | 20 |
| **Model /method evaluated** | Electronic communication (telephone or computer) | Psychological intervention delivered via remote communication | Personal medical services, GP-led telephone consultations, nurse-led telephone consultations/triage in general practice, nurse-led care in general practice, walk-in centres, NHS Direct and pharmacist-led care in the community | Mass media (for example, radio, television, newspapers and leaflets) | Telerehabilitation | Information giving prior to consultation | Easy-to-read written material, videotapes, CD-ROM, computer programs, interactive videodiscs and in-person instruction |
| **Comparison** | Control | Control; conventional face-to-face therapy; different types of remote therapy | No direct comparison | No direct comparison | Control (face-to-face or usual care) | Control (for example, usual care, leaflets, general discussion) | No intervention. Literature at a standard level |

| Outcome | Service user satisfaction, appointment keeping | Ability to increase access to services | Use of healthcare services | Objective (not self-reported) utilisation of healthcare services by healthcare professionals and individuals | Attendance and adherence to programmes, service user accessability to programmes, service user satisfaction and healthcare utilisation | Question asking, individuals' anxiety, knowledge and satisfaction | Health knowledge, health behaviours and use of healthcare services |
|---|---|---|---|---|---|---|---|
| **Participant characteristics** | General population | ICD-10 or DSM diagnoses of mood or functional (non-organic) mental health problem – that is, depression, anxiety or anxiety-related disorders | Vulnerable groups (BME groups; older people) | General population | General population | General population | People with low literacy skills |
| **Review quality** | Adequate | Adequate | Adequate | Adequate | Included study quality is assessed but not reported | Adequate | Adequate |
| **Pooled effect sizes or summary of findings** | Interventions resulted in: • higher service user satisfaction • fewer unkept appointments • higher utilisation of preventative healthcare by elderly individuals | Versus control: • depression: 0.44 (95% CI, 0.29 to 0.59; seven comparisons, N = 726) • anxiety-related disorders: 1.15 (95% CI, 0.81 to 1.49; three comparisons, N = 168) | Overall evidence is insufficient to make recommendations, but first-wave personnel medical-services pilots showed evidence of improved access to primary care in under-served areas/populations | Mass media can have an impact on healthcare service utilisation, but evidence is methodologically flawed and should be viewed with caution | Interventions resulted in: • greater attendance • greater adherence • higher service user satisfaction • healthcare utilisation was rarely measured in included studies and the results are inconclusive | Interventions resulted in: • significant increase in question asking (0.27, 95% CI, 0.19 to 0.36) • individuals' satisfaction (0.09, 95% CI, 0.03 to 0.16) • non-significant changes in individuals' anxiety before and after consultation, individuals' knowledge, length of consultation | Effectiveness of interventions inconclusive |

[1]Mental healthcare-specific.

73

CHAPMAN2004 included papers conducted in the UK only. BALAS1997, GRILLI2002, and KAIRY2009 were not UK-focused and included studies from a number of different of countries. BEE2008 and KINNERSLEY2008 were not limited to specific countries, but were notably conducted by UK-based groups and included a number of studies conducted in the UK. PIGNONE2005 was limited to developed countries only, in order to include research most applicable to the US.

### 4.3.4    Clinical evidence

A summary of the individual review findings can be found in Table 9, with further explanation below.

*Systematic reviews assessing mental healthcare for the general population*
BEE2008 conducted a meta-analysis evaluating the effectiveness of a psychological therapy (any therapy) delivered via remote communication rather than face-to-face, for increasing access to services. The study reported that psychotherapy via remote communication was more effective than control (pooled control groups consisting of usual care, waitlist and no treatment) for both depressive disorders (effect size = 0.44; 95% confidence interval [CI], 0.29 to 0.59) and anxiety-related disorders (effect size = 1.15; 95% CI, 0.81 to 1.49). However, only two studies included in the review evaluated the effectiveness of remote communication psychotherapy versus face-to-face psychotherapy and the results of the sub-group analyses were found to be non-significant.

*Systematic reviews assessing the general population (non-mental healthcare-specific)*
GRILLI2002 reported that planned mass media interventions, such as educational campaigns, for physical health issues such as cancer screening and immunisation programmes had a positive effect on healthcare utilisation. However, there was insufficient evidence to evaluate the most effective mass media intervention for increasing healthcare utilisation.

KAIRY2009 evaluated telerehabilitation (physiotherapy via remote communication) for individuals with spinal cord injuries requiring neurological, cardiac and speech/language impairment rehabilitation. Telerehabilitation was associated with good attendance of treatment programmes, as well as good adherence. Telerehabilitation was also associated with high service user and therapist satisfaction. Outcomes assessing healthcare utilisation were conflicted, with some studies reporting greater utilisation and some reporting less utilisation. However, it must be noted that the intention of the interventions was not always to increase the utilisation of healthcare. For example, studies might report fewer hospitalisations or visits to healthcare professionals as a positive impact on healthcare utilisation.

In keeping with this, BALAS1997 evaluated various electronic communication methods and reported that telephone follow-up and counselling was more effective than control for individuals keeping appointments, and was rated higher for service user satisfaction. In addition, a telephone reminder system was effective in persuading older people to receive preventative care and for appointment keeping. Pre-recorded messages and computer-generated reminder messages were significantly effective in increasing visits to healthcare services, and after-hours telephone access was also associated with higher service user satisfaction.

KINNERSLEY2008 assessed the effectiveness of information giving prior to a consultation on various outcomes that related to both access and uptake of treatment. The results of the meta-analyses indicated that information giving prior to consultation significantly increased question asking (effect size = 0.27; 95% CI, 0.19 to 0.36) and individuals' satisfaction (effect size = 0.09; 95% CI, 0.03 to 0.16). No significant effects on the anxiety of the individual either before or after consultations were observed.

*Systematic reviews assessing vulnerable groups*

CHAPMAN2004[5] and PIGNONE2005 investigated the effectiveness of various adaptations to existing services and interventions (for example, telephone consultations, walk-in centres, NHS Direct, CD-ROMs and interactive videodisks) for improving clinical outcomes and access to general healthcare for vulnerable groups (see study information in Table 9 for a list of models/methods evaluated). In a qualitative review of recent innovations in UK-based services, CHAPMAN2004 reported that personal medical services, which allow primary healthcare teams to target services for specific population groups and enhance services in under-developed areas, have been found to improve the quality of mental healthcare, the care of older people and care in deprived areas. This evidence is based on the findings of pilot studies of personal medical services across the UK. GP-led telephone consultations were also found to be effective in increasing the availability and use of primary care services. However, this method cannot help improve access to healthcare for people who do not have a telephone or language difficulties and hence may not be appropriate for certain vulnerable groups. CHAPMAN2004 reported that walk-in centres were effective in increasing access to healthcare for a minority of the general population. However, this was not the case for BME groups and other vulnerable groups, rather for white middle-class individuals and young and middle-aged men who are not considered a vulnerable group with limited access to healthcare. Furthermore, NHS Direct was also found to have good onward referral rates, but again does not address inequalities or improve access for vulnerable groups and is underused by older people.

PIGNONE2005 investigated interventions to address factors that aim to promote access through the use of healthcare information for people with poor literacy with the intention of improving understanding of health, health behaviours and use of healthcare services. In one study, the use of a combined intervention comprising a short video, a coaching tool, a verbal recommendation and a brochure improved utilisation of a healthcare service. This review found no other studies that investigated interventions to improve access to healthcare services for people with poor literacy from BME groups or other vulnerable groups.

---

[5]This review also identified other service delivery methods with outcomes not relevant to this chapter (see paper for more details).

## 4.4 SERVICE DEVELOPMENTS AND INTERVENTIONS SPECIFICALLY DESIGNED TO PROMOTE ACCESS

### 4.4.1 Introduction

The alternative approach to improving access to healthcare for target groups is to specifically develop novel methods of engaging individuals and delivering therapy.

### 4.4.2 Clinical review protocol

The review aimed to perform a narrative synthesis of the evidence relating to services, and the development of services that are focused on community outreach and engagement, with the aim of improving access to healthcare for hard-to-reach groups (for example, BME groups and older people). The review protocol including the review question, information about databases searched and the eligibility criteria used in this section of the guideline can be found in Table 10. A search for systematic reviews published since 1995 was conducted. The GDG decided that systematic reviews conducted before 1995 would not be useful in evaluating access to healthcare, therefore these were excluded. Furthermore, due to the large volume of literature retrieved from the search, the GDG decided to evaluate papers from the last 7 years alone. The GDG conducted an additional search for RCTs published between 2004 and 2010 with the aim of identifying studies that may not have been captured by the included systematic reviews (searching for RCTs published in the last 6 years would identify the studies included in the majority of systematic reviews). Further information about the rationale for the method employed here can be found in Chapter 3 and the search strategy can be found in Appendix 6. The evidence was grouped according to the subquestions reflecting the content of the reviews. The three groups were individual-/practitioner-level interventions, system-level interventions and treatment-level interventions that aim to increase access or facilitate uptake of treatment. Individual-/practitioner-level interventions aim to change the behaviour of the healthcare professional or individual. System-level interventions refer to policies, organisational and structural factors or communication methods. Treatment-level interventions refer to the provision of new or adapted treatments that aim to increase access.

### 4.4.3 Studies considered[7]

The literature search for systematic reviews and RCTs yielded 7,534 papers[6]. Of these, six systematic reviews (ANDERSON2003 [Anderson *et al.*, 2003];

---

[6]The search strategy involved a general search covering all review questions addressed in this chapter.
[7]Here and elsewhere in the guideline, each study considered for review is referred to by a study ID in capital letters (primary author and date of study publication, except where a study is in press or has been submitted for publication, then a date is not used).

**Table 10:  Clinical review protocol for the review of service developments**

| Component | Description |
|---|---|
| Review question | In adults (18 years and older) at risk of depression or anxiety disorders* (in particular, BME groups and older people), do service developments and interventions that are specifically designed to promote access increase the proportion of people from the target group who access treatment, when compared with standard care? |
| Objectives | To perform a narrative synthesis of the evidence that assesses the effectiveness of service developments specifically designed to promote access |
| Subquestions | • Do new service developments targeted at changing the behaviour of the individual or the practitioner improve access to healthcare services? <br> • Do service developments targeted at the healthcare system improve access to healthcare services? <br> • Do specific treatments or interventions developed for vulnerable groups improve access to healthcare services? |
| Population | Adults (18 years and older) identified as at risk of depression or anxiety disorders* (in particular, BME groups and older people) |
| Intervention(s) | • Service developments that are specifically designed to promote access <br> • Specific models of service delivery (that is, community-based outreach clinics, clinics or services in non-healthcare settings) |
| Comparison | • Standard care |
| Critical outcomes | • Proportion of people from the target group who access treatment <br> • Uptake of treatment |
| Secondary outcomes | • Satisfaction, preference <br> • Anxiety about treatment <br> • Individual/practitioner communication |
| Electronic databases | Systematic reviews: CDSR, CINAHL, DARE, EMBASE, MEDLINE, PsycINFO <br> RCTs: CENTRAL |
| Date searched | Systematic reviews: 1 January 1995 to 10 September 2010 <br> RCTs: 1 January 2004 to 10 September 2010 |
| Study design | Systematic review and RCT |
| *Including GAD, panic disorder, social anxiety disorder, OCD, specific phobias and PTSD. | |

BEACH2006 [Beach *et al.*, 2006], FISHER2007 [Fisher *et al.*, 2007], FLORES2005 [Flores, 2005], MEGHANI2009 [Meghani *et al.*, 2009], VANCITTERS2004 [Van Citters & Bartels, 2004]) met the eligibility criteria for inclusion in the review. All included reviews were published in peer-reviewed journals between 2003 and 2009, and included a total of 148 studies identified from searches ranging from database inception to 2008. The characteristics of the reviews included in the narrative synthesis can be found in Table 11 and Table 12, with further information in Appendix 14.

In addition, ten studies were excluded from the narrative synthesis. Of these, seven were excluded because they were outside the scope (Bhui *et al.*, 2003; Gruen *et al.*, 2003; Jimison *et al.*, 2008; Ploeg *et al.*, 2005; Powell, 2002; Skultety & Zeiss, 2006; Warrilow & Beech, 2009) and three were excluded because they did not provide data on outcomes which evaluated access to healthcare (Bouman *et al.*, 2008; Cuijpers, 1998; Moffat *et al.*, 2009).

Of the six systematic reviews included, only one (VANCITTERS2004) was focused on improving access to mental healthcare services. All other included reviews were not specifically focused on mental health. However, BEACH2006 and FLORES2005 reported sub-analyses that focused on mental health. Four reviews focused on improving access for BME groups (ANDERSON2003, BEACH2006, FISHER2007, MEGHANI2009), one evaluated improving access for people with limited English proficiency (FLORES2005), and one review assessed interventions to improve access for older people (VANCITTERS2004).

ANDERSON2003 assessed individual-/practitioner-level interventions (cultural competency training, and use of interpreters and bilingual practitioners) as well as system-level interventions (a programme to recruit and retain staff who reflected the culture of the community served), compared against a control condition with no exposure to the intervention. BEACH2006 evaluated a number of interventions at the individual/practitioner level (for example, practitioner education), the system level (for example, tracking/reminder systems, culturally-specific healthcare settings, and linguistically- and culturally-appropriate health education materials) as well as treatment-level interventions (for example, culturally-tailored and multifaceted interventions) compared against a control condition with no exposure to the intervention. FISHER2007 reviewed interventions that were grouped into individual-level interventions, access interventions, and healthcare interventions compared against a control condition with no exposure to the intervention. FLORES2005 compared the effect of not using an interpreter when one was needed with the use of a trained or ad hoc translator, and the use of bilingual practitioners. MEGHANI2009 focused on the effectiveness of patient-practitioner 'race-concordance'[8], that is, the individual in need of healthcare and the practitioner are the same race. VANCITTERS2004 evaluated outreach methods designed to improve access for older people, as compared with traditional methods.

---

[8]Race is used in this context to describe the biological heritage of the individual and not their ethnicity, which refers to learned cultural behaviours and practices through geographical location.

**Table 11: Study information table for systematic reviews evaluating service developments that are specifically designed to promote access**

| Study ID | ANDERSON2003 | BEACH2006[1] | FISHER2007 | FLORES2005[1] | MEGHANI2009 | VANCITTERS2004 |
|---|---|---|---|---|---|---|
| Method used to synthesise evidence | Narrative | Narrative | Narrative | Narrative | Narrative | Narrative |
| Design of included studies | Not specified | RCTs | Various (not restricted to RCTs) | Various (not restricted to RCTs) | Qualitative and experimental studies | Various (not restricted to RCTs) |
| Dates searched | 1965 to 2001 | 1980 to 2003 | 1985 to 2006 | 1966 to 2003 | 1980 to 2008 | Database inception to 2004 |
| No. of included studies | 6 | 27 | 38 | 36 | 27 | 14 |
| Targeted | BME groups | BME groups | BME groups | Limited English-proficiency participants | BME groups | Older people |
| Review quality | The design and the quality of the included studies was unspecified | Adequate | Adequate | The quality of the included studies was unspecified | Adequate | The quality of the included studies was unspecified |
| Model/method evaluated | • Recruited members of staff who reflected the community culturally<br>• Use of interpreter or bilingual practitioners<br>• Cultural competence competence training<br>• Linguistically- and culturally-appropriate health education materials<br>• Culturally-specific healthcare settings | • Tracking/reminder systems<br>• Multifaceted interventions<br>• Bypassing the physician<br>• Practitioner education<br>• Structured questionnaire<br>• Remote simultaneous translation<br>• Culturally-tailored interventions | • Individual-level interventions to modify existing behaviour<br>• Interventions that increase access to existing healthcare environments<br>• Interventions that modify healthcare interventions | • Use of professional medical service interpreters<br>• Use of bilingual physicians<br>• Use of ad hoc interpreters | • Patient-practitioner race-concordance | • Gatekeeper model |
| Comparison | No exposure to intervention | No exposure to intervention | No exposure to intervention; pre- and post-intervention | Cross-comparisons; use of monolingual interpreter; no interpreter | Not applicable | Traditional referral sources (medical practitioners, family members and informal caregivers) |

[1]Some sub-analyses focused on mental healthcare are included.

**Table 12: Summary of findings for systematic reviews evaluating service developments that are specifically designed to promote access**

| Study ID | Outcome | Summary of findings |
|---|---|---|
| ANDERSON2003 | • Client satisfaction<br>• Racial/ethnic differentials in utilisation of healthcare services | • Insufficient evidence to evaluate effectiveness of culturally diverse staff reflecting the local community<br>• Use of bilingual practitioner resulted in patient being more likely to obtain a follow-up appointment than if interpreter used (OR = 1.92, 95% CI, 1.11 to 3.33).<br>• Interpreter not used – service user less likely to be given a follow-up appointment than those with language-concordant physician (OR = 1.79, 95% CI, 1.00 to 3.23). No difference in uptake of treatment<br>• Staff training about cultural awareness resulted in greater client satisfaction in African–American people (standard effect size = 1.6, p<0.001). Also more likely to return for more sessions (absolute difference = 33%, p<0.001)<br>• Only one out of four studies reported change in health behaviour due to use of signage and literature in individuals' language. Three out of four studies reported greater client satisfaction. Overall evidence is weak. |
| BEACH2006[1] | • Use of services<br>• Appropriateness of care<br>• Quality of practitioners<br>• Service user adherence<br>• Service user satisfaction<br>• Individual/practitioner communication | • Strong evidence to support the use of tracking/reminder systems<br>• Evidence is generally positive (but inconsistent across outcomes) for multi-faceted interventions<br>• Evidence supporting bypassing the physician for preventative services is fair<br>• Evidence supports education of practitioners because it had a positive effect on counselling behaviours<br>• Insufficient evidence to support the use of structured questionnaires in assessment<br>• Evidence for remote simultaneous translation shows favourable outcomes for accuracy of translation and practitioner/service user satisfaction; improved communication<br>• Evidence was weak and inconclusive for culturally-tailored interventions to improve quality of depression care |
| FISHER2007 | • Use of services<br>• Service user understanding<br>• Service user satisfaction | • Individual-level interventions resulted in general improvement in health, but no evidence for access outcomes<br>• Access-level interventions did not show any significant improvements in improving healthcare for BME groups<br>• Healthcare interventions (such as staff training in culturally-specific interventions) showed some evidence of improved service user understanding of disease, satisfaction, and some trends for improving behaviour |

| | |
|---|---|
| FLORES2005[1] | • Use of services<br>• Service user satisfaction<br>• Individual/practitioner communication | • Service user satisfaction – no difference between interpreter by telephone or in person; those who needed help but did not get an interpreter had lowest satisfaction; use of ad hoc interpreter lowest rating than use of professional interpreter<br>• Communication – 'no interpreter', service user had poor understanding of diagnosis/treatment plan; 'use of interpreter', service user more likely to incorrectly describe symptoms than those who did not need an interpreter; ad hoc interpreter, individuals not told medication side effects, misinterpretation and errors in translations, issues of confidentiality; mental health specifically, more open to misinterpretation, 'normalisation' of symptoms by interpreter or ad hoc interpreter such as family member<br>• Use of an interpreter – increased use of healthcare services; individuals with limited English-proficiency had a greater number of prescriptions written (adjusted mean difference = 1.4) and filled (adjusted mean difference = 1.3) than English-proficient individuals |
| MEGHANI2009 | • Utilisation of healthcare<br>• Individual preference (that is, normative expectations)<br>• Provision of healthcare<br>• Individual/practitioner communication<br>• Service user satisfaction<br>• Individual preference<br>• Perception of respect | • 'Race-concordance' had a positive impact on utilisation of healthcare<br>• Results for other outcomes are inconclusive |
| VANCITTERS2004 | • Use of mental healthcare services | • Gatekeeper model had more potential to reach individuals who were less likely to gain access to services (for example, those who lived alone, were widowed or divorced, or affected by economic and social isolation)<br>• At 1-year follow-up, no difference between two methods in service use or out-of-home placement |

[1]Some sub-analyses focused on mental healthcare are included.

All studies were narratively reviewed because the heterogeneity of interventions and outcomes reported across studies meant it was not possible to perform statistical meta-analyses. ANDERSON2003 was limited to countries with established market economies, as defined by the World Bank[9]. BEACH2006, FISHER2007 and MEGHANI2009 included only US-based papers in the review. FLORES2005 and VANCITTERS2004 did not limit studies by country. It should be noted that most studies evaluating new services and interventions were primarily focused on treatment outcomes (for example, symptoms, remission rates and so on), with outcomes evaluating access being of secondary importance.

### 4.4.4    Clinical evidence

*Individual-/practitioner-level interventions for black and minority ethnic groups*
ANDERSON2003 reported that individuals who had language-concordance with their healthcare practitioner were less likely to be discharged without a follow-up appointment than individuals who needed and used an interpreter (OR = 1.92, 95% CI, 1.11 to 3.33, k = 1). Furthermore, the same study found that people who needed but were not provided with an interpreter were more likely to be discharged without a follow-up appointment than those who had used language-concordant practitioners (OR = 1.79, 95% CI, 1.00 to 3.23, k = 1). However, there was no difference between groups in uptake of treatment. The review by FLORES2005 supports this conclusion because it found that individuals with limited English proficiency who did not have use of an interpreter were two times more likely to be discharged without an appointment than people who spoke the same language as the practitioner. However, no significant difference in knowledge of appointments and appointment attendance was observed between the three groups.

MEGHANI2009 found a positive association between individual-practitioner 'race-concordance' and healthcare utilisation, with fewer missed appointments for people in 'race-concordant' relationships with their healthcare practitioner. However, this was based on just two of the 27 studies included in the review and other studies found no significant effect of this on failure to use needed care or delay in using needed care. Furthermore, the review found a negative association between 'race-concordance' and the use of preventative and basic healthcare services, as well as retention in outpatient substance misuse treatment. Additionally, no significant effect of 'race-concordance' was observed for individual/practitioner communication, service user satisfaction and service user perception of respect, although a positive trend was observed for service user satisfaction (three out of five studies based on the same data source). Furthermore, across studies in this review, individuals' preference for a practitioner of their own race revealed mixed findings, with the majority of included studies finding no individual preference. It must be noted that some studies included

---

[9]Established market economies as defined by the World Bank are Andorra, Australia, Austria, Belgium, Bermuda, Canada, Channel Islands, Denmark, Faeroe Islands, Finland, France, Germany, Gibraltar, Greece, Greenland, Holy See, Iceland, Ireland, the Isle of Man, Italy, Japan, Liechtenstein, Luxembourg, Monaco, the Netherlands, New Zealand, Norway, Portugal, San Marino, Spain, St Pierre and Miquelon, Sweden, Switzerland, the UK and the US.

in this review assessed these outcomes by individual self-report and not objective measures of healthcare utilisation. This review concludes that primary language, a similar educational level for both the individual and the practitioner, how well the individual knew the practitioner and a sustained relationship with the practitioner were more important predictors of individual outcomes.

FLORES2005 evaluated communication issues, service user satisfaction with care and use of healthcare services among other outcomes for people with limited English proficiency. The results of the review revealed that individuals with limited English proficiency who had use of an interpreter had a greater number of prescriptions written (adjusted mean difference = 1.4) and collected (adjusted mean difference = 1.3) than those who were English proficient. People with limited English proficiency reported that understanding of diagnosis and treatment plans were worse for those who needed and did not get an interpreter than those who used an interpreter or were English proficient, as was service user satisfaction. However, some individuals found interpreters 'rude' and 'aggressive'. People with limited English proficiency who used an ad hoc interpreter (family members, friends, medical and non-medical staff not trained in translating, and strangers) were more likely to have not been informed about side effects of medication and to be less satisfied with care than English proficient individuals and those who used trained interpreters. Ad hoc interpreters were also found to make significant errors in translations that had potential clinical consequences.

FLORES2005 also reported that people seen by bilingual practitioners were more likely to accurately recall specific details about their diagnosis and treatment plan and to ask more questions than those seen by English-speaking monolingual practitioners. Individuals with limited English proficiency were also found to be more comfortable discussing embarrassing or sensitive details with a bilingual practitioner or when a family/friend translated than when alone with an English-speaking practitioner. However, it must be noted that this last assertion has no statistical basis.

The FLORES2005 review also evaluated the relationship between communication, interpreter services and mental healthcare, and contained conflicting findings from the studies included in the review. Some reported that people with limited English proficiency who had interpreters were significantly more likely to report satisfaction with their psychiatrist and the service they received. In addition, not having access to an interpreter was associated with an overestimation of the severity of impaired intellectual ability or thought disorders. However, other studies in the review found that use of ad hoc translators resulted in distortions because interpreters over-identified with the individuals. Psychiatrists also found it difficult to identify ambivalence in the individual when an interpreter was used. Distortions involved 'normalisations' of pathological symptoms by ad hoc interpreters and family member interpreters minimising or emphasising symptoms, sometimes speaking for the individual instead of translating their response.

Based on the findings of a single study within the FLORES2005 review that assessed counselling services, individuals who received a counselling intervention from staff who had participated in cultural competence training had significantly greater service user satisfaction than controls (standardised mean difference [SMD] = 1.6, $p < 0.001$). In addition to this finding, participants in the intervention group whose practitioners had received cultural competence training were returned for significantly more sessions than those in the control group (absolute difference = 33%, p <0.001). In keeping with this, BEACH2006 reported that practitioner education resulted in improvements in practitioner counselling behaviours for BME groups.

*System-level interventions for black and minority ethnic groups*
ANDERSON2003 aimed to assess the effectiveness of programmes to recruit and retain staff members who reflected the cultural diversity of the community. The reviewers did not identify sufficient literature to evaluate these programmes. ANDERSON2003 evaluated the use of culturally-specific health education materials for various outcomes. The review reported that the use of these materials had a positive effect on self-referral for screening (18% increase, p<0.01), as well as overall service user satisfaction with the materials. FISHER2007 evaluated the use of culturally-based interventions to improve access to healthcare for BME groups. The review did not find any evidence to support interventions such as the use of staff of the same culture as the individual, or culturally-specific messages (using community members to convey health information), materials or health-related practices aimed at changing individual behaviour among people from BME groups. Furthermore, although a number of studies that evaluated interventions aimed at matching the culture of the community with healthcare provisions were identified in this review (for example, lay educators, culturally-specific practitioners, public health nurses and small group sessions to educate the public), these studies did not show a significant benefit on the health behaviours and access to healthcare for BME groups.

BEACH2006 reported that the strategy of bypassing the physician and having a nurse or nurse practitioner screen individuals was found to be effective in the provision of preventative services for people from BME groups. There was insufficient evidence in this review to assess the added benefit of structured questionnaires to improve the assessment of BME groups and facilitate better communication between the individual and the practitioner (BEACH2006).

BEACH2006 identified a single study that evaluated the use of remote simultaneous translation[10], which reported an improvement in accuracy of translation, improved individual-practitioner communication, and greater service user and practitioner satisfaction.

BEACH2006 reported that there was strong evidence for the use of tracking/reminder systems in increased use of preventative healthcare services for BME groups.

*Treatment-level interventions for black and minority ethnic groups*
ANDERSON2003 did not identify any evidence that indicated the effectiveness of culturally- or ethnically-specific clinics or services located within the community served.

BEACH2006 identified a single study evaluating two types of culturally-specific interventions against a control (no treatment) for depression. The two interventions

---

[10]In which the interpreter translates simultaneously with the speaker but is not in the same room.

were QI-Meds and QI-Therapy[11] for treating depression in BME groups. There was insufficient evidence to assess the effectiveness of culturally-specific interventions on improving access for BME or other hard-to-reach groups; however, there was some evidence to support the use of multifaceted interventions for BME groups (BEACH2006).

FISHER2007 evaluated strategies (such as 'training of trainers', making culturally-specific adaptations to treatment interventions including CBT, and incorporating community workers into a standard intervention) and reported an improvement in individuals' understanding of disease, service user satisfaction and a trend for improving individual behaviours. However, no outcomes that assessed increased access or uptake of treatment were identified. It should be noted that the nature of the interventions and outcomes of the studies included in this review were highly variable.

*Interventions for older individuals*
VANCITTERS2004 reviewed the effectiveness of a community-based mental health outreach services for older people. The results of the review indicate that compared with traditional sources of referral (for example, medical practitioners, family members and informal caregivers), the use of the 'gatekeeper approach' (defined here as non-traditional community referral sources) reaches older people, who are less likely to gain access to mental healthcare and other services through traditional routes. However, at 1-year follow-up no significant difference was observed in service use or out-of-home placements between those referred using the gatekeeper model and those referred by traditional sources.

### 4.4.5 Clinical evidence summary

The above reviews have identified several potential factors that affect access to healthcare for the general population and the vulnerable groups that were the subject of specific reviews (BME groups and older people). The evidence base for the efficacy of mental healthcare interventions specifically is sparse and therefore evidence from the general healthcare literature was also drawn on.

*Factors affecting access*
For the purpose of this review, factors that may affect access have been categorised as individual-level factors, practitioner-level factors, system- and process-level factors and resource-based or practical factors.

---

[11]Quality improvement (QI) interventions were designed to take into account treatment choice and patient preference, as well as address language and cultural barriers, using culturally- and linguistically-appropriate educational and intervention materials when necessary. For the QI-Meds intervention, trained nurses were provided to support the patient with treatment adherence. For the QI-Therapy intervention, the patient was provided with eight to 12 sessions of CBT by specially trained therapists, and had access to other materials and resources. All patients had a choice of treatment and variability between groups was only for the availability of specialist resources (that is, the trained nurse in the QI-Meds group and the study-sponsored CBT therapists in the QI-Therapy group).

*Individual-level factors* identified in the review include:
● feelings of shame
● stigma and fear
● distrust of healthcare services
● masking and normalising of symptoms (especially mental health symptoms)
● limited English proficiency, resulting in communication problems
● lack of knowledge about mental health symptoms or services
● lack of support or encouragement to access healthcare services from families and community
● a belief in spirituality and self-reliance as a means of overcoming healthcare problems
● somatisation.

*Practitioner-level factors* identified in the review include:
● poor communication with patients and the wider community
● poor attitude to patients
● stereotyping of individuals by practitioners
● inadequate assessments arising from limited information about a range of issues (for example, cultural background)
● lack of secondary referral for those requiring further treatment or assessment
● minimisation or poor recognition of mental health symptoms.

*System- and service-level factors* identified in the review include:
● poor allocation of services and poor quality of services
● poor communication between services
● lack of flexibility in healthcare systems and practices to take into account individuals' cultural beliefs.
● use of standard procedures and practices that are unfamiliar or unexplained to vulnerable individuals.

*Resource-based or practical factors* identified in the review include:
● transportation issues
● poor appointment systems
● childcare issues.

*Adapting models of service delivery and therapeutic interventions*
Remote communication or other non face-to-face methods of treatment and communication were found to be effective in increasing access to mental healthcare and other healthcare services. However, these services may in turn create inequalities in access for those who may not have telephones or computers. They were also found to increase uptake and retention in treatment as well as have high service user satisfaction. The use of personal medical services targeting and enhancing service in underdeveloped areas was found to be effective in improving mental healthcare for older people and those in deprived areas. Information giving prior to consultations was also found to increase service user satisfaction and encourage question asking by individuals. The evidence suggests that walk-in centres and NHS Direct do not increase access for vulnerable groups. Mass media interventions and campaigns were found to be effective in promoting general healthcare utilisation.

*Service developments and interventions that are specifically designed to promote access*
Interventions designed to address the factors that affect access at the individual or practitioner level (for example, language concordance, cultural competence training for practitioners and use of interpreters) may increase access for vulnerable groups. There is some evidence (from a single review) to suggest that language-concordance between the individual and practitioner increases the number of individuals given follow-up appointments, although no evidence was found to indicate any increase in uptake of treatment. Negative effects were found when using interpreters on various outcomes, such as poor accuracy of translations by ad hoc translators, and 'normalisation' of clinically significant symptoms by ad hoc translators, especially for mental health symptoms. However, positive effects were identified on service user satisfaction and service user outcomes when qualified translators were used. The results of two systematic reviews found that cultural competence training and practitioner education resulted in greater service user satisfaction. It must be noted that only a small number of studies assessed these variables within the included systematic reviews.

System-level interventions targeted at BME groups were also evaluated in this review. The review did not identify sufficient evidence to assess the effectiveness of recruiting practitioners from the same culture as the individual in increasing access to services for BME groups. Although use of culturally-appropriate materials was found to have a positive impact on healthcare access and service user satisfaction with services in one review, other reviews could not support this assertion and hence the evidence of their effectiveness is inconclusive. There was strong evidence to support the use of tracking/reminder systems to increase the utilisation of healthcare by vulnerable people. There is no evidence to suggest that culturally adapted treatment interventions improve access for BME groups.

The evidence suggests that community-based outreach services such as the gatekeeper model were found to be more effective than traditional referral methods in reaching older people.

### 4.4.6    Health economic evidence

No studies were identified in the systematic literature review that considered the cost effectiveness of various methods and models adapted or designed to improve access to healthcare.

### 4.4.7    From evidence to recommendations

The evidence that informed the GDG's decisions on methods to improve access to mental health services for people with common mental health disorders was drawn from a number of sources. It included reviews of populations with a range of physical and mental disorders with severe mental illness (in some cases also including common mental health disorders), and populations where the only disorder was a common mental health disorder. The GDG considered it appropriate to use evidence

from such populations because the factors that might affect access in these populations (such as age or ethnicity) may exert their effect to a greater or lesser degree independent of the disorder itself. However, the GDG was mindful of the extrapolation
this required when drawing up the recommendations. The data reviewed also often
reported only improved access to services and not necessarily the impact on
outcomes, but the GDG took the view that this process measure (increased access)
was appropriate, particularly when other NICE guidelines (to which this guideline
relates) offer specific advice, where appropriate, on how interventions may be offered
or delivered to meet the needs of groups who are under-represented in services.

The evidence review suggests that there are a number of factors affecting access to
healthcare services for all people. For mental healthcare specifically, these factors
relate to factors such as stigma and fear along with a lack of knowledge about mental
healthcare services. For certain BME groups, this can further be extended to communication problems due to limited English proficiency and cultural views about mental
health problems that are not concordant with the conventional Western views in much
of the current healthcare system. The behaviour of a practitioner may also affect access
to mental healthcare through poor communication style, lack of cultural awareness,
lack of knowledge about available mental healthcare services and other poor practice
such as inadequate assessment and poor referral on to specialist services. The evidence
also suggests that there are systems and processes in place within healthcare provision
that can also negatively affect access to healthcare, for example rigid referral procedures and care pathways that do not account for individual variation in culture, poor
communication between services and a lack of quality mental healthcare services. In
addition, the literature also identified practical factors that affect access to healthcare,
such as lack of transportation, long waiting times and a lack of childcare.

The evidence suggests that modifications to existing methods and models can be
effective in addressing inequalities in healthcare provision across all groups, as well
as for targeted vulnerable groups. For example, the use of remote communication can
improve general access to mental healthcare services. Furthermore, adaptations to
existing services can also improve access for vulnerable groups. For example, the use
of bilingual therapists or qualified translators can improve access for certain BME
groups. These types of specific intervention were evaluated, and the evidence for
'race-concordance' between the individual and the practitioner was inconclusive.
Furthermore, although there was evidence to support the use of culturally appropriate
materials, there was no evidence to support the effectiveness of culturally-adapted
psychological interventions for improving access to mental healthcare services.

The GDG took into account the above factors and/or interventions that were associated with differential access to services. In doing so they were mindful of the lack of
evidence in some areas, the fact that some of the data drew on other areas of healthcare
and that the evidence for a direct impact on outcomes was often limited. Inevitably this
meant that the GDG drew on its expert opinion in formulating the recommendations.
The GDG also carefully considered the proper focus for the recommendations. For some,
the focus is on the behaviour of individual practitioners; for others, the focus is on the
service and on groups of healthcare professionals and managers working together to
develop and deliver improved methods to promote increased access to services.

## 4.5 RECOMMENDATIONS

4.5.1.1 Provide information about the services and interventions that constitute the local care pathway, including the:
- range and nature of the interventions provided
- settings in which services are delivered
- processes by which a person moves through the pathway
- means by which progress and outcomes are assessed
- delivery of care in related health and social care services.

4.5.1.2 When providing information about local care pathways to people with common mental health disorders and their families and carers, all healthcare professionals should:
- take into account the person's knowledge and understanding of mental health disorders and their treatment
- ensure that such information is appropriate to the communities using the pathway.

4.5.1.3 Provide all information about services in a range of languages and formats (visual, verbal and aural) and ensure that it is available from a range of settings throughout the whole community to which the service is responsible.

4.5.1.4 Primary and secondary care clinicians, managers and commissioners should collaborate to develop local care pathways (see also Section 7.5) that promote access to services for people with common mental health disorders by:
- supporting the integrated delivery of services across primary and secondary care
- having clear and explicit criteria for entry to the service
- focusing on entry and not exclusion criteria
- having multiple means (including self-referral) to access the service
- providing multiple points of access that facilitate links with the wider healthcare system and community in which the service is located.

4.5.1.5 Primary and secondary care clinicians, managers and commissioners should collaborate to develop local care pathways (see also Section 7.5) that promote access to services for people with common mental health disorders from a range of socially excluded groups including:
- black and minority ethnic groups
- older people
- those in prison or in contact with the criminal justice system
- ex-service personnel.

4.5.1.6 Support access to services and increase the uptake of interventions by:
- ensuring systems are in place to provide for the overall coordination and continuity of care of people with common mental health disorders
- designating a healthcare professional to oversee the whole period of care (usually a GP in primary care settings).

4.5.1.7 Support access to services and increase the uptake of interventions by providing services for people with common mental health disorders in a variety of settings. Use an assessment of local needs as a basis for the structure and distribution of services, which should typically include delivery of:

- assessment and interventions outside normal working hours
- interventions in the person's home or other residential settings
- specialist assessment and interventions in non-traditional community-based settings (for example, community centres and social centres) and where appropriate, in conjunction with staff from those settings
- both generalist and specialist assessment and intervention services in primary care settings.

4.5.1.8  Primary and secondary care clinicians, managers and commissioners should consider a range of support services to facilitate access and uptake of services. These may include providing:

- crèche facilities
- assistance with travel
- advocacy services.

4.5.1.9  Consider modifications to the method and mode of delivery of assessment and treatment interventions and outcome monitoring (based on an assessment of local needs), which may typically include using:

- technology (for example, text messages, email, telephone and computers) for people who may find it difficult to, or choose not to, attend a specific service
- bilingual therapists or independent translators.

4.5.1.10  Be respectful of, and sensitive to, diverse cultural, ethnic and religious backgrounds when working with people with common mental health disorders, and be aware of the possible variations in the presentation of these conditions. Ensure competence in:

- culturally sensitive assessment
- using different explanatory models of common mental health disorders
- addressing cultural and ethnic differences when developing and implementing treatment plans
- working with families from diverse ethnic and cultural backgrounds[12].

4.5.1.11  Do not significantly vary the content and structure of assessments or interventions to address specific cultural or ethnic factors (beyond language and the cultural competence of staff), except as part of a formal evaluation of such modifications to an established intervention, as there is little evidence to support significant variations to the content and structure of assessments or interventions.

---

[12]Adapted from *Depression* (NICE, 2009a).

# 5    CASE IDENTIFICATION AND FORMAL ASSESSMENT

## 5.1    INTRODUCTION

### 5.1.1    Recognition of depression

As was described in Chapter 2, most people with depression who consult their GP are not recognised as depressed, in large part because most such service users are consulting for a somatic symptom and do not consider themselves as depressed despite the presence of symptoms of depression (Kisely *et al.*, 1995). Symptoms such as fatigue, insomnia and chronic pain, which are associated with depression, may be missed because they are attributed to a physical disorder (a disorder that is actually comorbid with depression).

It has been shown that only around 30% of people presenting with depressive disorder are diagnosed and offered treatment (Marks *et al.*, 1979). This is a source of concern, although it is probably more likely for mild rather than more severe disorders (Kessler *et al.*, 2002a). The consequences of this poor recognition are uncertain. In a large multicentre WHO study of mental disorders, episodes of depression that were either untreated by the GP or missed entirely had the same outlook as treated episodes of depression; however, they were milder at initial consultation (Goldberg *et al.*, 1998). A smaller UK study (Kessler *et al.*, 2002b) found that the majority of people with undetected depression either recovered or were diagnosed during the follow-up period; however, almost 20% of individuals included in the study remained undetected by a healthcare professional and unwell after 3 years.

People with depression with more severe disorders or who present with psychological symptoms are more likely to be recognised as depressed. This is an undesirable state of affairs as large numbers of people experience depression each year, which has major implications for primary care.

### 5.1.2    Recognition of anxiety disorders

As with depression, anxiety symptoms are also often not recognised by primary healthcare professionals because service users may not complain of them directly (Tylee & Walters, 2007). Modes of presentations for anxiety disorders, which initially may not be recognised as being due to anxiety, include frequent attendance with multiple symptoms that may initially be considered as possible symptoms of a physical disorder (Blashki *et al.*, 2007).

Given that anxiety disorders are often associated with physical symptoms, it is not surprising to find that they are also commonly found among people receiving care in non-psychiatric secondary care settings. As in primary care, these frequently go unrecognised unless clinicians specifically look out for these disorders during routine consultations (Kroenke *et al.*, 1997).

Based upon surveys in hospital settings, OCD is also common among people with chronic physical health problems. For example 20% of UK dermatology outpatients (Fineberg *et al.*, 2003) and 32% of people presenting to rheumatologists and dermatologists with systemic lupus erythematosis (Slattery *et al.*, 2004) met criteria for OCD.

The nature of some symptoms of panic attacks, such as palpitations, tachycardia, shortness of breath and chest pain, may lead some individuals to think that they are experiencing a potentially life threatening illness such as a heart attack. This often results in presentation to accident and emergency departments. It has been estimated that between 18 and 25% of patients who present to emergency or outpatient cardiology settings meet the criteria for panic disorder (Huffman & Pollack, 2003), which is often not recognised.

The problem of under-recognition for anxiety disorders has recently been highlighted by evidence that the prevalence of PTSD is significantly under-recognised in primary care (Ehlers *et al.*, 2009). Many individuals will consult their GP shortly after experiencing a traumatic event, but will not present a complaint or request for help specifically related to the psychological aspects of the trauma; for example, an individual who has been physically assaulted, or involved in a road traffic accident or an accident at work might present requiring attention to the physical injuries sustained. Similarly, individuals who have been involved in traumatic life events often present at local emergency departments, notification of which is sent to GPs.

In both anxiety and depressive disorders, the initial presentation and complaint may take the form of somatic symptoms alone, such as lethargy or poor sleep in the case of depression and palpitations or muscular tension in the case of anxiety disorders. In light of this fact, consideration should be given to these symptoms as possible indicators of a common mental health disorder, in particular where no physical cause of these symptoms is apparent. Finally, as was also noted in Chapter 2, one major reason for poor recognition of common mental health disorders has been found to be a lack of effective consultation skills on the part of some GPs.

## 5.2    CASE IDENTIFICATION

### 5.2.1    Introduction

The first NICE guideline on depression, *Depression: Management of Depression in Primary and Secondary Care* (NICE, 2004b; NCCMH, 2004a), in addition to other NICE mental health guidelines, considered the case for general population screening for a number of mental health disorders, and concluded that it should only be undertaken for specific high-risk populations where benefits of early identification outweigh the downsides, such as people with a history of depression, significant physical illnesses causing disability or other mental health problems such as dementia. The criteria by which NICE judged the value of this approach was set out by the UK NHS National Screening Committee. Additional experience on the use of case identification strategies for depression has emerged since this approach was endorsed and incentivised under the NHS primary care QOF (British Medical Association & NHS Employers, 2006).

Recently, the updated edition of the *Depression: the Treatment and Management of Depression in Adults* guideline (NCCMII, 2010b) and the guideline on *Depression in Adults with a Chronic Physical Health Problem* (NCCMH, 2010a) reviewed available case identification instruments for depression. These guidelines recommended that healthcare professionals should be alert to possible depression (particularly in people with a past history of depression or a chronic physical health problem with associated functional impairment) and consider asking people who may have depression two questions, known as the 'Whooley questions':

1. During the last month, have you often been bothered by feeling down, depressed or hopeless?
2. During the last month, have you often been bothered by having little interest or pleasure in doing things?

If a person answers 'yes' to either of these questions, then the guidelines recommend that a practitioner who is competent to perform a mental health assessment should review the person's mental state and associated functional, interpersonal and social difficulties. Furthermore, when assessing a person with suspected depression, the guidelines recommend that practitioners should consider using a validated measure (for example, for symptoms, functions and/or disability) to inform and evaluate treatment.

Compared with depression, the case for the routine identification of anxiety has received less attention. Nevertheless, the epidemiology and unmet needs attributable to anxiety are similar to that of depression. There has been less experience to draw upon relating to the use of routine case identification measures in primary care in the UK, since their use has not previously been endorsed by the UK QOF. A decision was taken when formulating the scope of this guideline that the use of brief anxiety questionnaires should be considered alongside depression questionnaires. The classification of anxiety disorders is more complex compared with depressive disorders; however, the view of the GDG was that the development of separate case identification questions for each type of anxiety disorder would very likely be impractical and have no utility for routine use in primary care. The GDG's preference was to explore the possibility that a small number of case identification questions with general applicability to a range of anxiety disorders should be the starting point for a review in this area. As with depressive disorders, a potentially positive response would then prompt a further assessment.

Given that case identification instruments were recently reviewed for the two guidelines on depression, the present review will focus on case identification instruments for anxiety or GAD.

*Definition*

Case identification instruments were defined, for the purposes of this review, as validated psychometric measures that were used to identify people with anxiety. The review was limited to instruments likely to be used in UK clinical practice, that is, 'ultra-brief instruments' (defined as those with one to three items) or 'longer instruments' (defined as those with four to 12 items). The identification instruments were assessed in consultation samples (which included primary care and general medical services) and community populations. 'Gold standard' diagnoses were defined as DSM or *International Classification of Diseases* (ICD) diagnosis of anxiety; studies were sought that compared case identification with an ultra-brief or longer instrument with a gold standard. Studies that did not clearly state the comparator to be diagnosis by DSM or ICD, used a scale with greater than 12 items, or did not provide sufficient data to be included in the review were excluded.

### 5.2.2 Clinical review protocol

The review protocol, including the review questions, information about the databases searched, and the eligibility criteria used for this section of the guideline, can be found in Table 13 (further information about the search strategy can be found in Appendix 6).

### 5.2.3 Studies considered

The literature search for observational studies yielded 3,849 papers. Further inspection of these identified a total of 20 studies (N = 15,344) that met the eligibility criteria for this review: BYRNE2011 (Byrne & Pachana, 2011), CAMPBELL2009 (Campbell-Sills *et al.*, 2009), DENNIS2007 (Dennis *et al.*, 2007), EACK2006 (Eack *et al.*, 2006), GILL2007 (Gill *et al.*, 2007), HALL1999 (Hall *et al.*, 1999), HAWORTH2007 (Haworth *et al.*, 2007), KRASUCKI1999 (Krasucki *et al.*, 1999), KREFETZ2004 (Krefetz *et al.*, 2004), KROENKE2007 (Kroenke *et al.*, 2007), LANG2009 (Lang *et al.*, 2009), LOVE2002 (Love *et al.*, 2002), MEANS-C2006 (Means-Christensen *et al.*, 2006), NEWMAN2002 (Newman *et al.*, 2002), POOLE2006 (Poole & Morgan, 2006), SMITH2006 (Smith *et al.*, 2006), STARK2002 (Stark *et al.*, 2002), WEBB2008 (Webb *et al.*, 2008), WHELAN2009 (Whelan-Goodinson *et al.*, 2009) and WILLIAMSON2005 (Williamson *et al.*, 2005). Of the 20 studies, five were conducted using a sample of older people, 15 were conducted using consultation samples (six of these were in primary care), five were conducted using a community sample and eight were conducted using people with chronic physical health problems. All studies were published in journals between 1999 and 2010. Of the excluded studies, a number did not meet one or more eligibility criteria (112 were about depression only, 30 did not use an appropriate gold standard, 74 were about an instrument with more than 12 items and 294 reported data for a non-English language instrument) or could not be evaluated (438 reported insufficient data and 53 were not available as full text). Further information about both included and excluded studies can be found in Appendix 14.

### 5.2.4 Evaluating identification instruments for anxiety

Review Manager Version 5.0 (Cochrane Collaboration, 2008) was used to summarise diagnostic accuracy data from each study using forest plots and summary ROC plots.[13] Where more than two studies reported appropriate data, a bivariate diagnostic

---

[13]LANG2009 reported sensitivity and specificity, but did not report information to calculate true positives, false positives, true negatives and false negatives, and therefore is not included in the figures.

**Table 13:  Clinical review protocol for the review of case identification tools**

| Component | Description |
|---|---|
| Review question(s) | 1.  In adults (18 years and older) with a suspected anxiety disorder at first point of contact, what ultra-brief identification tools (one to three items) when compared with a gold standard diagnosis (based on DSM or ICD criteria) improve identification (that is, sensitivity, specificity, LR+, LR–, diagnostic OR) of people with an anxiety disorder? |
|  | 2.  In adults (18 years and older) with a suspected anxiety disorder at first point of contact, what longer identification tools (four to 12 items) when compared with a gold standard diagnosis (based on DSM or ICD criteria) improve identification (that is, sensitivity, specificity, LR+, LR–, diagnostic OR) of people with an anxiety disorder? |
| Objectives | To determine whether there are any case identification instruments that could be recommended for use in primary care. |
| Population | Adults (18 years and older) |
| Intervention(s) | Case identification instruments (≤12 items) |
| Comparison | DSM or ICD diagnosis of anxiety or GAD |
| Critical outcomes | Sensitivity, specificity, positive predictive value, negative predictive value, AUC |
| Electronic databases | CINAHL, EMBASE, MEDLINE, PsycINFO |
| Date searched | Inception to 10 September 2010 |
| Study design | Cross sectional |

accuracy meta-analysis was conducted using Stata 10 (StataCorp, 2007) with the MIDAS (Module for Meta-analytical Integration of Diagnostic Test Accuracy Studies; Dwamena, 2007) command to obtain pooled estimates of sensitivity, specificity, likelihood ratios and diagnostic OR (for further details, see Chapter 3). To maximise the available data, the most consistently reported and recommended cut-off points for each of the scales were extracted (see Table 14).

Heterogeneity is usually much greater in meta-analyses of diagnostic accuracy studies compared with RCTs (Cochrane Collaboration, 2008; Gilbody *et al.*, 2007). Therefore

**Table 14: Cut-off points used for each of the case identification instruments**

| Instrument | Details | Cut-off point |
|---|---|---|
| Anxiety and Depression Detector (ADD) (GAD item) | Five yes/no items, one of which is used to detect GAD | 1 |
| Anxiety Disorder Scale – Generalised Anxiety Subscale (ADS-GA) | 11 yes/no items, which are added together to produce a score from 0 to 11 | 2 to 3+ |
| ADS-GA (three items) | Three items from the ADS-GA | 1 to 2+ |
| ADS-GA (four items) | Four items from the ADS-GA | 1 to 2+ |
| Beck Anxiety Inventory – Fast Screen (BAI-FS) | Seven items (subjective, non-somatic symptoms) from the BAI | 4+ |
| Brief Symptom Inventory (BSI) – Anxiety subscale | Six items, rated on a five-point scale of distress, ranging from not at all (0) to extremely (4). The two-item version consists of items 1 and 4. | 63+ (T score) |
| BSI-Anxiety (two items) | Items 1 and 4 from the BSI-Anxiety, rated on a five-point scale of distress, ranging from not at all (0) to extremely (4) | 2.5+ |
| Eysenck Personality Questionnaire – Neuroticism Scale (EPQ-N) | Neuroticism scale from the EPQ | 0.37 |
| Generalized Anxiety Disorder scale – 2 items (GAD-2) | Two items from the GAD-7 | 3+ |
| Generalized Anxiety Disorder scale – 7 items (GAD-7) | A seven-item self-report scale measuring symptoms of GAD over the previous 2 weeks on a four-point Likert-type scale | 8+ |
| Generalized Anxiety Disorders Questionnaire, 4th Edition (GAD-Q-IV) | Nine-item self-report measure, designed for use as an initial screen to diagnose GAD | 4.5+ |
| Geriatric Anxiety Inventory – Short Form (GAI-SF) | Five items from the GAI | 3+ |
| General Health Questionnaire – 12 item version (GHQ-12) | 12 items from the GHQ-28 | 2 to 3+ |

*(Continued)*

**Table 14:** *(Continued)*

| | | |
|---|---|---|
| Hospital Anxiety and Depression Scale – Anxiety subscale (HADS-A) | Seven items from the HADS, measuring anxiety symptoms over the previous week on a seven-point Likert-type scale | 7 to 8+ |
| Mental Health Component Summary scale (MCS-12) | Mental Health Component Summary Scale of the SF-12 | ≤50 |
| Overall Anxiety Sensitivity and Impairment Scale (OASIS) | A five-item self-report measure. Responses are coded 0 to 4 | 8+ |
| Patient Health Questionnaire (PHQ-A) | Anxiety module from the PHQ. Responses are scored on a three-point Likert-type scale, ranging from 'Not at all' to 'More than half the days' | Not relevant |
| Penn State Worry Questionnaire (PSWQ-A) | An abbreviated version of the PSWQ developed for older adults | 22+ |
| Rotterdam Symptom Checklist (RSCL) | A self-report scale to measure symptoms of psychological distress reported by people attending primary care services | 7+ |
| Visual Analogue Scale (VAS) | A 20-centimetre line divided into ten equal-sized parts ranging from 'No anxiety' to 'Most anxiety'. Participants draw a vertical line through where they feel their anxiety over the past week is best represented | 10 to 11 centimetres |

a higher threshold for acceptable heterogeneity in such meta-analyses is required. However when pooling studies resulted in $I^2$ >90%, meta-analyses were not conducted.

Only three instruments were evaluated for diagnostic accuracy by more than one study (HADS-A, eight studies; GHQ-12, two studies; GAD-Q-IV, two studies), but only the HADS-A studies could be meta-analysed. Table 15 and Figure 4 summarise the diagnostic accuracy data for each of the ultra-brief instruments. Figure 3 shows a forest plot of the sensitivity and specificity for the ultra-brief instruments. Table 16, Figure 5, Figure 6 and Figure 7 summarise the diagnostic accuracy data for each of the longer instruments. Figure 8 and Figure 9 summarise the results of the meta-analysis of the HADS-A.

### 5.2.5    Clinical evidence summary

Only the HADS-A had enough evidence to synthesise the results using meta-analysis, although it should be noted that no studies were conducted in primary care. Therefore, the clinical utility of all instruments should be interpreted with some caution.

**Table 15: Evidence summary table for ultra-brief instruments (one to three items)**

| Instrument (sample) | Target condition | No. of items | Included studies | Sensitivity/ specificity | LR+ LR– | Diagnostic OR |
|---|---|---|---|---|---|---|
| ADD (GAD item) (consultation sample [primary care], adults) | GAD | 1 | MEANS-C2006 | 1.00* 0.56 | 2.25 0.02 | 126.00 |
| GAD-Q-IV – item 2 (consultation sample [primary care], older adults) | GAD | 1 | WEBB2008 | 0.78 0.69 | 2.52 0.32 | 7.89 |
| VAS (consultation sample, older adults) | Anxiety | 1 | DENNIS2007 | 0.50 0.61 | 1.27 0.82 | 1.54 |
| BSI-Anxiety (2 items) (consultation sample [primary care], adults) | Anxiety | 2 | LANG2009 | 0.55 0.85 | 3.67 0.53 | 6.93 |
| GAD-2 (consultation sample [primary care], adults) | Anxiety | 2 | KROENKE2007 | 0.65 0.88 | 5.42 0.40 | 13.62 |
| GAD-2 (consultation sample [primary care], adults) | GAD | 2 | KROENKE2007 | 0.86 0.83 | 5.06 0.17 | 29.99 |
| BSI-Anxiety (2 items) (consultation sample [primary care], adults) | Anxiety | 2 | LANG2009 | 0.55 0.85 | 3.67 0.53 | 6.93 |
| ADS-GA (3 items) (consultation sample [primary care], older adults) | GAD | 3 | KRASUCKI1999 | 0.77 0.83 | 4.53 0.28 | 16.35 |

*Reported as 1.00, but converted to 0.99 so that LR and diagnostic OR could be calculated.

## Figure 3: Forest plot of sensitivity and specificity for ADD (GAD item), GAD-Q-IV item 2, VAS, GAD-2 and ADS-GA (three items)

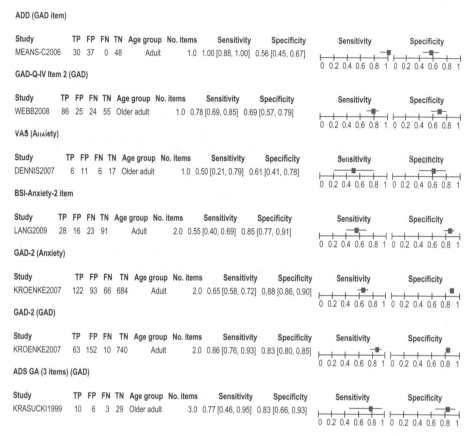

ADD (GAD item)

| Study | TP | FP | FN | TN | Age group | No. items | Sensitivity | Specificity |
|---|---|---|---|---|---|---|---|---|
| MEANS-C2006 | 30 | 37 | 0 | 48 | Adult | 1.0 | 1.00 [0.88, 1.00] | 0.56 [0.45, 0.67] |

GAD-Q-IV Item 2 (GAD)

| Study | TP | FP | FN | TN | Age group | No. items | Sensitivity | Specificity |
|---|---|---|---|---|---|---|---|---|
| WEBB2008 | 86 | 25 | 24 | 55 | Older adult | 1.0 | 0.78 [0.69, 0.85] | 0.69 [0.57, 0.79] |

VAS (Anxiety)

| Study | TP | FP | FN | TN | Age group | No. items | Sensitivity | Specificity |
|---|---|---|---|---|---|---|---|---|
| DENNIS2007 | 6 | 11 | 6 | 17 | Older adult | 1.0 | 0.50 [0.21, 0.79] | 0.61 [0.41, 0.78] |

BSI-Anxiety-2 item

| Study | TP | FP | FN | TN | Age group | No. items | Sensitivity | Specificity |
|---|---|---|---|---|---|---|---|---|
| LANG2009 | 28 | 16 | 23 | 91 | Adult | 2.0 | 0.55 [0.40, 0.69] | 0.85 [0.77, 0.91] |

GAD-2 (Anxiety)

| Study | TP | FP | FN | TN | Age group | No. items | Sensitivity | Specificity |
|---|---|---|---|---|---|---|---|---|
| KROENKE2007 | 122 | 93 | 66 | 684 | Adult | 2.0 | 0.65 [0.58, 0.72] | 0.88 [0.86, 0.90] |

GAD-2 (GAD)

| Study | TP | FP | FN | TN | Age group | No. items | Sensitivity | Specificity |
|---|---|---|---|---|---|---|---|---|
| KROENKE2007 | 63 | 152 | 10 | 740 | Adult | 2.0 | 0.86 [0.76, 0.93] | 0.83 [0.80, 0.85] |

ADS GA (3 items) (GAD)

| Study | TP | FP | FN | TN | Age group | No. items | Sensitivity | Specificity |
|---|---|---|---|---|---|---|---|---|
| KRASUCKI1999 | 10 | 6 | 3 | 29 | Older adult | 3.0 | 0.77 [0.46, 0.95] | 0.83 [0.66, 0.93] |

With regard to ultra-brief instruments (defined as those with one to three items), for the identification of any anxiety disorder or GAD in adults the GAD-2 had the best diagnostic accuracy for use in primary care. For the identification of GAD in older adults, the three-item version of the ADS-GA had the best accuracy. In secondary care only the VAS has been evaluated, but diagnostic accuracy was poor.

With regard to longer instruments (defined as those with four to 12 items), for the identification of GAD in adults, the GAD-7 had the best diagnostic accuracy for use in primary care. For the identification of GAD in older adults, the four-item version of the ADS-GA had the best accuracy for use in primary care. In secondary care, the GAI-SF has adequate accuracy for the identification of GAD in older people. In a community sample, the GAD-Q-IV had good accuracy for the identification of GAD in adults. No other instrument had adequate accuracy, including the HADS-A, although, as can be seen in Figure 9, the HADS-A may have better diagnostic accuracy when used with older adults.

**Figure 4: Summary ROC plot of tests for ultra-brief instruments**

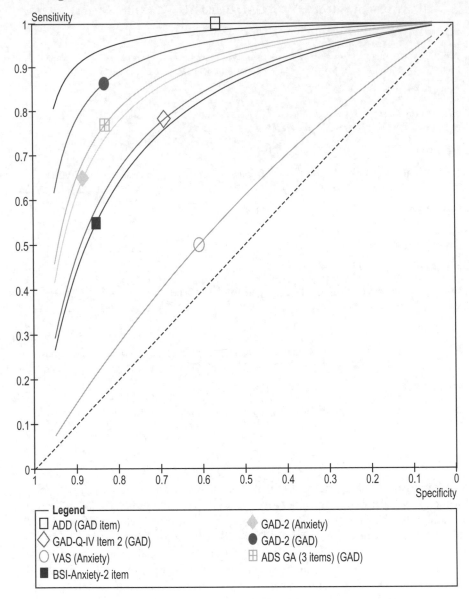

### 5.2.6    Health economic evidence

The systematic search of the economic literature undertaken for the guideline identified only one eligible study on identification methods of postnatal depression (Hewitt *et al.*, 2009). This was an HTA and the validity (diagnostic accuracy), acceptability,

**Table 16: Evidence summary table for longer instruments (four to 12 items)**

| Instrument (sample) | Target condition | No. of items | Included studies | Sensitivity/ specificity | LR+ LR− | Diagnostic OR |
|---|---|---|---|---|---|---|
| ADS-GA (4 items) (consultation sample [primary care], older adults) | GAD | 4 | KRASUCKI1999 | 0.77 0.83 | 4.53 0.28 | 16.35 |
| OASIS (consultation sample [primary care], adults) | Anxiety | 5 | CAMPBELL-SILLS2009 | 0.89 0.71 | 3.07 0.15 | 19.81 |
| GAI-SF (community sample, older adults) | GAD | 5 | BYRNE2011 | 0.75 0.87 | 5.77 0.29 | 20.08 |
| BSI-Anxiety (6 items) (consultation sample [primary care], adults) | Anxiety | 6 | LANG2009 | 0.47 0.91 | 5.22 0.58 | 8.97 |
| BAI-FS (consultation sample, adults, chronic health problems) | Anxiety | 7 | KREFETZ2004 | 0.82 0.59 | 2.00 0.31 | 6.55 |
| GAD-7 (consultation sample [primary care], adults) | Anxiety | 7 | KROENKE2007 | 0.77 0.82 | 4.28 0.28 | 15.25 |
| GAD-7 (consultation sample [primary care], adults) | GAD | 7 | KROENKE2007 | 0.92 0.76 | 3.83 0.11 | 36.42 |
| HADS-A (consultation sample, adults and older adults, chronic health problems) | Anxiety | 7 | DENNIS2007 HALL1999 HAWORTH2007 LOVE2002 | 0.77 (0.62 to 0.88) $I^2 = 85\%$ 0.72 | 2.8 (2.0 to 3.9) 0.32 | 9 (4 to 22) |

*(Continued)*

**Table 16** (*Continued*)

| Instrument (sample) | Target condition | No. of items | Included studies | Sensitivity/ specificity | LR+ LR– | Diagnostic OR |
|---|---|---|---|---|---|---|
| | | | POOLE2006 SMITH2006 STARK2002 WHELAN2009 | (0.65 to 0.78) $I^2 = 86\%$ | (0.17 to 0.58) | |
| PHQ-A (community sample, adults) | Anxiety | 7 | EACK2006 | 0.42 0.85 | 2.80 0.68 | 4.10 |
| RSCL (consultation sample, chronic health problems) | Anxiety | 8 | HALL1999 | 0.85 0.67 | 2.58 0.22 | 11.51 |
| PSWQ-A (consultation sample [primary care], older adults) | GAD | 8 | WEBB2008 | 0.79 0.63 | 2.14 0.33 | 6.41 |
| GAD-Q-IV (consultation sample [primary care], older adults) | GAD | 9 | WEBB2008 | 0.68 0.72 | 2.43 0.44 | 5.46 |
| GAD-Q-IV (community sample, adults) | GAD | 9 | NEWMAN2002 | 0.83 0.89 | 7.55 0.19 | 39.50 |
| ADS-GA (consultation sample [primary care], older adults) | GAD | 11 | KRASUCKI1999 | 0.85 0.71 | 2.93 0.21 | 13.87 |
| EPQ-N (consultation sample, adults) | GAD | 12 | WILLIAMSON 2005 | 0.82 0.80 | 4.10 0.23 | 18.22 |
| GHQ-12 (community sample, adults) | GAD | 12 | WILLIAMSON 2005 | 0.76 0.78 | 3.45 0.31 | 11.23 |
| MCS-12 (community sample, adults) | Anxiety | 12 | GILL2007 | 0.81 0.73 | 3.00 0.26 | 11.53 |

**Figure 5: Forest plots of sensitivity and specificity for ADS-GA (four items), OASIS, GAI-SF, BSI-Anxiety – six item, BAI-FS and GAD-7**

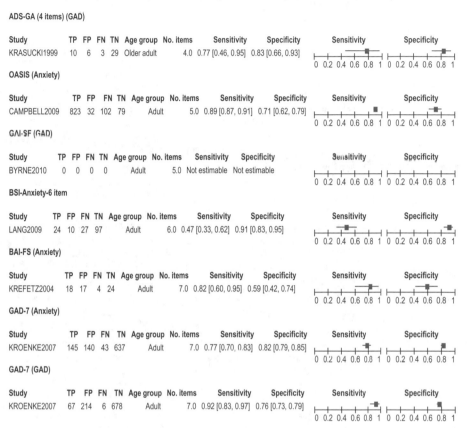

clinical effectiveness and cost effectiveness of methods to identify postnatal depression were assessed. Although Hewitt and colleagues (2009) conducted an extensive systematic literature review, none of the studies retrieved comprised a full economic evaluation of a postnatal depression identification method. A model was therefore constructed to assess the costs and outcomes of different identification strategies. The analysis was conducted from the NHS/personal social services (PSS) perspective. Although Hewitt and colleagues (2009) found 14 different strategies to have been validated in the literature, a review analysis of the validity of the diagnostic accuracy of the different identification methods was conducted in the HTA report and those results were used to determine the identification strategies considered in the economic analysis. Specifically the analysis considered the Edinburgh Postnatal Depression Scale (EPDS) (cut-off points seven to 16) and the BDI (cut-off point ten), which were compared with current practice (that is, routine case identification without the formal use of a diagnostic instrument). The model consisted of two parts: (1) an identification model reflecting the diagnostic performance and administration costs of the alter-

## Figure 6: Forest plots of sensitivity and specificity for PHQ-A, RSCL, PSWQ-A, GAD-Q-IV, ADS-GA, EPQ-N, GAD-12 and MCS-12

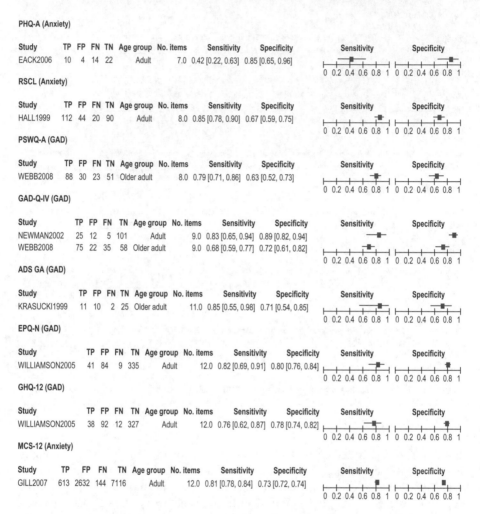

native identification strategies; and (2) a treatment model that evaluated the subsequent costs and outcomes, expressed in quality-adjusted life years (QALYs).

Women were assumed to enter the model at 6 weeks postnatally. The source of clinical effectiveness data was a systematic review and meta-analysis. Resource use estimates were based on assumptions and the NICE *Antenatal and Postnatal Mental Health* guideline (NCCMH, 2007). National unit costs were used and were expressed in 2006–07 prices.

The analysis estimated that routine care was the least costly and least effective strategy. Strategies were ranked in terms of costs (from the least expensive to the most expensive); the EPDS cut-off points 7 and 13 and the BDI cut-off point 10 were dominated

**Figure 7: Summary ROC plot of tests for longer instruments**

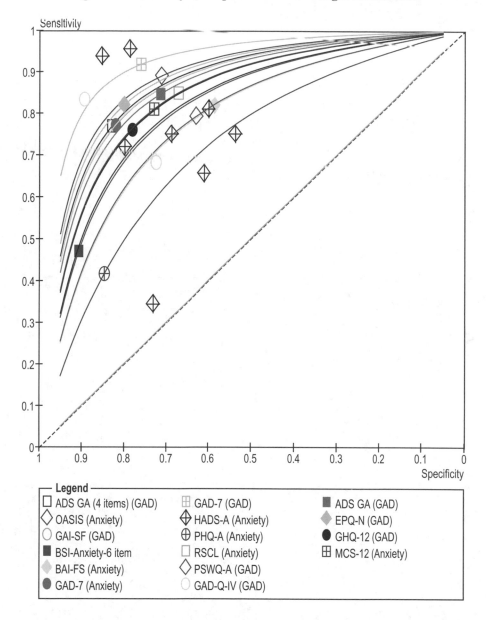

because they were more expensive and less effective than the previous strategies and were excluded. The incremental cost-effectiveness ratios (ICERs) of the non-dominant strategies were calculated and the ICER for the EPDS cut-off point 15 was found to be higher than that of the next more effective strategy on the ranked list, and thus was excluded due to extended dominance. Of the remaining non-dominated identification

**Figure 8: Forest plot of sensitivity and specificity for HADS-A**

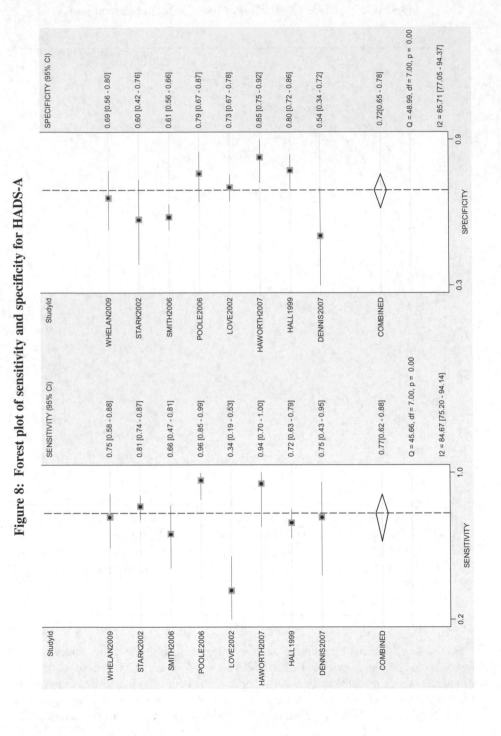

## Figure 9:  Summary ROC plot of tests for HADS-A, by age group

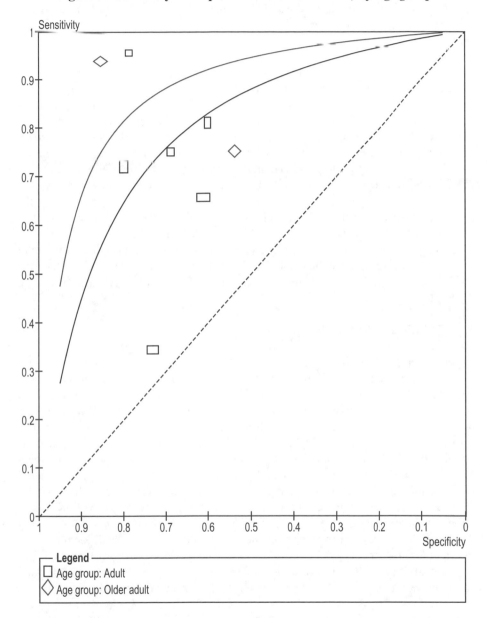

strategies, the EPDS at a cut-off point of 16 when compared with routine care resulted in an ICER of £41,103 per QALY. The ICER of the EPDS at a cut-off point of 14 was £49,928 per QALY compared with the EPDS cut-off point of 16. The ICER of the EPDS at lower cut-off points (for example, eight, nine to 11) exceeded £100,000 per QALY. At each of the three willingness-to-pay thresholds examined, namely £20,000, £30,000 and

£40,000, the strategy with the highest individual probability of being cost effective was routine current practice, with probability reaching 88%, 59% and 39%, respectively. Formal identification strategies had a combined probability of being cost effective that increased with higher willingness to pay; this combined probability exceeded the respective probability of routine current practice at a willingness-to-pay between £30,000 and £40,000 per QALY. However, individual probabilities of each strategy were low, indicating a high uncertainty among the different formal identification strategies as to which is the optimal strategy in terms of cost effectiveness. The extensive sensitivity analyses performed demonstrated that the results were sensitive to the cost of treating false positive cases. This economic study has also been reported elsewhere (Paulden *et al.*, 2010) and limitations of the model, and consequently the validity of the conclusions drawn, have been pointed out (Pilling & Mavranezouli, 2010) including the assumptions that a positive response to the case identification questions leads directly to the provision of a psychological intervention; the use in the model of only one type of intervention (the most costly); and the fact that the model assumes zero false positives in routine practice when the actual rate is likely to be nearer 15% (Mitchell *et al.*, 2009).

Details on the methods used for the systematic review of the economic literature are described in Chapter 3; the evidence table with details of the study is presented in Appendix 10. The completed methodology checklist of the study is provided in Appendix 12.

### 5.2.7    Economic modelling

*Introduction: the objective of economic modelling*
The cost effectiveness of different identification methods for anxiety disorders was considered by the GDG as an area with likely significant resource implications. In addition, it was an area where available clinical data were adequate to allow the development of an economic model. Therefore, an economic model was constructed to assess the relative cost effectiveness of identification methods for people with anxiety disorders in the UK. In constructing this model, the GDG was concerned to model an element of the case identification and assessment pathway. Specifically, the model was designed to test whether the use of a brief case identification tool (the GAD-2), followed by the use of a more formal assessment method (the GAD-7), was more cost effective than standard care in the identification and initial assessment of anxiety disorders. In this case 'formal assessment' refers to the use of an additional psychometric measure (the GAD-7). 'Further assessment' refers to the routine clinical assessments that healthcare professionals would undertake to arrive at an informed and consensual decision with the person about the choice of treatment.

*Economic modelling methods*
**Interventions assessed**
The choice of interventions assessed in the economic analysis was determined after reviewing available relevant clinical data included in the guideline systematic literature review and the expert opinion of the GDG. Based on these, the following identification methods were assessed in the economic analysis: the use of the GAD-2

(cut-off point of three or more) followed by GAD-7 (cut-off point of eight or more), compared with GP assessment (that is, routine case identification without the formal use of a diagnostic instrument)[14]. It should be noted that the economic model focused on GAD because there were better data available relative to other anxiety disorders and it is one of the more commonly presenting anxiety disorders.

**Model structure**

A decision-analytic model in the form of a decision-tree was constructed using Microsoft Office Excel 2007 (Microsoft, 2007). According to the model structure, two hypothetical cohorts of people with GAD were initiated on one of the two identification strategies. People found positive for GAD with the GAD-2 were further assessed using the GAD-7. Depending on whether people undertaking the test did or did not have GAD and the outcome of the identification test, four groups of people were formed: true positive, true negative, false positive and false negative. Each of the four groups was assigned to a care pathway and followed up for 34 weeks. The care pathways for people identified as having GAD reflect the pathways described in the NICE *Generalised Anxiety Disorder in Adults* guideline (NCCMH, 2011a). People who were found to be true positive for GAD were assumed to receive one of the following treatment options, in proportions determined by the expert opinion of the GDG: (1) active monitoring (10%); (2) low-intensity psychological interventions (55%); (3) high-intensity psychological interventions (24.5%); and (4) pharmacological treatment (10.5%). Based on the *Generalised Anxiety Disorder in Adults* guideline (NCCMH, 2011a), low-intensity psychological interventions consisted of non-facilitated self-help, guided self-help and psychoeducational groups in equal proportions; high-intensity interventions consisted of CBT and applied relaxation; drug treatment consisted of sertraline for 8 weeks followed by 26 weeks of maintenance therapy with sertraline. Based on the duration required for pharmacological treatment, the time horizon of the analysis was 34 weeks. People who were found to be false positive for GAD received the same treatments in the same proportions as described for those who were found to be true positive, but were assumed to stop treatment earlier, and hence consumed only 20% of the healthcare resources (and consequently incurred 20% of the respective costs). People who were found to be false negative were assumed to receive no formal treatment, but incurred health and social care costs. People who were found to be true negative were assumed to receive no treatment and incur no health or social care costs. A schematic diagram of the model is presented in Figure 10.

The economic analysis adopted the perspective of the NHS and PSS, as recommended by NICE (2009d). Costs consisted of identification costs (GP time), treatment costs for those identified as having GAD (low- and high-intensity psychological interventions as well as pharmacological interventions), and health and social care costs incurred by people with GAD that were not identified by one of the alternative strategies, or that were identified but did not respond to treatment. The measure of outcome was the QALY.

---

[14]The rationale for choosing the GAD-2 can be found in Section 5.2.10.

**Figure 10: Schematic diagram of decision-tree constructed for the assessment of the relative cost effectiveness of different identification strategies for people with GAD – costs and outcomes considered in the analysis**

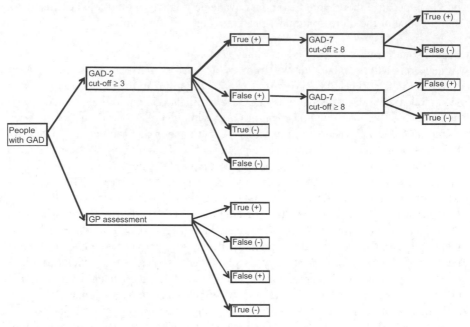

*Clinical input parameters of the economic model*

Clinical input parameters of the identification model included the sensitivity and specificity of the identification methods (GP assessment, GAD-2 and GAD-7). Sensitivity and specificity of the two formal identification methods were obtained from KROENKE2007, while the sensitivity of the GP assessment was obtained from Wittchen and colleagues (2002), and Davidson and colleagues (2010). The respective specificity of the GP assessment was a conservative estimate based on the expert opinion of the GDG. It must be noted that the model assumed that diagnostic characteristics of GAD-2 and GAD-7 were independent from each other, although administration of GAD-7 followed that of GAD-2. Regarding treatment, response rates were obtained from studies included in the systematic review and meta-analysis conducted for the *Generalised Anxiety Disorders in Adults* guideline (NCCMH, 2011a). Response rates for psychological interventions were estimated using an intention-to-treat approach. This means that response estimates accounted for the total number of people receiving psychological therapy, including dropouts. In contrast, response rates for people receiving pharmacological treatment did not account for people who discontinued treatment due to intolerable side effects, in accordance with the respective network meta-analysis undertaken for the *Generalised Anxiety Disorders in Adults* guideline. Given that the proportion of people receiving pharmacological therapy in the model is relatively low (10.5%), non-consideration of discontinuation due to intolerable side effects following pharmacological treatment was not expected to have significantly affected the results of the economic analysis. People under active monitoring (10% of people identified as GAD positive) were all assumed to improve because the GDG considered that initially a higher proportion of people who were identified as GAD positive would be assigned to active monitoring in UK routine clinical practice; however, some people would not improve and would, in reality, be offered one of the other treatment options described in the model. For simplicity, the model assumed that a lower percentage of people were offered active monitoring compared with routine practice, but all of them improved. The remaining people, who in routine practice would be transferred from active monitoring to other treatments following non-improvement, were assumed in the model to be initiated on other treatment options immediately following the identification of GAD.

*Utility data and estimation of QALYs*

To express outcomes in the form of QALYs, the health states of the economic model needed to be linked to appropriate utility scores. Utility scores represent the HRQoL associated with specific health states on a scale from 0 (death) to 1 (perfect health); they are estimated using preference-based measures that capture people's preferences on the HRQoL experienced in the health states under consideration. The utility scores for specific health states associated with GAD were obtained from Allgulander and colleagues (2007), consistent with the *Generalised Anxiety Disorder in Adults* guideline (NCCMH, 2011a).

*Cost data*

Costs associated with the identification methods were calculated by combining resource use estimates (GP time) with respective national unit costs (Curtis, 2009). It was assumed that administration of GAD-2 and GAD-7 required 10 and 15 minutes, respectively, whereas routine GP assessment required on average one GP visit.

Costs of psychological treatments (low- and high-intensity psychological interventions) were estimated using average estimates of the respective costs from the *Generalised Anxiety Disorder in Adults* guideline (NCCMH, 2011a). Costs of pharmacological treatment were also based on the NICE guideline (NCCMH, 2011a), using treatment with sertraline as reference. People who were falsely detected as having GAD were assumed to incur 20% of the treatment cost of a true positive person, according to the GDG's estimate. Health and social care costs of people falsely negative (that is, people having GAD but not identified by the methods assessed in the model), as well as the respective costs of people not responding to treatment, were taken from the NICE guideline (NCCMH, 2011a), based on resource use data reported in the most recent adult psychiatric morbidity survey in England (McManus *et al.*, 2009), further expert opinion (GDG for the *Generalised Anxiety Disorder in Adults* guideline) and national unit costs (Curtis, 2009).

All costs were expressed in 2009 prices. Discounting of costs and outcomes was not necessary since the time horizon of the analysis was shorter than 1 year.

Table 17 reports the values of all input parameters utilised in the economic model, and provides details on the sources of data and methods that were used at the estimation of input parameters.

**Table 17: Input parameters utilised in the economic model of pharmacological treatments for people with GAD**

| Input parameter | Deterministic value | Source of data – comments |
|---|---|---|
| **Sensitivity of identification methods:** | | |
| GAD-2 (cut off ≥3) | 0.86 | KROENKE2007 |
| GAD-7 (cut off ≥8) | 0.92 | KROENKE2007 |
| GP assessment | 0.34 | Wittchen and colleagues (2002); Davidson and colleagues (2010) |
| **Specificity of identification methods:** | | |
| GAD-2 (cut off ≥3) | 0.83 | KROENKE2007 |
| GAD-7 (cut off ≥8) | 0.76 | KROENKE2007 |
| GP assessment | 0.9 | GDG assumption |
| **Probability of treatment response:** | | |
| Active monitoring | 1.00 | GDG estimate – see text for more details |
| Low-intensity interventions | 0.635 | Titov and colleagues (2009) – CCBT (low-intensity intervention) for people with GAD |
| High-intensity intervention | 0.40 | NCCMH (2011a) – guideline meta-analysis |
| Drug therapy with sertraline | 0.63 | NCCMH (2011a) – network meta-analysis of data included in the guideline systematic review of pharmacological treatments |
| **Utilities:** | | |
| Response | 0.760 | Allgulander and colleagues (2007) |
| Non-response | 0.630 | Allgulander and colleagues (2007) |
| No relapse following response (remission) | 0.790 | Allgulander and colleagues (2007) |

| | | |
|---|---|---|
| **Identification costs:** | | Based on 10 minutes of surgery/clinic GP consultation for administration of the GAD-2, 15 minutes for administration of the GAD-7 and one visit for GP assessment (GDG expert opinion); combined with national unit costs (Curtis, 2009) |
| GAD-2 | £30 | |
| GAD-7 | £45 | |
| GP assessment | £35 | |
| **Cost of low-intensity psychological interventions:** | | NCCMH (2011a) – non-facilitated self-help estimated to consist of one 15-minute session with a mental health nurse (band 5) plus the use of a booklet costing £4; guided self-help estimated to comprise three to six sessions with a mental health nurse (band 5), with the first session lasting 45 minutes and the rest 30 minutes, plus the use of a booklet costing £4; psychoeducational group estimated to consist of six sessions of 2 hours each, provided by two mental health nurses (band 5) to groups of ten to 30 people. Unit cost of mental health nurse (band 5) £44 per hour of face-to-face contact (Curtis, 2009) |
| Non-facilitated self-help | £15 | |
| Guided self-help | £117 | |
| Psychoeducational group | £72 | |
| **Mean cost:** | £68 | |
| **Cost of high-intensity psychological interventions:** | | NCCMH (2011a) – each session lasting 1 hour, provided by clinical psychologists. Unit cost of clinical psychologist: £75 per hour of client contact (Curtis, 2009) |
| CBT or applied relaxation (12 sessions) | £900 | |
| Three booster sessions for responders only | £225 | |
| **Cost of pharmacological treatment:** | | NCCMH (2011a) – based on use of sertraline at a daily dosage of 100 mg and GP monitoring visits, comprising one visit at initiation of treatment, two more visits over the first 8 weeks of |
| Acute phase (8 weeks) | £108.18 | |
| Maintenance treatment (26 weeks) | £45.34 | |

*(Continued)*

**Table 17** (*Continued*)

| Input parameter | Deterministic value | Source of data – comments |
|---|---|---|
| | | treatment and another visit during maintenance treatment. Cost of sertraline based on *BNF* 59 (British Medical Association & the Royal Pharmaceutical Society of Great Britain, March 2010); cost of GP visit based on national sources (Curtis, 2009) |
| **Weekly health and social care cost incurred by people with GAD** | £15.47 | NCCMH (2011a) – weekly cost incurred by people with GAD (true positive) not responding to treatment and by people with GAD who failed to be diagnosed (false negative). Estimate based on resource use data reported in the most recent adult psychiatric morbidity survey in England (McManus *et al.*, 2009), further expert opinion and national unit costs (Curtis, 2009) |

*Data analysis and presentation of the results*

A sensitivity analysis was undertaken where data were analysed as point estimates; results were presented as mean total costs and QALYs associated with each identification method. Subsequently, the ICER is calculated, which expresses the additional cost per additional unit of benefit associated with one identification method relative to its comparator. Estimation of such a ratio allows consideration of whether the additional benefit is worth the additional cost when choosing one treatment option over another.

One-way sensitivity analyses explored:

- The impact of the uncertainty characterising the sensitivity and specificity of the identification methods assessed. A scenario of 10%, 15% and 25% change in these estimates was tested to investigate whether the conclusions of the analysis would change. Furthermore, two-way sensitivity analyses on sensitivity and specificity was also performed to further investigate uncertainty around those parameters. A scenario of 10% and 20% simultaneous change in those parameters was tested.
- The impact of changes in the consultation time necessary for the performance of the GAD-2 and GAD-7, respectively. A scenario of 25% change in these estimates was tested to investigate whether the conclusions of the analysis would change.
- The impact of the cost incurred by those falsely detected as having anxiety. A scenario of 25% change of the estimate used was tested to investigate whether the conclusions of the analysis would change.
- The impact of uncertainty characterising treatment costs was assessed. A scenario of 10%, 15% and 25% change of the estimates was tested to investigate whether the conclusions of the analysis would remain robust.
- Last extreme scenarios were tested as to the percentage of those who were true positive for GAD who received the different treatment options. Holding the percentage of those under active monitoring stable, the percentage that followed low-intensity psychological interventions, high-intensity psychological interventions and pharmacological treatment varied between 15 and 60%.

### 5.2.8    Economic modelling results

According to deterministic analysis, accounting for both identification and treatment costs, identification of anxiety using formal identification methods (namely GAD-2 and GAD-7), was estimated to be a cost-effective option because it resulted in a higher number of QALYs gained and lower total costs when compared with GP assessment without using a formal identification tool. Therefore, there was no need to estimate an ICER.

Table 18 provides mean costs and QALYs for every identification option assessed in the economic analysis.

Results were robust under all scenarios examined in one-way and two-way sensitivity analyses: formal identification of anxiety using GAD-2 and GAD-7 either remained the dominant strategy or resulted in a ICER when compared against GP assessment without an identification, which was well below £20,000 per QALY, the lower cost effectiveness threshold set by NICE (NICE, 2009d).

**Table 18: Mean costs and QALYs for each identification option for people with GAD assessed in the economic analysis – results per 1000 people**

| Identification method | Mean total QALYs | Mean total costs | ICER |
|---|---|---|---|
| GAD-2/ GAD-7 | 513.29 | £65,439 | GAD-2/GAD-7 dominant |
| GP assessment | 511.25 | £67,812 | |

*Discussion – limitations of the analysis*

The results of the economic analysis suggest that the use of GAD-2 followed by GAD-7 as a tool for the identification of people with anxiety is a cost-effective option when compared with GP assessment alone (without using any formal identification tools). The cost effectiveness of the identification methods is mainly attributed to their diagnostic accuracy combined with the fact that they can be easily and quickly performed by GPs, resulting in relatively low intervention costs.

One of the limitations of the economic analysis is that, due to lack of available evidence, a number of the estimates used were based on GDG assumptions. Despite the fact that impact of their variability was assessed in sensitivity analysis, further research is required to compare the diagnostic performance of different identification tools for anxiety, case finding questions and generic anxiety measures, and to evaluate their impact on costs, resource use and health outcomes. As the treatment model was adopted from the *Generalised Anxiety Disorder in Adults* guideline, it is subject to the same limitations reported there (NCCMH, 2011a), along with the limitation that although GAD is one of the most commonly presenting anxiety disorders in primary care, the treatment outcomes that informed the model will be different for other disorders.

### 5.2.9 Overall conclusions from economic evidence

Existing economic evidence is particularly limited in the area of identification methods for people with common mental health disorders. The economic analysis undertaken for this guideline suggests that the use of formal identification tools (GAD-2 followed by GAD-7) comprises a cost-effective option when compared with GP assessment alone (without using formal identification tools) for people with GAD (as a proxy for the anxiety disorders), because it appears to result in better outcomes (more people identified and higher number of QALYs) and lower total costs.

### 5.2.10 From evidence to recommendations

The GDG agreed that diagnostic accuracy would be assessed using sensitivity, specificity, ROC curves, negative and positive likelihood ratios, and diagnostic

ORs. Based on the approach taken for the updated editions of the *Depression* guidelines (NCCMH, 2010a and 2010b), when describing the sensitivity and specificity of the different instruments, the GDG defined values above 0.9 as 'excellent', 0.8 to 0.9 as 'good', 0.5 to 0.7 as 'moderate', 0.3 to 0.5 as 'low' and less than 0.3 as 'poor'. For likelihood ratios, a value of LR+ >5 and LR– <0.3 suggests the test is relatively accurate. For diagnostic ORs, a value of 20 or greater suggests a good level of accuracy.

The GDG aimed to develop recommendations that promoted the cost-effective identification of individuals with anxiety and depressive disorders. The recently completed NICE *Depression* guideline performed a systematic review of case identification methods for depression, and the GDG adapted the recommendations from the guideline for case identification (see NCCMH, 2010b, for a full description and discussion of the relevant evidence). In contrast, none of the other NICE guidelines that focused on anxiety disorders had developed recommendations for the identification of anxiety. In developing the recommendations for case identification for anxiety disorders, the GDG was mindful that the main focus of this guideline was on primary care services and the requirement to develop a method that not only had good sensitivity and specificity for all anxiety disorders but one that was also feasible (that is, had good clinical utility). The GAD-2 instrument performed best, and was the one measure that met the two key criteria of good diagnostic accuracy and feasibility. The GDG concluded that, although some of the longer instruments had good diagnostic accuracy, these instruments would not be feasible in the context of primary care. The GDG therefore decided to adopt the GAD-2 as the recommended measure. However, the GDG was concerned that the GAD-2 focused on anxiety and worry and that a number of people with an established phobic disorder would not be identified. This was thought possible because those with an established phobic disorder may avoid phobic objects or situations and, as a consequence of the avoidance, would not experience significant anxiety or worry and would therefore score low on the GAD-2. The GDG took the view that it was important to ask a subsidiary question for those people where the practitioner had a significant suspicion of an anxiety disorder but had returned a GAD score of less than three. The question, 'Do you find yourself avoiding places or activities and does this cause you problems?', was designed to detect a number of people with phobia whose functioning was impaired but who otherwise would not be identified by the two GAD questions. The GDG also undertook health economic modelling of the use of the two GAD questions. This modelled a larger part of the care pathway than was covered by the case identification questions alone and included the use of the GAD-7 (see Section 5.3) as part of the assessment subsequent to a positive response to the case identification questions. The economic model suggested that the combination of the case identification questions with the use of a formal assessment tool (the GAD-7) was cost effective and further supports the GDG's view that a recommendation for the case identification of anxiety disorders was appropriate. The recommendations set out below were developed in conjunction with the recommendations for assessment set out in Section 5.3.8 of this chapter.

### 5.2.11 Recommendations

5.2.11.1 Be alert to possible depression (particularly in people with a past history of depression, possible somatic symptoms of depression or a chronic physical health problem with associated functional impairment) and consider asking people who may have depression two questions, specifically:
- During the last month, have you often been bothered by feeling down, depressed or hopeless?
- During the last month, have you often been bothered by having little interest or pleasure in doing things?

If a person answers 'yes' to either of the above questions consider depression and follow the recommendations for assessment (see Section 5.3.8)[15].

5.2.11.2 Be alert to possible anxiety disorders (particularly in people with a past history of an anxiety disorder, possible somatic symptoms of an anxiety disorder or in those who have experienced a recent traumatic event). Consider asking the person about their feelings of anxiety and their ability to stop or control worry, using the 2-item Generalized Anxiety Disorder scale (GAD-2; see Appendix 13).
- If the person scores three or more on the GAD-2 scale, consider an anxiety disorder and follow the recommendations for assessment (see Section 5.3.8).
- If the person scores less than three on the GAD-2 scale, but you are still concerned they may have an anxiety disorder, ask the following: 'Do you find yourself avoiding places or activities and does this cause you problems?'. If the person answers 'yes' to this question consider an anxiety disorder and follow the recommendations for assessment (see Section 5.3.8).

5.2.11.3 For people with significant language or communication difficulties, for example people with sensory impairments or a learning disability, consider using the Distress Thermometer[16] and/or asking a family member or carer about the person's symptoms to identify a possible common mental health disorder. If a significant level of distress is identified, offer further assessment or seek the advice of a specialist.[15]

### 5.2.12 Research recommendations

5.2.12.1 In people with suspected anxiety disorders. What is the clinical utility of using the GAD-2 compared with routine case identification to accurately

---

[15]Adapted from *Depression* (NICE, 2009a).
[16]The Distress Thermometer is a single-item question screen that will identify distress coming from any source. The person places a mark on the scale answering: 'How distressed have you been during the past week on a scale of 0 to 10?' Scores of 4 or more indicate a significant level of distress that should be investigated further (Roth *et al.*, 1998).

identify different anxiety disorders? Should an avoidance question be added to improve case identification? (See Appendix 11 for further details.)

## 5.3 FORMAL ASSESSMENT OF THE NATURE AND SEVERITY OF COMMON MENTAL HEALTH DISORDERS

### 5.3.1 Introduction

*Assessment of depression*

Since April 2006, the UK GP contract QOF has incentivised GPs to measure the severity of depression at the outset of treatment in all diagnosed cases using validated questionnaires (British Medical Association & NHS Employers, 2006). The aim is to improve the targeting of treatment of diagnosed cases, particularly antidepressant prescribing, to those with moderate to severe depression, in line with the NICE guidelines.

The three recommended severity measures are the PHQ-9 (Kroenke *et al.*, 2001), the depression subscale of the HADS (Wilkinson & Barczak, 1988; Zigmond & Snaith, 1983) and the BDI-II (Beck, 1996; Arnau *et al.*, 2001). In general, a higher score on these measures indicates greater severity requiring greater intervention. However, the QOF guidance, again in line with the NICE guidance, also recommends that clinicians consider the degree of associated disability, previous history and patient preference when assessing the need for treatment rather than relying completely on the questionnaire score (British Medical Association & NHS Employers, 2006).

Data on the completion of the measures from the NHS Information Centre showed that they were used in a mean of 91% of diagnosed cases across all UK practices in 2007–08, up from 81% in 2006–07 (NHS Information Centre, 2008). The accuracy and utility of the measures has been questioned by GPs, however, suggesting that even if they use the questionnaires they may ignore the scores when deciding about treatment or referral (Jeffries, 2006).

Analysis of anonymous record data showed that prescriptions for antidepressants and referrals for psychiatric, psychological or social care were significantly associated with higher severity measure scores. However, overall rates of treatment and referral were very similar for service users assessed with different questionnaire measures, despite the fact that the different measures categorised differing proportions of service users as having major depression. These results suggested that practitioners (as would be expected given that factors such as associated functional impairment, duration of symptoms, patient preference and previous treatment) do not decide on drug treatment or referral on the basis of severity questionnaire scores alone (Kendrick *et al.*, 2009).

Furthermore, qualitative interviews with GPs participating in the same study (Kendrick *et al.*, 2009) showed that they were generally cautious about the validity and utility of identification tools, and sceptical about the motives for their introduction. The practitioners considered their practical wisdom and clinical judgement to be more important than identification tools and were concerned that the latter reduced the 'human element' of the consultation. Some even avoided coding patients' symptoms as depression in favour of other diagnostic labels, to avoid completing the severity measures and to save time in the consultation (Dowrick *et al.*, 2009b). This emphasises the importance of ensuring that the introduction of new diagnostic techniques is done in such a way that it fits with existing practice and systems of care, and takes into account possible developmental or training needs of the practitioners expected to use the techniques.

Moreover, the recent *Depression* guidelines (NICE, 2009a and 2009b) have attempted to move away from focusing on any one aspect of the disorder, such as symptom severity, which can have the unwanted effect of leading to an over-simplified categorisation of depression, and influencing treatment choice, on a single factor such as symptom count. An important consideration was to provide a strong steer away from only using symptom counting to make the diagnosis of depression and by extension to emphasise that the use of symptom severity rating scales by themselves should not be used to make a diagnosis, although they can be important as an aid in assessing severity and response to treatment.

To make a diagnosis of depression requires assessment of three linked but separate factors: (i) severity, (ii) duration and (iii) impairment. The diagnosis of 'major depression' is based not only on the severity of depression, but also on its persistence, the presence of other symptoms and the degree of functional and social impairment. Individual symptoms should be assessed for severity and impact on function, and be present for most of every day. Service users who fulfil criteria for major depression of recent onset may improve spontaneously, and for those with mild depression or others whose symptom trajectory is showing improvement, it may be appropriate to ask the service user to come back for a review of symptoms in 1 to 2 weeks because a proportion will respond within a few weeks following some reassurance, psychoeducation and support from primary care staff without recourse to a formal intervention.

It is also important to emphasise that there appears to be no hard-and-fast 'cut off' between 'clinically significant' and 'normal' degrees of depression; the greater the severity of depression, the greater the morbidity and adverse consequences (Kessing, 2007; Lewinsohn *et al.*, 2000). When taken together with other aspects that need to be considered, such as duration, stage of illness and treatment history, there are considerable challenges when attempting to classify depression into simple categories.

In recent years there has been a greater recognition of the need to consider depression that is 'subthreshold', that is, depression that does not meet the full criteria for a depressive/major depressive episode. Persistent subthreshold depressive symptoms – the preferred term in the *Depression* guidelines (NICE, 2009a and 2009b) – can cause considerable morbidity, and human and economic costs, and are more common in those with a history of major depression as well as being a risk factor for future major depression (Rowe & Rapaport, 2006).

Diagnosis using the three aspects listed above (severity, duration and impairment) provides a partial characterisation of the individual experience of depression. Depressed people vary in the pattern of symptoms they experience, their family history, personalities, pre-morbid difficulties (for example, sexual abuse), psychological mindedness, and current relational and social problems – all of which may significantly affect outcomes. It is also common for depressed people to have a comorbid psychiatric diagnosis, such as GAD, social anxiety disorder, panic disorder and various personality disorders (Brown *et al.*, 2001), and physical comorbidity.

Depression is often accompanied by anxiety, and in these circumstances one of three diagnoses can be made: (i) depression (with anxiety symptoms), (ii) depression comorbid with a diagnosed anxiety disorder, or (iii) mixed depression and anxiety symptoms when the severity of symptoms for both depression and anxiety are below the threshold for either disorder.

*Assessment of anxiety disorders*
Compared with depression, the diagnosis, classification and epidemiology of anxiety disorders are inevitably more complex given the number of anxiety disorders. This raises particular challenges when developing simple but robust case identification and assessment strategies in this area, compared with depression.

According to the DSM-IV-TR (APA, 2000), there are six main types of anxiety disorders in adults: specific phobia, social phobia, PTSD, GAD, panic disorder (with or without agoraphobia) and OCD. Other defined anxiety disorders in adults include acute stress disorder and anxiety disorder not otherwise specified. ICD-10 (ICD, 10th revision, WHO, 1992) currently classifies disorders as phobic anxiety disorders, other anxiety disorders (including GAD and panic disorder), OCD, and reaction to severe stress and adjustment disorders. Despite their different classifications, there is consensus that the common theme throughout anxiety disorders is the overestimation of threat with anxiety that is characterised by fear and avoidance behaviour.

In the National Comorbidity Survey – Revised, the lifetime prevalence of anxiety disorders was 28.8% compared with 20.8% for mood disorders (Kessler *et al.*, 2005a) and the median age of onset was 11 years old (compared with 30 years old for mood disorders). Specific and social phobias had the highest lifetime prevalence rate (12.5% and 12.1%, respectively), with agoraphobia without panic disorder having the lowest lifetime prevalence at 1.4% followed by OCD at 1.6%.

Unlike other disorders within DSM-IV, there are no 'trumping' rules within the main anxiety disorders hence it is possible to have co-occurring multiple anxiety disorders, and this is the case for a substantial minority of service users (Kessler *et al.*, 2005b). In addition to the significant associations between the individual anxiety disorders, anxiety and mood disorders commonly co-occur (Rush *et al.*, 2004). Approximately 50% of all people with depression meet criteria for at least one anxiety disorder and half of these individuals meet criteria for multiple anxiety disorders (Zimmerman *et al.*, 2000). Co-occurring depression and anxiety can impact on treatment decisions (Petersen *et al.*, 2009) and may also negatively affect treatment outcome (Brown *et al.*, 1996).

This chapter considers the clinical utility of more formal assessments of the nature and severity of common mental health disorders (including problem specification or diagnosis). The following chapter covers the assessment of risk associated with the disorder – factors associated with response to treatment, including characteristics of the service user and their disorder, informing initial treatment choices – and also addresses the related issue of ROM.

### 5.3.2 Clinical review protocol

The aim of this review was to perform a narrative synthesis of existing NICE guidelines, and to supplement that synthesis using existing systematic reviews and recent RCTs that were not included in existing reviews, examining the clinical utility of more formal assessments of the nature and severity of common mental health disorders (including problem specification or diagnosis). In addition, the longer instruments reviewed for the identification of anxiety (see Section 5.2) were considered for use during formal assessment of anxiety disorders. The review protocol, including the review question, information about databases searched and the eligibility criteria used in this section of the guideline can be found in Table 19. Although the search was conducted for the period 1995 to 2010, the focus was only on systematic reviews published since 2003 (further information about the rationale for the method employed here can be found in Chapter 3 and the search strategy can be found in Appendix 6).

### 5.3.3 Studies considered

Five existing NICE guidelines that were relevant to common mental health disorders were utilised:
- *Depression* (NCCMH, 2010b; NICE, 2009a)
- *Generalised Anxiety Disorder and Panic Disorder (With or Without Agoraphobia) in Adults* (NICE, 2011a) and *Generalised Anxiety Disorder in Adults* (NCCMH, 2011a)
- *Obsessive-compulsive Disorder* (NCCMH, 2006; NICE, 2005a)
- *Post-traumatic Stress Disorder* (NCCMH, 2005; NICE, 2005b)
- *Antenatal and Postnatal Mental Health* (NCCMH, 2007; NICE, 2007a).

In addition, the literature search for systematic reviews yielded 5,231 papers. Scanning titles/abstracts identified 34 potentially relevant reviews[17]; however, further inspection found none that met the eligibility criteria for inclusion. Evidence from supplementary searches identified one recent clinical guideline that specifically reviewed the evidence for formal assessment in people with a common mental health disorder in primary care (New Zealand Guidelines Group, 2008), and a case identification algorithm developed by the IAPT programme to support staff working in IAPT services to structure the form and content of a brief mental state review in primary care and related settings (IAPT, 2010). A list of included and excluded studies with reason for exclusion can be found in Appendix 14.

### 5.3.4 Summary of evidence from existing NICE guidelines

Evidence from existing NICE guidelines relevant to common mental health disorders were synthesised in two ways. The first utilised text from the body of each full guideline, while the second utilised recommendations from each guideline. For evidence

---

[17]This includes reviews potentially relevant to the assessment topics covered in Chapter 6.

**Table 19:    Clinical review protocol for the review of formal assessments**

| Component | Description |
|---|---|
| Review question | In adults (18 years and older) identified with depression (including subthreshold disorders) or an anxiety disorder*, what is the clinical utility of more formal assessments of the nature and severity of common mental health disorders (including problem specification or diagnosis) when compared with another management strategy? |
| Objectives | To perform a narrative synthesis of NICE guidelines and systematic reviews |
| Population | Adults (18 years and older) identified with depression (including subthreshold disorders) or an anxiety disorder* |
| Intervention(s) | Formal assessments of the nature and severity of common mental health disorders (including problem specification or diagnosis) |
| Comparison | Another management strategy |
| Critical outcomes | Clinical utility outcomes |
| Electronic databases | Systematic reviews: CDSR, CINAHL, DARE, EMBASE, MEDLINE, PsycINFO RCTs: CENTRAL |
| Date searched | Systematic reviews: 1 January 1995 to 10 September 2010 RCTs: 1 January 2008 to 10 September 2010 |
| Study design | Systematic review and RCT |
| *Including GAD, panic disorder, social anxiety disorder, OCD, specific phobias and PTSD. | |

from guideline text, a member of the technical team extracted any text that appeared to be relevant to assessment. As can be seen in Table 20, tabulation was then used to categorise relevant text from each guideline as relating to the clinical utility of formal assessment, as other information relevant to assessment, or as not relevant (text not shown). For recommendations, each guideline was examined for potentially relevant recommendations and these were tabulated (see Table 21). Recommendations that were specific to risk assessment were removed from the table and can be found in the section on risk assessment in Chapter 6. Recommendations and associated text from existing guidelines were then used to develop recommendations that were either common to all common mental health disorders or disorder specific.

**Table 20: Preliminary summary and synthesis of relevant text (by guideline)**

| Guideline | Clinical utility of formal assessment |
|---|---|
| *Generalised Anxiety Disorder and Panic Disorder (with or without Agoraphobia) in Adults* (NCCMH, 2011a) | Topic not specifically reviewed. |
| | **Other information relevant to assessment** |
| | Be alert for GAD in people with repeated presentation with worries about different issues. |
| | Factors that are important to assess and relevant for treatment choices: Duration of GAD, degree of distress, functional impairment, diagnostic comorbidities and past mental health history and response to treatment. |
| | Key comorbidities: Other anxiety and depressive disorders, alcohol and drug misuse and chronic physical health problems. |
| | In line with *Depression* (NCCMH, 2010b), the GDG considered practitioners need to make a clinical judgement where the GAD is comorbid with other anxiety disorders or a depressive disorder and first treat the disorder that is primary in terms of severity and likelihood that treatment will impact overall functioning. |
| | With the high comorbidity between GAD and alcohol misuse, the GDG considered a recommendation about when to first treat the GAD and when first to manage the alcohol misuse to be important for practitioners. |
| *Antenatal and Postnatal Mental Health* (NCCMH, 2007) (For common mental health disorders only) | **Clinical utility of formal assessment** |
| | Topic not specifically reviewed. |
| | **Other information relevant to assessment** |
| | After identifying a possible mental disorder in a woman during pregnancy or the postnatal period, further assessment should be considered, in consultation with colleagues if necessary. |
| | The woman's GP should be informed in all cases in which a possible current mental disorder or a history of significant mental disorder is detected, even if no further assessment or referral is made. |

**Table 20:** (*Continued*)

| Depression (NCCMH, 2010b) | **Clinical utility of formal assessment** |
|---|---|
| | Topic not specifically reviewed. |
| | **Other information relevant to assessment** |
| | Assessment and co-ordination of care |
| | Given the low detection and recognition rates, it is essential that primary care and mental health practitioners have the required skills to assess the patients with depression, their social circumstances and relationships, and the risk they may pose to themselves and to others. This is especially important in view of the fact that depression is associated with an increased suicide rate, a strong tendency for recurrence, and high personal and social costs. The effective assessment of a patient, including risk assessment and the subsequent co-ordination of their care (through the use of the Care Programme Approach in secondary care services), is highly likely to improve outcomes and should therefore be comprehensive. |
| *Obsessive-compulsive Disorder* (NCCMH, 2006) | **Clinical utility of formal assessment** |
| | Three instruments have been developed for use in the non-specialist as well as the psychiatric setting. |
| | The computerised Symptom Driven Diagnostic System for Primary Care (Weissman *et al.*, 1998) – comparison of the results of this test with those from a reliable structured clinical interview. Structured Clinical Interview for DSM-IV (SCID-IV) gave poor overall agreement ($\kappa = 0.28$) and the test cannot therefore be recommended (Taylor *et al.*, 2002). |
| | Computerised telephone-administered version of the Primary Care Evaluation of Mental Disorders (PRIME-MD) (Kobak *et al.*, 1997) – compared with the SCID-IV, the PRIME-MD provided reliability in diagnosing OCD ($\kappa = 0.64$). The screening instrument is disadvantaged by requiring a specialised computer programme and the system is not widely available in the UK. |
| | Zohar-Fineberg Obsessive Compulsive Screen (devised by J. Zohar for the International Council on OCD in 1995. It consists of five brief questions designed to be administered |

(*Continued*)

**Table 20:** (*Continued*)

| | |
|---|---|
| | by a doctor or a nurse and takes less than 1 minute to administer) (Fineberg & Roberts, 2001) – it was validated against the Mini International Neuropsychiatric Interview in a relatively small population of UK dermatology outpatients (Lecrubier *et al.*, 1997) where it was found to have good patient acceptability as well as satisfactory sensitivity (94.4%) and specificity (85.1%) (Fineberg *et al.*, 2003). Its psychometric properties are undergoing further evaluation in a range of psychiatric and non-psychiatric settings. In view of its brevity and utility, it can be considered as a possible screening tool for further evaluation. |
| | A variety of self-report questionnaires have been developed for OCD that may be useful for detection (Taylor, 1995; Taylor *et al.*, 2002) – self-report versions of the Yale-Brown Obsessive Compulsive Scale, both paper and computer administered, have been developed (Rosenfeld *et al.*, 1992; Steketee *et al.*, 1996) and have equivalent properties to the clinician-administered Yale-Brown Obsessive Compulsive Scale. |
| | **Other information relevant to assessment** |
| | It should not be underestimated how difficult it can be for people with OCD to first disclose their symptoms to family and friends and to the medical profession (Newth & Rachman, 2001). |
| *Post-traumatic Stress Disorder* (**NCCMH, 2005**) | **Clinical utility of formal assessment** |
| | Well-validated, structured clinical interviews that facilitate the diagnosis of PTSD include the SCID-IV (First *et al.*, 1997), the Clinician-Administered PTSD Scale (Blake *et al.*, 1995) and the PTSD Symptom Scale – Interview version (Foa *et al.*, 1993). All these instruments are based on the DSM-IV definition of PTSD. |
| | There is a range of useful self-report instruments of PTSD symptoms, including: Impact of Event Scale (Horowitz *et al.*, 1979) and Impact of Event Scale – Revised (Weiss & Marmar, 1997), Post-traumatic Diagnostic Scale (Foa *et al.*, 1997), Davidson Trauma Scale (Davidson *et al.*, 1997) and PTSD Checklist (Weathers & Ford, 1996). |
| | Good practice point checklists of common traumatic experiences and symptoms may be helpful for some patients who find it hard to name them. Both the Clinician-Administered |

**Table 20:** (*Continued*)

| | |
|---|---|
| | PTSD Scale (Blake *et al.*, 1995) and the Post-traumatic Diagnostic Scale (Foa *et al.*, 1997) include checklists. |
| | **Other information relevant to assessment** |
| | Epidemiological research has shown that the diagnosis of PTSD is greatly underestimated if the interviewer does not directly ask about the occurrence of specific traumatic events (Solomon & Davidson, 1997).<br><br>Primary care staff should consider that PTSD can arise not simply from single events such as an assault or a road traffic accident but also from the repeated trauma associated with childhood sexual abuse, domestic violence or the repeated trauma associated with being a refugee. A small proportion of PTSD cases have delayed onset (probably less than 15%; McNally, 2003). The assessment of such presentations is essentially the same as for non-delayed presentations. |

**Table 21: Preliminary summary and synthesis of relevant recommendations (by guideline)**

| Guideline | Recommendation |
|---|---|
| *Generalised Anxiety Disorder and Panic Disorder (with or without Agoraphobia) in Adults* (**NICE, 2011a**) | For people who may have GAD, conduct a comprehensive assessment that does not rely solely on the number, severity and duration of symptoms, but also considers the degree of distress and functional impairment.<br><br>As part of the comprehensive assessment, consider how the following factors might have affected the development, course and severity of the person's GAD:<br>• presence of a comorbid depressive disorder or other anxiety disorder<br>• presence of comorbid substance misuse<br>• any comorbid medical condition<br>• history of mental health disorders. |
| *Antenatal and Postnatal Mental Health* (**NICE, 2007a**) (**For common mental health disorders only**) | After identifying a possible mental disorder in a woman during pregnancy or the postnatal period, further assessment should be considered, in consultation with colleagues if necessary:<br>• If the healthcare professional or the woman has significant concerns, the woman should normally be referred for further assessment to her GP. |

(*Continued*)

**Table 21:** (*Continued*)

| | |
|---|---|
| | • If the woman has, or is suspected to have, a severe mental illness (for example, bipolar disorder or schizophrenia), she should be referred to a specialist mental health service, including, if appropriate, a specialist perinatal mental health service. This should be discussed with the woman and preferably with her GP.<br><br>The woman's GP should be informed in all cases in which a possible current mental disorder or a history of significant mental disorder is detected, even if no further assessment or referral is made. |
| ***Depression*** **(NICE, 2009a)** | Be respectful of, and sensitive to, diverse cultural, ethnic and religious backgrounds when working with people with depression, and be aware of the possible variations in the presentation of depression. Ensure competence in:<br>• culturally sensitive assessment.<br><br>When assessing a person who may have depression, conduct a comprehensive assessment that does not rely simply on a symptom count. Take into account both the degree of functional impairment and/or disability associated with the possible depression and the duration of the episode.<br><br>In addition to assessing symptoms and associated functional impairment, consider how the following factors may have affected the development, course and severity of a person's depression:<br>• any history of depression and comorbid mental health or physical disorders<br>• any past history of mood elevation (to determine if the depression may be part of bipolar disorder[18]<br>• any past experience of, and response to, treatments<br>• the quality of interpersonal relationships<br>• living conditions and social isolation.<br><br>*Learning disabilities*<br>When assessing a person with suspected depression, be aware of any learning disabilities or acquired cognitive impairments and, if necessary, consider consulting with a relevant specialist when developing treatment plans and strategies. |

---

[18]Refer if necessary to *Bipolar Disorder* (NICE, 2006).

**Table 21:** (*Continued*)

| | |
|---|---|
| *Obsessive-compulsive Disorder* (**NICE, 2005a**) | When assessing people with OCD or body dysmorphic disorder, healthcare professionals should sensitively explore the hidden distress and disability commonly associated with the disorders, providing explanation and information wherever necessary. In particular, people with OCD who are distressed by their obsessive thoughts should be informed that such thoughts are occasionally experienced by almost everybody and, when frequent and distressing, are a typical feature of OCD.<br><br>For people known to be at higher risk of OCD (such as individuals with symptoms of depression, anxiety, alcohol or substance misuse, body dysmorphic disorder or an eating disorder), or for people attending dermatology clinics, healthcare professionals should routinely consider and explore the possibility of comorbid OCD by asking direct questions about possible symptoms such as the following:<br>• Do you wash or clean a lot?<br>• Do you check things a lot?<br>• Is there any thought that keeps bothering you that you would like to get rid of but cannot?<br>• Do your daily activities take a long time to finish?<br>• Are you concerned about putting things in a special order or are you very upset by mess?<br>• Do these problems trouble you?<br><br>Each primary care trust, mental healthcare trust and children's trust that provides mental health services should have access to a specialist OCD/body dysmorphic disorder multidisciplinary team offering age-appropriate care. This team would perform the following functions: increase the skills of mental health professionals in the assessment and evidence-based treatment of people with OCD or body dysmorphic disorder, provide high-quality advice, understand family and developmental needs, and, when appropriate, conduct expert assessment and specialist cognitive-behavioural and pharmacological treatment. |
| *Post-traumatic Stress Disorder* (**NICE, 2005b**) | For PTSD sufferers presenting in primary care, GPs should take responsibility for the initial assessment and the initial coordination of care. This includes the determination of the need for emergency medical or psychiatric assessment.<br><br>Assessment of PTSD sufferers should be conducted by competent individuals and be comprehensive including physical, psychological and social needs and a risk assessment. |

(*Continued*)

**Table 21:** (*Continued*)

| | Where management is shared between primary and secondary care, there should be clear agreement among individual healthcare professionals about the responsibility for monitoring patients with PTSD. This agreement should be in writing (where appropriate, using the Care Programme Approach) and should be shared with the patient and, where appropriate, their family and carers. |
| --- | --- |
| | People who have lost a close friend or relative due to an unnatural or sudden death should be assessed for PTSD and traumatic grief. In most cases, healthcare professionals should treat the PTSD first without avoiding discussion of the grief. |

### 5.3.5    Summary of clinical evidence from other sources

The New Zealand guideline on identification of common mental health disorders (New Zealand Guidelines Group, 2008) systematically reviewed the evidence for assessment instruments that were brief (less than 5 minutes) to administer. Included in their review was the first *Depression* guideline (NCCMH, 2004a), a review of screening for depression in adults (Pignone *et al.*, 2002), two reviews of screening for alcohol problems (Aertgeerts *et al.*, 2004; Fiellin *et al.*, 2000) and 27 primary studies (some of which were included in the NICE guideline and/or the other included systematic reviews). The New Zealand guideline review concluded that the PHQ-9 appeared to have the best clinical utility for the assessment of depression, being reliable and valid for identifying depression, and sensitive to change. In addition, it was reported that other instruments with acceptable clinical utility were the GHQ-12 (Von Korff *et al.*, 1987; Schmitz *et al.*, 1999) and the Common Mental Disorder Questionnaire (CMDQ; Christensen *et al.*, 2005). It was also stated that other brief tools, such as the Center for Epidemiological Studies Depression scale (CES-D; Fechner-Bates *et al.*, 1994), the World Health Organization Wellbeing Index (WHO-5; Henkel *et al.*, 2003) and Duke-Anxiety-Depression scale (Parkerson & Broadhead, 1997) are less accurate for routine use in primary care. The GAD-7 and the two-item version, GAD-2, (Kroenke *et al.*, 2007; Spitzer *et al.*, 2006) were described as valid for detecting anxiety disorders, and the GAD-7 was included as a potentially useful assessment tool. The Kessler-10 questionnaire was included as a potentially useful assessment tool, but described as only validated in secondary care (Andrews & Slade, 2001).

The IAPT screening prompts tool (IAPT, 2010) was developed on the basis of the diagnostic criteria contained in ICD-10 and also makes explicit links to the use of formal measures such as the PHQ-9. It sets out a stepwise approach to questions about the experience, duration of the symptoms and impact on functioning based on

ICD-10 criteria. It is intended to be brief and can be integrated into a broader assessment of the presenting problem. It also drew on the algorithm for the differential diagnosis of anxiety and depressive disorders in the NICE *Anxiety* guideline (2004a). It was explicitly designed to aid IAPT staff and others working in primary care to differentiate between depression and the anxiety disorders.

### 5.3.6 Health economic evidence

The health economic evidence in support of the recommendations is contained in Section 5.2.6 to 5.2.9 of this chapter, using a model that was developed for the case identification questions (GAD-2) and the use of the GAD 7. The model was disorder-specific (focused on GAD). The model suggested that the combined case identification (GAD-2) and further formal assessment strategy (GAD-7) was likely to be cost effective.

### 5.3.7 From evidence to recommendations

The GDG aimed to provide appropriate and feasible advice for the assessment of common mental health disorders primarily focusing on primary care settings. The primary evidence source for these recommendations was drawn from existing NICE guidelines because no systematic reviews that met eligibility criteria for inclusion were found. Given the recent publication of the two *Depression* guidelines (NICE, 2009a and 2009b), and their recommendation for case identification and formal assessment, the GDG did not review those recommendations. However, given that there is reasonable evidence of the uptake of those recommendations (supported by the QOF), the GDG bore in mind the nature and structure of those recommendations when developing the recommendations for anxiety disorders. The recommendations drawn from individual guidelines drew on a range of different evidence sources including, where available, primary studies and systematic reviews, but also in many cases the expert advice of the GDG as high quality evidence was often lacking in this area. Therefore, the GDG took the view that the evidence developed by a range of expert groups on the best evidence available was the appropriate source from which to develop advice for assessment for this guideline. In doing so, the GDG aimed to develop recommendations that were feasible and that wherever possible had applicability across the full range of common mental health disorders, in particular the anxiety disorders. This meant that the GDG restricted their recommendations to self-completion questionnaires as the basis for any recommendations about formal rating scales because the increased time associated with the use of a clinician-rated measure would significantly detract from the use of the measure in routine care.

A number of key areas emerged where consensus and agreement was found across the five relevant guidelines. These included the manner in which the assessment should be undertaken, the content of the assessment (including the focus on the severity of symptoms), the associated functional impairment, the duration of symptoms, the use of formal rating scales (see Chapter 7), and also the previous experience of treatment and the impact on psychological factors. The GDG also considered the important area of comorbidity recognising that this is often high across the range of common mental health disorders. Taken together, this approach led to the development of recommendations about the methods by which to engage clients in the assessment process; to assess and evaluate their mental state; and the factors that may be taken into account, including previous treatment and any associated psychological and social factors. In doing so, the GDG was keen to develop recommendations that informed primary care staff on the important issue of immediate treatment and/or referral for further treatment. The GDG was also aware that they were drawing on existing evidence sources (NICE guidelines), the evidence for which had not been reviewed by the GDG. It was therefore important that the precise meaning of the recommendations drawn from other guidelines were not altered, although some re-wording and restructuring of those recommendations was required to produce a coherent, clear and comprehensible set of recommendations for this guideline. The GDG was also conscious of the need to develop systems that might support the use of ROM and this was a further factor that influenced the structure and content of the assessment (again see Chapter 7 for a discussion of formal rating scales). The GDG took the view that the IAPT screening prompts tool could be of help to staff beyond those working in primary care as a way of structuring an assessment of mental state and therefore included it in the recommendations.

The GDG also considered that it was important to examine the cost effectiveness of these measures. As can be seen in Chapter 6 (Sections 6.2.6 and 6.3.6) the GDG chose to focus on the cost effectiveness of the case identification and assessment for GAD. This is one of the more commonly presenting, although under-recognised, common mental health disorders in primary care. Two key elements of the care pathway were assessed: the initial case identification for GAD and the use of the GAD-7 in addition to the standard clinical assessment. The model clearly indicated that such an approach may well be cost effective. The available data for other anxiety disorders were of poorer quality and so no other models were developed for other anxiety disorders. Given the broadly similar performance of the GAD-7 (in terms of sensitivity and specificity), and the fact that the treatment outcomes for the other anxiety disorders are also broadly comparable with, if not better than, those for GAD (NICE, 2011a and 2005b), the GDG took the view that an extrapolation from this model to other anxiety disorders was warranted. For depression, no model was developed because the approach used for case identification of depression is already well-established in the NHS and the evidence reviewed in the recent *Depression* guidelines (NICE, 2009a and 2009b) did not suggest any changes to current practice.

When drafting the recommendations, the GDG recognised that a number of key areas required further research. In particular, uncertainty remains about the accuracy and consequent identification of appropriate treatment by para-professionals in primary care. An assessment by a mental health professional will probably result in more accurate identification of problems and appropriate treatment, but is likely to entail greater cost and potentially significantly longer waiting times for interventions, both of which can have deleterious effects on care. In addition, a number of different ratings scales for depression and anxiety disorders are in current use, both in research studies and clinical practice. This makes obtaining comparative estimates of clinical outcomes at the individual level difficult when moving between research and clinical settings, and also between different clinical settings. A method that allows for prompt and easy 'walking across' between assessment instruments would have a potentially significant clinical benefit in routine care.

## 5.4 RECOMMENDATIONS

### 5.4.1 Clinical recommendations

5.4.1.1 If the identification questions (see Section 5.2.11) indicate a possible common mental health disorder, but the practitioner is not competent to perform a mental health assessment, refer the person to an appropriate healthcare professional. If this professional is not the person's GP, inform the GP of the referral[19].

5.4.1.2 If the identification questions (see Section 5.2.11) indicate a possible common mental health disorder, a practitioner who is competent to perform a mental health assessment should review the person's mental state and associated functional, interpersonal and social difficulties[19].

5.4.1.3 When assessing a person with a suspected common mental health disorder, consider using:
- a diagnostic or problem identification tool or algorithm, for example, the Improving Access to Psychological Therapies (IAPT) screening prompts tool[20]
- a validated measure relevant to the disorder or problem being assessed, for example, the 9-item Patient Health Questionnaire (PHQ-9), the Hospital Anxiety and Depression Scale (HADS) or the 7-item Generalized Anxiety Disorder scale (GAD-7) to inform the assessment and support the evaluation of any intervention.

5.4.1.4 All staff carrying out the assessment of suspected common mental health disorders should be competent to perform an assessment of the presenting problem in line with the service setting in which they work, and be able to:
- determine the nature, duration and severity of the presenting disorder
- take into account not only symptom severity but also the associated functional impairment
- identify appropriate treatment and referral options in line with relevant NICE guidance.

---

[19]Adapted from *Depression* (NICE, 2009a).
[20]For further information, see *The IAPT Data Handbook* (IAPT, 2010; Appendix C, 'IAPT provisional diagnosis screening prompts'; available from: www.iapt.nhs.uk/services/measuring-outcomes).

5.4.1.5 All staff carrying out the assessment of common mental health disorders should be competent in:

- relevant verbal and non-verbal communication skills, including the ability to elicit problems, the perception of the problem(s) and their impact, tailoring information, supporting participation in decision-making and discussing treatment options
- the use of formal assessment measures and routine outcome measures in a variety of settings and environments.

5.4.1.6 In addition to assessing symptoms and associated functional impairment, consider how the following factors may have affected the development, course and severity of a person's presenting problem:

- a history of any mental health disorder
- a history of a chronic physical health problem
- any past experience of, and response to, treatments
- the quality of interpersonal relationships
- living conditions and social isolation
- a family history of mental illness
- a history of domestic violence or sexual abuse
- employment and immigration status.

If appropriate, the impact of the presenting problem on the care of children and young people should also be assessed, and if necessary local safeguarding procedures followed[21].

5.4.1.7 When assessing a person with a suspected common mental health disorder, be aware of any learning disabilities or acquired cognitive impairments, and if necessary consider consulting with a relevant specialist when developing treatment plans and strategies[21].

5.4.1.8 If the presentation and history of a common mental health disorder suggest that it may be mild and self-limiting (that is, symptoms are improving) and the disorder is of recent onset, consider providing psychoeducation and active monitoring before offering or referring for further assessment or treatment. These approaches may improve less severe presentations and avoid the need for further interventions.

5.4.1.9 Always ask people with a common mental health disorder directly about suicidal ideation and intent. If there is a risk of self-harm or suicide:

- assess whether the person has adequate social support and is aware of sources of help
- arrange help appropriate to the level of risk (see Section 6.2.9)
- advise the person to seek further help if the situation deteriorates[21].

5.4.1.10 During pregnancy or the postnatal period, women requiring psychological interventions should be seen for treatment normally within 1 month of initial assessment, and no longer than 3 months afterwards. This is because of the lower threshold for access to psychological interventions during

---

[21]Adapted from *Depression* (NICE, 2009a).

pregnancy and the postnatal period arising from the changing risk–benefit ratio for psychotropic medication at this time[22].

5.4.1.11　When considering drug treatments for common mental health disorders in women who are pregnant, breastfeeding or planning a pregnancy, consult *Antenatal and Postnatal Mental Health* (NICE, 2007a) for advice on prescribing.

### 5.4.2　Research recommendations

5.4.2.1　For people with a suspected common mental health disorder, what is the clinical and cost effectiveness of using a comprehensive assessment (conducted by a mental health professional) versus a brief assessment (conducted by a paraprofessional)? (See Appendix 11 for further details.)

5.4.2.2　What methodology should be used to allow 'walking across' from one assessment instrument for common mental health disorders to another? (See Appendix 11 for further details.)

---

[22]Adapted from *Antenatal and Postnatal Mental Health* (NICE, 2007a).

# 6 FURTHER ASSESSMENT OF RISK AND NEED FOR TREATMENT, AND ROUTINE OUTCOME MONITORING

## 6.1 INTRODUCTION

This chapter is focused on the further assessment and decision making that follows on from an initial assessment, the primary purpose of which is to identify and characterise the nature of the presenting problem, as discussed in Chapter 5. A further task of this chapter is to advise on how the information gained from the assessment can be used to inform the choice of appropriate treatment. This will be informed by a number of factors including patient characteristics, the patient's previous experience of treatment, the presence of other mental and physical disorders, the nature of the treatment and the setting in which it is delivered. The degree of risk that the patient faces can also significantly affect both the nature of the treatment and the setting in which it is provided, and this may, to a greater or lesser extent, be independent of the nature of the disorder.

Finally, this chapter considers ROM and the role it has to play in the delivery of effective interventions for people with common mental health disorders.

## 6.2 RISK ASSESSMENT

### 6.2.1 Introduction

Common mental health disorders are associated with an increased risk of suicide; this is most marked in depression, which is the single greatest cause of death by suicide (Moscicki, 2001), but an increased risk of suicide is also found across the range of anxiety disorders (Khan *et al.*, 2002). Identifying those with common mental health disorders at risk of suicide is therefore of considerable importance. A number of methods have been developed to assess risk of suicide and all tend to focus on a number of common issues, including suicidal ideation, intent and planning, past history of suicide attempts and protective factors (for example, presence of supportive family or close friends), and risk factors (such as drug or alcohol misuse). Suicide prevention strategies tend to focus on the delivery of protocols to ensure that appropriate information is obtained and systems are in place for the effective management and monitoring of identified risks (for example, National Patient Safety Agency, 2009). However, these approaches tend to be focused on secondary care mental health services and inpatient services in particular. Primary care-focused initiatives tend to focus more on staff training to improve identification and detection, for example through improved questioning techniques and communication skills (for example, Gask *et al.*, 2008). However, it should be noted that a review of suicide prevention schemes concluded that the proper recognition and treatment of depression were probably effective but that evidence for other strategies was limited or inconclusive (Mann *et al.*, 2005).

In common mental health disorders there has been much less focus on harm to others or harm to self from neglect, but both risks can and do occur in people with common mental health disorders. Neglect of self is more frequent in people with more severe disorders.

*Current practice*

Risk assessment protocols are now standard in all secondary care mental health services and often with systems in place for monitoring their implementation. Such systems usually require explicit questioning and reporting about certain thoughts or behaviours such as suicidal ideation, plans or intent. Other risk areas, such as risk to children, are also highly specified with all healthcare professionals under a statutory obligation to report suspected child abuse or maltreatment. Responsibilities are also placed on healthcare professionals in relation to vulnerable adults. These responsibilities apply as much to primary as to secondary care services. Some primary care-based services, such as those IAPT services based in primary care, will have routine protocols in place, but for other primary care practitioners, including GPs, it is less likely to be the case that common protocols exist and this may lead to greater variation in practice (Bajaj *et al.*, 2008).

### 6.2.2    Clinical review protocol

The aim of this review was to perform a narrative synthesis of existing NICE guidelines and published systematic reviews addressing risk assessment for people with a common mental health disorder. The review protocol, including the review question, information about databases searched and the eligibility criteria used in this section of the guideline can be found in Table 22. Although the search was conducted for the period 1995 to 2010, the focus was on systematic reviews published since 2003. Further information about the rationale for the method employed here can be found in Chapter 3 and about the search strategy in Appendix 6.

### 6.2.3    Studies considered

Five existing NICE guidelines that were relevant to common mental health disorder were utilised:
- *Depression* (NCCMH, 2010b; NICE, 2009a)
- *Generalised Anxiety Disorder and Panic Disorder (With or Without Agoraphobia) in Adults* and *Generalised Anxiety Disorder in Adults* (NCCMH, 2011a)
- *Obsessive-compulsive Disorder* (NCCMH, 2006; NICE, 2005a)

**Table 22: Clinical review protocol for the review of risk assessment**

| Component | Description |
|---|---|
| Review question | In adults (18 years and older) identified with depression (including subthreshold disorders) or an anxiety disorder*, what is the definition, delivery and value (or otherwise) of risk assessment? |
| Objectives | To perform a narrative synthesis of existing NICE guidelines and systematic reviews addressing risk assessment for people with a common mental health disorder |
| Population | Adults (18 years and older) identified with depression (including subthreshold disorders) or an anxiety disorder* |
| Intervention(s) | Risk assessment |
| Comparison | Standard management strategy |
| Critical outcomes | Clinical utility |
| Electronic databases | Systematic reviews: CDSR, CINAHL, DARE, EMBASE, MEDLINE, PsycINFO<br>RCTs: CENTRAL |
| Date searched | Systematic reviews: 1 January 1995 to 10 September 2010<br>RCTs: 1 January 2008 up to 10 September 2010 |
| Study design | Systematic review and RCTs |
| *Including GAD, panic disorder, social anxiety disorder, OCD, specific phobias and PTSD. | |

- *Post-traumatic Stress Disorder* (NCCMH, 2005; NICE, 2005b)
- *Antenatal and Postnatal Mental Health* (NCCMH, 2007; NICE, 2007).

In addition, the literature search for systematic reviews yielded 5,231 papers. Scanning titles/abstracts identified 34 potentially relevant reviews[23]. Further inspection of each paper revealed only one systematic review, MCMILLAN2007 (McMillan *et al.*, 2007), that met eligibility criteria. This review focused on whether the Beck Hopelessness Scale (BHS) could be utilised to identify people at risk of deliberate, non-fatal self-harm and suicide. The characteristics of this review can be found in Table 23. Further information about both included and excluded studies can be found in Appendix 14.

---

[23]This includes reviews potentially relevant to the assessment topics covered in the previous chapter.

**Table 23: Study information table for systematic reviews of risk assessment**

| Study ID | MCMILLAN2007 |
| --- | --- |
| Method used to synthesise evidence | Meta-analysis |
| Design of included studies | Cohort |
| Evidence search | CINAHL, EMBASE, MEDLINE (1950 to January 2006) and PsycINFO. |
| No. of included studies | 19 (ten studies included in the diagnostic accuracy meta-analysis) |
| Review quality | Moderate risk of bias (quality of included studies not assessed/reported) |
| Instrument/method of assessment reviewed | BHS |
| Reference standard used by primary studies | Number of people with the outcome (suicide or self-harm) |

### 6.2.4    Summary of evidence from existing NICE guidelines

The method used to review existing NICE guidelines relevant to common mental health disorders can be found in the review of formal assessment reported in the previous chapter (see Section 5.3). The *Depression*, *Obsessive-compulsive Disorder* and *Post-traumatic Stress Disorder* guidelines (NICE, 2009a, 2005a and 2005b, respectively) contained recommendations about risk assessment, and these are summarised in Table 24. These recommendations were used to inform the development of recommendations that were either common to all common mental health disorders or disorder specific.

### 6.2.5    Clinical evidence from existing systematic reviews

MCMILLAN2007 assessed the ability of the BHS to predict non-fatal self-harm and suicide by systematically searching for studies that used a cohort design. The review identified ten studies (four on suicide and six on self-harm), with varying lengths of follow-up. All but one study used adult samples. Random-effects meta-analysis was used to synthesise data to obtain pooled estimates of sensitivity, specificity, LR+ and LR−, and a summary diagnostic OR.

**Table 24: Preliminary summary and synthesis of relevant recommendations (by guideline)**

| Guideline | Recommendation |
|---|---|
| *Depression* (NICE, 2009a) | Always ask people with depression directly about suicidal ideation and intent. If there is a risk of self-harm or suicide:<br>• assess whether the person has adequate social support and is aware of sources of help<br>• arrange help appropriate to the level of risk<br>• advise the person to seek further help if the situation deteriorates.<br><br>If a person with depression presents considerable immediate risk to themselves or others, refer them urgently to specialist mental health services.<br><br>Advise people with depression of the potential for increased agitation, anxiety and suicidal ideation in the initial stages of treatment; actively seek out these symptoms and:<br>• ensure that the person knows how to seek help promptly<br>• review the person's treatment if they develop marked and/or prolonged agitation.<br><br>Advise a person with depression and their family or carer to be vigilant for mood changes, negativity and hopelessness, and suicidal ideation, and to contact their practitioner if concerned. This is particularly important during high-risk periods, such as starting or changing treatment and at times of increased personal stress.<br><br>If a person with depression is assessed to be at risk of suicide:<br>• take into account toxicity in overdose if an antidepressant is prescribed or the person is taking other medication; if necessary, limit the amount of drug(s) available<br>• consider increasing the level of support, such as more frequent direct or telephone contacts<br>• consider referral to specialist mental health services. |
| *Obsessive-compulsive Disorder* (NICE, 2005a) | In people who have been diagnosed with OCD, healthcare professionals should assess the risk of self-harm and suicide, especially if they have also been diagnosed with depression. Part of the risk assessment should include the impact of their compulsive behaviours on themselves or others. Other comorbid conditions and psychosocial factors that may contribute to risk should also be considered. |

*Continued*

**Table 24:** **(*Continued*)**

| | |
|---|---|
| ***Post-traumatic Stress Disorder* (NICE, 2005b)** | For PTSD sufferers presenting in primary care, GPs should take responsibility for the initial assessment and the initial coordination of care. This includes the determination of the need for emergency medical or psychiatric assessment. |
| | Assessment of PTSD sufferers should be conducted by competent individuals and be comprehensive, including physical, psychological and social needs and a risk assessment. |
| | For PTSD sufferers whose assessment identifies a high risk of suicide or harm to others, healthcare professionals should first concentrate on management of this risk. |

*Using the Beck Hopelessness Scale to predict suicide*
Based on four studies, and using a cut-off score of at least 9, the pooled sensitivity of the BHS was 0.80 (95% CI, 0.68 to 0.90, $I^2 = 57\%$) and specificity was 0.42 (95% CI, 0.41 to 0.44, $I^2 = 76\%$). Likelihood ratios for positive and negative tests were 1.55 (95% CI, 1.31 to 1.83, $I^2 = 44\%$) and 0.45 (95% CI, 0.20 to 1.03, $I^2 = 49\%$), respectively. The pooled diagnostic OR was 3.39 (95% CI, 1.29 to 8.88, $I^2 = 37\%$). The pooled AUC was 0.70 (95% CI, 0.59 to 0.85).

*Using the Beck Hopelessness Scale to predict non-fatal self-harm*
Based on six studies and using a cut-off score of at least 9, the pooled sensitivity of the BHS was 0.78 (95% CI, 0.74 to 0.82, $I^2 = 0\%$) and specificity was 0.42 (95% CI, 0.38 to 0.45, $I^2 = 90\%$). Likelihood ratios for positive and negative tests were 1.29 (95% CI, 1.09 to 1.52, $I^2 = 74\%$) and 0.58 (95% CI, 0.47 to 0.71, $I^2 = 0\%$) respectively. The pooled diagnostic OR was 2.27 (95% CI, 1.53 to 3.37, $I^2 = 35\%$), regardless of setting, length of follow-up and baseline risk. The pooled AUC was 0.63 (95% CI, 0.57 to 0.70). After removing the study that used an adolescent population, the results remained similar.

**6.2.6     Clinical evidence summary of existing systematic reviews**

Using the standard cut-off point of at least 9, the evidence suggests that the BHS has limited clinical utility for identifying people at increased risk of suicide or non-fatal self-harm.

### 6.2.7 Health economic evidence

No studies were identified in the systematic literature review that considered the cost effectiveness of risk assessment for people with a common mental health disorder.

### 6.2.8 From evidence to recommendations

As can be seen from the review of risk assessment, very little evidence from existing systematic reviews was identified that was directly relevant to the clinical question. In developing the recommendations about risk, the GDG therefore had to rely on the existing recommendations relevant to risk identified from current NICE mental health guidelines on depressive and anxiety disorders. As can be seen from the table of relevant recommendations (Table 24) there is a significant focus on depression, which is not surprising given that depression is the single greatest cause of suicide. However, as noted in the introduction there is an elevated risk in populations with anxiety disorders compared with non-anxious populations. In addition, there are risks arising from harm to others (not commonly associated with common mental health disorders and the risk of self-neglect), which may be higher in other disorders (for example, in OCD). The GDG carefully considered these recommendations; while it was recognised that it was important for the focus to remain on depression, clear recommendations were needed for the other disorders. The GDG was also aware that they were drawing on existing evidence sources (NICE guidelines), the evidence for which had not been reviewed by them. It was therefore important that the precise meaning of the recommendations drawn from other guidelines was not altered, although some re-wording and restructuring of those recommendations was required in order to produce a coherent, clear and comprehensible set of recommendations for this guideline. The GDG therefore took the view that it was appropriate to reproduce the most important recommendations concerning risk assessment from the *Depression* guidelines, with minor amendments as described above. These were supplemented by recommendations for the other common mental health disorders. In developing these recommendations the GDG was also mindful that risk assessment is not a one off activity, and should not only be focused on the risk of self-harm but, where appropriate, on harm to others and self-neglect. Risk assessment should also relate to the overall process of the assessment, management and monitoring of person's care.

### 6.2.9 Recommendations

6.2.9.1   If a person with a common mental health disorder presents a high risk of suicide or potential harm to others, a risk of significant self-neglect, or severe functional impairment, assess and manage the immediate problem first and then refer to specialist services. Where appropriate inform families and carers.

6.2.9.2    If a person with a common mental health disorder presents considerable and immediate risk to themselves or others, refer them urgently to the emergency services or specialist mental health services[24].

6.2.9.3    If a person with a common mental health disorder, in particular depression, is assessed to be at risk of suicide:

- take into account toxicity in overdose, if a drug is prescribed, and potential interaction with other prescribed medication; if necessary, limit the amount of drug(s) available
- consider increasing the level of support, such as more frequent direct or telephone contacts
- consider referral to specialist mental health services[24].

## 6.3    FACTORS THAT PREDICT TREATMENT RESPONSE

### 6.3.1    Introduction

A considerable number of people with a common mental health disorder do not respond adequately to initial treatment and may require further treatment of a different or more intensive kind. While the response to treatment also varies by disorder (see, for example, Westen & Morrison, 2001), there is no doubt that people experience increased distress if an inappropriate or ineffective treatment is offered. The first stage in this process is an accurate diagnosis or characterisation of a person's problems. This is important because NICE guidelines are condition- or diagnosis-specific. However, this is unlikely to be sufficient because a number of other factors are known or are hypothesised to be predictive of treatment response. In some cases this has focused on attempts to 'subtype' or further categorise a disorder. This has perhaps been most notable in the case of depression where there has been a long tradition of developing subtypes of depressive disorders, including, for example, reactive and endogenous depression, atypical depression and melancholia. However, these categories have not yielded much interesting data about the likely response to treatment (NICE, 2009a and 2009b). Other approaches have focused on characteristics such as severity and chronicity, which have pan-diagnostic elements to them and have been shown to be associated with differential outcomes, although at times it has been difficult to distinguish between predictors of the response to treatment from predictors of the course of illness.

Given the current limited knowledge about which factors are associated with better antidepressant or psychotherapy response, most individual treatment decisions rely upon clinical judgement and patient preference. Clinical guidelines explicitly address this issue and aim to support clinicians and patients in arriving at the right choice for them, in terms of initial treatment and for subsequent treatment if the initial treatment has had limited or no benefit. The intention is that this will lead to treatment strategies that could be tailored to the individual (Dodd & Berk, 2004). However, for

---

[24]Adapted from *Depression* (NICE, 2009a).

a clinician meeting with a patient for the first time, particularly one with a significant history of problems and with limited benefit from treatment, pulling together a range of recommendations from across a number of guidelines is challenging.

The GDG also recognised that when developing a set of recommendations about predictors of treatment response, these would have to be compatible with the existing NICE guidelines. (Note that a number of these guidelines had directly and indirectly addressed the question of treatment response.) Identifying novel data or reviews, which pointed to different treatment options than were set out in existing NICE guidelines, was inherently problematic. First, it may only be possible to properly evaluate these new data by comparing the findings against existing treatment recommendations, and this could imply a revision of the existing treatment recommendations of current guidelines. This was simply not possible; the group lacked the resources and competence to do so and no proper structures were in place to meet the consultation requirements for the development or updating of another NICE guideline. In light of this, the GDG decided to concentrate primarily on existing NICE guidance in developing their treatment recommendations for this section using the evidence from any new studies to inform the process of adaptation of the existing guidelines rather than supplant them.

Thus, the objective of this section of the guideline was to synthesise recommendations from existing NICE guidelines relevant to common mental health disorders and extract those factors that modify recommendations for treatment. This was supplemented by published systematic reviews addressing treatment response factors for people with common mental health disorders.

In developing recommendations based on existing NICE guidelines, key principles were formulated to guide the process, namely that in developing this guideline the meaning and intent of the original recommendations should be preserved. In practice this means that the recommendations in this guideline should properly express the information provided by the original evidence-based reviews and also be supportive, or not contradict, the actions specified in the original recommendations.

Based on these principles a decision was made to either adopt or adapt a recommendation. Adoption involved the simple transfer of a recommendation to this guideline from another guideline; no changes to wording or structure were to be made. Adaptation involved making a number of changes to the recommendation, while still preserving meaning and intent[25]. These adaptations to a guideline recommendation take a number of forms:

- Changes in terminology – this involved the replacement of the original wording of a guideline with new wording, to facilitate understanding (for example, using the term 'facilitated self-help' to cover terms such as 'guided self-help').
- Changes in the structure and wording of a recommendation – to properly express the meaning and intent of the original recommendation in a form that was compatible with a recommendation about referral.
- Changes involving the combination of a number of recommendations from either a single guideline, or more than one guideline – for example, recommendations

---

[25]In the final version of the guideline all recommendations from other NICE mental health guidelines were adapted rather than adopted.

for the treatment of persistent subthreshold depressive symptoms and mild to moderate depression from the two *Depression* guidelines (NICE, 2009a and 2009b) were combined to facilitate understanding for healthcare professionals. Of course, such recommendations could also involve changes in terminology as well as structure.

Guided by the above principles, relevant recommendations from the NICE guidelines were extracted as detailed in Section 6.3.2. The new recommendations were then synthesised from a review of existing relevant NICE guidelines, and these recommendations were organised within a stepped-care framework and presented to the GDG for review. The GDG was asked to focus on the value of the recommendations as treatment and referral recommendations, and asked to ensure that, where possible, the meaning and intent of the recommendations had been preserved. The recommendations were then sent for further review by senior members of the original GDGs who had developed the recommendations, who were also asked to consider whether the original meaning and intent had been preserved.

### 6.3.2 Clinical review protocol

The aim of this review was to perform a narrative synthesis of existing NICE guidelines and published systematic reviews addressing which factors predict treatment response and/or treatment failure in people with a common mental health disorder. The review protocol, including the review question, information about databases searched and the eligibility criteria used in this section of the guideline can be found in Table 25. The search was restricted to systematic reviews published since 2003 only. Further information about the rationale for the method employed here can be found in Chapter 3 and the search strategy can be found in Appendix 6.

### 6.3.3 Studies considered

Nine existing NICE guidelines that were relevant to common mental health disorders were utilised:

- *Depression* (NICE, 2009a; NCCMH, 2010b)
- *Depression in Adults with a Chronic Physical Health Problem* (NICE, 2009b; NCCMH, 2010a)
- *Generalised Anxiety Disorder and Panic Disorder (With or Without Agoraphobia) in Adults* (NICE, 2011a and *Generalised Anxiety Disorder in Adults* (NCCMH, 2011a))
- *Obsessive-Compulsive Disorder* (NICE, 2005a; NCCMH, 2006)
- *Post-traumatic Stress Disorder* (NICE, 2005b; NCCMH, 2005)
- *Antenatal and Postnatal Mental Health* (NICE, 2007a; NCCMH, 2007)
- *Alcohol-use Disorders* (NICE, 2011b; NCCMH, 2011b)
- *Drug Misuse: Psychosocial Interventions* (NICE, 2007b; NCCMH, 2008a)
- *Drug Misuse: Opioid Detoxification* (NICE, 2007c; NCCMH, 2008b).

**Table 25: Clinical review protocol for the review of predictors of response**

| Component | Description |
|---|---|
| Review question | In adults (18 years and older) identified with depression (including subthreshold disorders) or an anxiety disorder*, which factors predict treatment response and/or treatment failure? |
| Objectives | To perform a narrative synthesis of existing NICE guidelines and published systematic reviews addressing treatment response factors for people with common mental health disorder. |
| Population | Adults (18 years and older) identified with depression (including subthreshold disorders) or an anxiety disorder* |
| Intervention(s) | Not applicable |
| Comparison | Not applicable |
| Critical outcomes | Association between predictor and treatment response/ failure |
| Electronic databases | Systematic reviews: CINAHL, CDSR, DARE, EMBASE, MEDLINE, PsycINFO |
| Date searched | 1 January 2003 to 10 January 2011 |
| Study design | NICE guidelines, systematic reviews |
| *Including GAD, panic disorder, social anxiety disorder, OCD, specific phobias and PTSD. | |

In addition, the literature search for systematic reviews yielded 2,343 papers. Scanning titles/abstracts identified 34 potentially relevant reviews[26]; however, further inspection found only six systematic reviews that met the eligibility criteria: DODD2004 (Dodd & Berk, 2004), FEKADU2009 (Fekadu *et al.*, 2009), HARDEVELD2010 (Hardeveld *et al.*, 2010), MITCHELL2005 (Mitchell & Subramaniam, 2005), NELSON2009 (Nelson *et al.*, 2009) and POMPILI2009 (Pompili *et al.*, 2009). Of the included reviews, two focused on predictors of treatment response (DODD2004, NELSON2009), one on predictors of non-adherence to antidepressant medication (POMPILI2009), two on risk factors for depression recurrence (FEKADU2009, HARDEVELD2010) and one on prognosis of depression in mid-life and older people (MITCHELL2005). The characteristics of the studies included in the narrative synthesis can be found in Table 26. Further information about both included and excluded studies can be found in Appendix 14.

---

[26]This includes reviews potentially relevant to the assessment topics covered in the previous chapter.

**Table 26: Study information table for systematic reviews of predictors of response**

| Study ID | DODD2004 | FEKADU2009 | HARDEVELD2010 | MITCHELL2005 | NELSON2009 | POMPILI2009 |
|---|---|---|---|---|---|---|
| **Predictor** | Biological, psychosocial, clinical factors | Clinical factors | Psychosocial and clinical factors | Age | Presence of anxiety | Psychosocial and clinical factors |
| **Outcome** | Response to antidepressant treatment | Treatment response/ readmission | Recurrence of major depressive disorder (MDD) | Treatment response and remission/ recurrence of depression | Response to second generation antidepressant treatment | Medication adherence |
| **Method used to synthesise evidence** | Narrative | Narrative | Narrative | Narrative | Meta-analysis | Narrative |
| **Design of included studies** | Preference for clinically relevant primary research articles | Observational and longitudinal (minimum follow-up 6 months) | Naturalistic longitudinal study (minimum follow-up 6 months and sample size of 50) | Comparative studies of mid- and late-life first-epsiode depression (minimum sample size of 20 in each group) | Randomised, double-blind placebo-controlled trials | Primary research, review articles and descriptive papers that measured adherence |
| **Dates searched** | 1966 to 2004 | Inception to 2008 | 1980 to 2008 | 1966 to 2004 | 1966 to 2006 | 1975 to 2009 |
| **Diagnosis** | Depression | Treatment-resistant depression | MDD | Depression | Late-life depression | Unipolar and bipolar depression |
| **No. of included studies** | 95 | 9 (4 with relevant data) | 27 | 36 primary articles | 10 | 104 |
| **Review quality** | High risk of bias (only MEDLINE searched, quality of included studies not assessed/ reported, poor description of methodology) | Low risk bias | Low risk of bias | Low risk of bias | Low risk of bias | Moderate risk of bias (quality of included studies not assessed/reported) |

### 6.3.4 Summary of evidence from existing NICE guidelines

Recommendations from existing NICE guidelines relevant to common mental health disorders were summarised for the purposes of the GDG and synthesised using tabulation. Each guideline was examined for potentially relevant recommendations and these were categorised into the following themes: illness severity, duration and response to treatment (Table 27), disorder subtype (Table 28), comorbidities (Table 29), previous illness (Table 30), previous response to treatment (Table 31), personal characteristics (Table 32) and service user preference (Table 33). Some of the recommendations have been reproduced as they appeared in the original guidelines; others have been condensed and summarised for the purposes of this review and to aid the GDG. The synthesis was then used to inform the method of adoption and adaptation of existing NICE guideline recommendations.

**Table 27: Preliminary summary and synthesis of recommendations relating to illness severity, duration or response to treatment (by guideline) to support the process of adoption and adaptation**

| Guideline | Selected text from recommendations |
|---|---|
| *Alcohol-use Disorders* (NICE, 2011b) | None identified |
| *Antenatal and Postnatal Mental Health* (NICE, 2007a) (For common mental health disorders only) | For women with symptoms of depression and/or anxiety that do not meet diagnostic criteria but significantly interfere with personal and social functioning, consider: <br>• individual brief psychological treatment (four to six sessions), IPT or CBT for women with a previous episode of anxiety/depression <br>• social support for example, regular informal individual or group-based support for women who have not had a previous episode of depression or anxiety. <br><br>Mild-moderate depression during pregnancy/the postnatal period, consider: <br>• self-help strategies <br>• non-directive counselling at home <br>• brief CBT <br>• IPT. <br><br>*Mild depression* <br>If a woman is taking an antidepressant for current mild depression, the medication should be withdrawn gradually and monitoring considered. If intervention is then needed, consider: <br>• self-help approaches <br>• brief psychological treatment. |

*Continued*

**Table 27:** (*Continued*)

| | |
|---|---|
| | ***Moderate depression***<br>If a woman is taking an antidepressant for current moderate depression, consider:<br>• switching to psychological therapy<br>• switching to an antidepressant with lower risk.<br><br>***Severe depression***<br>If a woman is currently taking an antidepressant for severe depression, consider:<br>• combining drug treatment with psychological treatment, but switching to an antidepressant with lower risk<br>• switching to psychological treatment. |
| ***Depression*** (**NICE, 2009a**) | For persistent subthreshold depressive symptoms or mild to moderate depression, consider offering:<br>• individual guided self-help<br>• CCBT<br>• a structured group physical activity programme.<br><br>For people with depression who decline an antidepressant, CBT, IPT, behavioural activation and behavioural couples therapy, consider:<br>• counselling for people with persistent subthreshold depressive symptoms or mild to moderate depression<br>• short-term psychodynamic psychotherapy for people with mild to moderate depression.<br><br>Discuss with the person the uncertainty of the effectiveness of counselling and psychodynamic psychotherapy in treating depression.<br><br>Do not use antidepressants routinely unless symptoms have been present for a long period or if they persist after other interventions.<br><br>For moderate or severe depression, provide a combination of antidepressant medication and a high-intensity psychological intervention (CBT or IPT).<br><br>For people with long-standing moderate or severe depression who would benefit from additional social or vocational support, consider:<br>• befriending as an adjunct to pharmacological or psychological treatments<br>• a rehabilitation programme if a person's depression has resulted in loss of work or disengagement from other social activities over a longer term. |

*Continued*

**Table 27:** (*Continued*)

| Guideline | Selected text from recommendations |
|---|---|
| | For people with severe depression and those with moderate depression and complex problems, consider: <br>• referring to specialist mental health services for a programme of coordinated multiprofessional care. <br><br>Consider electroconvulsive therapy (ECT) for acute treatment of severe depression that is life threatening and when a rapid response is required, or when other treatments have failed. <br><br>Do not use ECT routinely for people with moderate depression but consider it if their depression has not responded to multiple drug treatments and psychological treatment. <br><br>Consider inpatient treatment for people with depression who are at significant risk of suicide, self-harm or self-neglect. <br><br>People with depression who have residual symptoms should be offered one of the following psychological interventions: <br>• individual CBT <br>• mindfulness-based cognitive therapy. <br><br>For people with severe depression and those with moderate depression and complex problems, consider: <br>• providing collaborative care if the depression is in the context of a chronic physical health problem with associated functional impairment. <br><br>People who are considered to be at significant risk of relapse (including those who have relapsed despite antidepressant treatment or who are unable or choose not to continue antidepressant treatment) should be offered one of the following: <br>• individual CBT <br>• mindfulness-based cognitive therapy. |
| ***Depression in Adults with a Chronic Physical Health Problem* (NICE, 2009b)** | Persistent subthreshold depressive symptoms or mild to moderate depression and a chronic physical health problem, consider: <br>• low intensity psychosocial interventions <br>• medication <br>• referral for further assessment and interventions. |

*Continued*

**Table 27:** *(Continued)*

| | |
|---|---|
| | Moderate and severe depression, offer:<br>• high-intensity psychological interventions<br>• combined treatments<br>• collaborative care<br>• referral for further assessment and interventions.<br><br>Severe and complex depression, risk to life and severe self-neglect, offer:<br>• medication<br>• high-intensity psychological interventions<br>• ECT<br>• crisis service<br>• combined treatments<br>• multi-professional and inpatient care.<br><br>Consider medication, high-intensity psychological interventions, combined treatments, collaborative care and referral for further assessment and interventions when:<br>• persistent subthreshold depressive symptoms or mild to moderate depression persist after initial interventions.<br><br>Consider collaborative care for moderate to severe depression when:<br>• depression has not responded to initial high-intensity psychological interventions and/or medication. |
| ***Drug Misuse: Opioid Detoxification* (NICE, 2007c)** | None identified. |
| ***Drug Misuse: Psychosocial Interventions* (NICE, 2007b)** | None identified. |
| ***Generalised Anxiety Disorder and Panic Disorder (with or without Agoraphobia) in Adults* (NICE, 2011a)** | Offer an individual high-intensity psychological intervention or a pharmacological intervention to people with GAD with marked functional impairment or those whose symptoms have not adequately responded to Step 2 interventions.<br><br>Offer CBT or applied relaxation to people with GAD with marked functional impairment or those whose symptoms have not adequately responded to Step 2 interventions. |

*Continued*

**Table 27:** (*Continued*)

| Guideline | Selected text from recommendations |
|---|---|
| *Obsessive-compulsive Disorder* (**NICE, 2005a**) | In initial treatment, low-intensity psychological treatments should be offered if the degree of functional impairment is mild. |
| | Adults with moderate functional impairment should be offered the choice of either a course of an SSRI or more intensive CBT. |
| | For adults with OCD who are housebound, unable or reluctant to attend a clinic, or have significant problems with hoarding, a period of home-based treatment may be considered. |
| | For adults with OCD who are housebound and unable to undertake home-based treatment because of the nature of their symptoms, a period of CBT by telephone may be considered. |
| | For adults with OCD, if there has been no response to a full trial of at least one SSRI alone, a full trial of combined treatment with CBT (including ERP) and an SSRI, and a full trial of clomipramine alone, the patient should be referred to a multidisciplinary team with specific expertise in the treatment of OCD/body dysmorphic disorder for assessment and further treatment planning. |
| | For OCD associated with severe risk to life, reassess and discuss options. Consider:<br>• care coordination<br>• SSRI or clomipramine<br>• CBT (including ERP)<br>• combination of SSRI or clomipramine and CBT (including ERP)<br>• augmentation strategies<br>• admission<br>• special living arrangements. |
| | A small minority of adults with long-standing and disabling obsessive-compulsive symptoms that interfere with daily living and have prevented them from developing a normal level of autonomy may, in addition to treatment, need suitable accommodation in a supportive environment that will enable them to develop life skills for independent living. |

*Continued*

**Table 27:** (*Continued*)

| | |
|---|---|
| ***Post-traumatic Stress Disorder* (NICE, 2005b)** | The severity of the initial traumatic response is reasonable indicator of the need for early a intervention. |
| | Where symptoms are mild and have been present for less than 4 weeks after the trauma, watchful waiting, as a way of managing the difficulties presented by people with PTSD, should be considered. A follow-up contact should be arranged within 1 month |
| | Trauma-focused CBT should be offered to those with severe post traumatic symptoms or with severe PTSD in the first month after the traumatic event. These treatments should normally be provided on an individual outpatient basis |
| | Trauma-focused CBT should be offered to those with severe post-traumatic symptoms or with severe PTSD in the first month after the traumatic event. These treatments should normally be provided on an individual outpatient basis. |
| | Consider extending the duration of treatment beyond 12 sessions if several problems need to be addressed in the treatment of PTSD, particularly after multiple traumatic events, traumatic bereavement, or where chronic disability resulting from the trauma, significant comorbid disorders or social problems are present. |
| | For people with PTSD who have no or only limited improvement with a specific trauma-focused psychological treatment, healthcare professionals should consider the following options:<br>• an alternative form of trauma-focused psychological treatment with a course of pharmacological treatment. |
| | For people with PTSD whose assessment identifies a high risk of suicide or harm to others, healthcare professionals should first concentrate on management of this risk |

**Table 28: Preliminary summary and synthesis of selected text from recommendations relating to disorder subtype (by guideline) to support the process of adoption and adaptation**

| Guideline | Recommendation |
|---|---|
| *Alcohol-use Disorders* **(NICE, 2011b)** | None identified |
| *Antenatal and Postnatal Mental Health* **(NICE, 2007a)** **(For common mental health disorders only)** | None identified |
| *Depression* **(NICE, 2009a)** | Do not routinely vary the treatment strategies for depression described in this guideline by depression subtype (for example, atypical depression or seasonal depression) as there is no convincing evidence to support such action. Advise people with winter depression that follows a seasonal pattern and who wish to try light therapy in preference to antidepressant or psychological treatment that the evidence for the efficacy of light therapy is uncertain. |
| *Depression in Adults with a Chronic Physical Health Problem* **(NICE, 2009b)** | None identified |
| *Drug Misuse: Opioid Detoxification* **(NICE, 2007c)** | None identified |
| *Drug Misuse: Psychosocial Interventions* **(NICE, 2007b)** | None identified |
| *Generalised Anxiety Disorder and Panic Disorder (with or without Agoraphobia) in Adults* **(NICE, 2011a)** **(GAD)** | None identified |
| *Obsessive-compulsive Disorder* **(NICE, 2005a)** | For adults with obsessive thoughts who do not have overt compulsions, CBT (including exposure to obsessive thoughts and response prevention of mental rituals and neutralising strategies) should be considered. |
| *Post-traumatic Stress Disorder* **(NICE, 2005b)** | None identified |

**Table 29:  Summary of selected text from recommendations relating to comorbidities (by guideline)**

| Guideline | Recommendation |
|---|---|
| *Alcohol-use Disorders* (NICE, 2011b) | For people who misuse alcohol and have comorbid depression or anxiety disorders, treat the alcohol misuse first as this may lead to significant improvement in the depression and anxiety. If depression or anxiety continues after 3 to 4 weeks of abstinence from alcohol, assess the depression or anxiety and consider referral and treatment in line with the relevant NICE guideline for the particular disorder (*Depression* [NICE, 2009a] and *Generalised Anxiety Disorder and Panic Disorder [With or Without Agoraphobia] in Adults* [NICE, 2011a]). |
| *Antenatal and Postnatal Mental Health* (NICE, 2007a)<br><br>(For common mental health disorders only) | None identified |
| *Depression* (NICE, 2009a) | When depression is accompanied by symptoms of anxiety, the first priority should usually be to treat the depression. When the person has an anxiety disorder and comorbid depression or depressive symptoms, consider treating the anxiety disorder first. |
| *Depression in Adults with a Chronic Physical Health Problem* (NICE, 2009b) | When depression is accompanied by symptoms of anxiety, the first priority should usually be to treat the depression. When the patient has an anxiety disorder and comorbid depression or depressive symptoms, consult the NICE guideline for the relevant anxiety disorder and consider treating the anxiety disorder first.<br><br>When an antidepressant is to be prescribed for a patient, take into account:<br>• the presence of additional physical health disorders. |
| *Drug Misuse: Opioid Detoxification* (NICE, 2007c) | None identified |
| *Drug Misuse: Psychosocial Interventions* (NICE, 2007b) | Evidence-based psychological treatments (in particular, CBT) should be considered for the treatment of comorbid depression and anxiety disorders in line with existing NICE guidance for people who misuse cannabis or stimulants, and for those who have achieved abstinence or are stabilised on opioid maintenance treatment. |
| *Generalised Anxiety Disorder and Panic Disorder (With or Without Agoraphobia) in Adults* (NICE, 2011a) (GAD) | Consider referral to secondary care if the person with GAD has severe anxiety with marked functional impairment in conjunction with:<br>• a risk of self-harm or suicide<br>• significant comorbidity<br>• complex physical health problems<br>• self-neglect. |

*Continued*

**Table 29:** (*Continued*)

| Guideline | Recommendation |
|---|---|
| | When providing treatment for people with GAD and a mild learning disability or mild acquired cognitive impairment provide the same interventions as for other people with GAD, or adjust the method of delivery or duration. |
| | When assessing or providing an intervention for people with GAD and a moderate to severe learning disability or moderate to severe acquired cognitive impairment, consider consulting with a relevant specialist. |
| | If a person with GAD also has a comorbid depressive or other anxiety disorder, treat the primary disorder first. |
| | Non-harmful alcohol misuse should not be a contraindication to active treatment of GAD. For people with GAD with harmful and dependent alcohol misuse, treat the alcohol misuse first as this alone may lead to significant improvement in the symptoms of GAD. |
| | Specialist mental health services should conduct a thorough, holistic reassessment of: <br>• substance use <br>• the role of agoraphobic and other avoidant symptoms <br>• comorbidities. |
| *Obsessive-compulsive Disorder* (**NICE, 2005a**) | Adults with OCD with mild functional impairment who are unable to engage in low intensity CBT, or for whom low intensity treatment has proved to be inadequate, should be offered the choice of either a course of SSRI or more intensive CBT when OCD is associated with significant comorbidity or severe impairment, consider: <br>• SSRI or clomipramine <br>• CBT (including ERP) <br>• combination of SSRI or clomipramine and CBT (including ERP) <br>• care coordination <br>• augmentation strategies <br>• admission <br>• social care. |
| *Post-traumatic Stress Disorder* (**NICE, 2005b**) | When a patient presents with PTSD and depression, healthcare professionals should consider treating the PTSD first. |
| | For people with PTSD who are so severely depressed that this makes initial psychological treatment of PTSD very difficult, healthcare professionals should treat the depression first. |
| | For people with PTSD with drug or alcohol problems, healthcare professionals should treat the drug or alcohol problem first. |
| | When offering trauma-focused psychological interventions to people with PTSD with comorbid personality disorder, healthcare professionals should consider extending the duration of treatment. |
| | Where sleep is a major problem for an adult with PTSD, hypnotic medication may be appropriate for short-term use. |

156

**Table 30: Preliminary summary and synthesis of selected text from recommendations relating to previous illness (by guideline) to support the process of adoption and adaptation**

| Guideline | Recommendation |
|---|---|
| *Alcohol-use Disorders* (NICE, 2011b) | None identified |
| *Antenatal and Postnatal Mental Health* (NICE, 2007a)<br><br>(For common mental health disorders only) | None identified |
| *Depression* (NICE, 2009a) | Consider antidepressants for people with a past history of moderate or severe depression.<br><br>For people with depression who are at significant risk of relapse or have a history of recurrent depression, discuss with them treatments to reduce the risk of recurrence, including continuing medication, augmentation of medication or psychological treatment (CBT). Treatment choice should be influenced by previous treatment history, including the consequences of a relapse, residual symptoms, response to previous treatment and any discontinuation symptoms. |
| *Depression in Adults with a Chronic Physical Health Problem* (NICE, 2009b) | Consider medication, when:<br>• there is a history of moderate to severe depression<br>• mild depression complicates the care of the physical health problem<br>• subthreshold depressive symptoms have been present for a long period<br>• subthreshold depressive symptoms or mild depression persist(s) after other interventions. |
| *Drug Misuse: Opioid Detoxification* (NICE, 2007c) | None identified |
| *Drug Misuse: Psychosocial Interventions* (NICE, 2007b) | None identified |
| *Generalised Anxiety Disorder and Panic Disorder (with or without Agoraphobia) in Adults* (NICE, 2011a) | None identified |
| *Obsessive-compulsive Disorder* (NICE, 2005a) | None identified |
| *Post-traumatic Stress Disorder* (NICE, 2005b) | None identified |

**Table 31: Preliminary summary and synthesis of selected text from recommendations relating to previous response to treatment (by guideline) to support the process of adoption and adaptation**

| Guideline | Recommendation |
|---|---|
| *Alcohol-use Disorders* (**NICE, 2011b**) | None identified |
| *Antenatal and Postnatal Mental Health* (**NICE, 2007a**)<br><br>(**For common mental health disorders only**) | None identified |
| *Depression* (**NICE, 2009a**) | Support and encourage a person who has bene-fited from taking an antidepressant to continue medication for at least 6 months after remission of an episode of depression. |
| *Depression in Adults with a Chronic Physical Health Problem* (**NICE, 2009b**) | The choice of intervention should be influenced by the previous course of depression and response to treatment. |
| *Drug Misuse: Opioid Detoxification* (**NICE, 2007c**) | None identified |
| *Drug Misuse: Psychosocial Interventions* (**NICE, 2007b**) | None identified |
| *Generalised Anxiety Disorder and Panic Disorder (with or without Agoraphobia) in Adults* (**NICE, 2011a**) | The following must be taken into account when deciding which medication to offer:<br>• previous treatment response<br>• tolerability<br>• the possibility of interactions with concomitant medication. |
| *Obsessive-compulsive Disorder* (**NICE, 2005a**) | None identified |
| *Post-traumatic Stress Disorder* (**NICE, 2005b**) | None identified |

**Table 32: Preliminary summary and synthesis of selected text from recommendations relating to personal characteristics (by guideline) to support the process of adoption and adaptation**

| Guideline | Recommendation |
|---|---|
| *Alcohol-use Disorders* (NICE, 2011b) | None identified |
| *Antenatal and Postnatal Mentol Health* (NICE, 2007a) **(For common mental health disorders only)** | When prescribing a drug for a woman with a mental disorder who is planning a pregnancy, pregnant or breastfeeding, prescribers should:<br>• choose drugs with lower-risk profiles for the mother and the fetus or infant<br>• start at the lowest effective dose, and slowly increase it; this is particularly important where the risks may be dose related<br>• use monotherapy in preference to combination treatment<br>• consider additional precautions for preterm, low birth weight or sick infants. |
| *Depression* (NICE, 2009a) | Do not routinely vary the treatment strategies for depression described in this guideline by personal characteristics (for example, sex or ethnicity) as there is no convincing evidence to support such action. |
| *Depression in Adults with a Chronic Physical Health Problem* (NICE, 2009b) | None identified |
| *Drug Misuse: Opioid Detoxification* (NICE, 2007c) | None identified |
| *Drug Misuse: Psychosocial Interventions* (NICE, 2007b) | None identified |
| *Generalised Anxiety Disorder and Panic Disorder (with or without Agoraphobia) in Adults* (NICE, 2011a) | The following must be taken into account when deciding which medication to offer:<br>• the age of the person<br>• risks<br>• the likelihood of accidental overdose<br>• the likelihood of deliberate self-harm, by overdose or otherwise. |
| *Obsessive-compulsive Disorder* (NICE, 2005a) | Obsessive-compulsive symptoms may sometimes involve a person's religion, such as religious obsessions and scrupulosity, or cultural practices. When the boundary between religious or cultural practice and obsessive-compulsive symptoms is unclear, healthcare professionals should, with the patient's consent, consider seeking the advice and support of an appropriate religious or community leader to support the therapeutic process.<br><br>For adults with OCD living with their family or carers, involving a family member or carer as a co-therapist in ERP should be considered where appropriate and acceptable. |
| *Post-traumatic Stress Disorder* (NICE, 2005b) | None identified |

**Table 33: Prelimiary summary and synthesis of selected text from recommendations relating to service user preference (by guideline) to support the process of adoption and adaptation**

| Guideline | Recommendation |
|---|---|
| *Alcohol-use Disorders* (NICE, 2011b) | None identified |
| *Antenatal and Postnatal Mental Health* (NICE, 2007a) **(For common mental health disorders only)** | Consider antidepressant treatment if the woman has expressed a preference for it. |
| *Depression* (NICE, 2009a) | For people with depression who decline an antidepressant, CBT, IPT, behavioural activation and behavioural couples therapy, consider: <br>• counselling for people with persistent subthreshold depressive symptoms or mild to moderate depression <br>• short-term psychodynamic psychotherapy for people with mild to moderate depression. <br><br>For people with depression who are at significant risk of relapse or have a history of recurrent depression, discuss with the person treatments to reduce the risk of recurrence, including continuing medication, augmentation of medication or psychological treatment (CBT). Treatment choice should be influenced by the person's preference. |
| *Depression in Adults with a Chronic Physical Health Problem* (NICE, 2009b) | The choice of intervention should be influenced by the patient's treatment preference and priorities. |
| *Drug Misuse: Opioid Detoxification* (NICE, 2007c) | None identified |
| *Drug Misuse: Psychosocial Interventions* (NICE, 2007b) | None identified |
| *Generalised Anxiety Disorder and Panic Disorder (with or without Agoraphobia) in Adults* (NICE, 2001a) | Inform people with GAD who have not received or have refused treatment offered in Steps 1 to 3 of the potential benefits of such treatments. Offer them whichever treatments have not been tried. |

*Continued*

160

**Table 33:** (*Continued*)

|  | The following must be taken into account when deciding which medication to offer:<br>• the preference of the person being treated. |
| --- | --- |
| *Obsessive-compulsive Disorder* (**NICE, 2005a**) | In initial treatment low-intensity psychological treatments should be offered if the patient expresses a preference for a low-intensity approach.<br><br>When adults request psychological therapy other than cognitive and/or behavioural therapies as a specific treatment they should be informed that there is as yet no convincing evidence for a clinically important effect of these treatments.<br><br>Neurosurgery is not recommended for OCD unless it is specifically requested by the patient because they have severe OCD that is refractory to other forms of treatment. |
| *Post-traumatic Stress Disorder* (**NICE, 2005b**) | Drug treatments (paroxetine or mirtazapine for general use, and amitriptyline or phenelzine for initiation only by mental health specialists) should be considered for the treatment of PTSD in adults who express a preference not to engage in trauma-focused psychological treatment.<br><br>Patient preference should be an important determinant of the choice among effective treatments. People with PTSD should be given sufficient information about the nature of these treatments to make an informed choice. |

### 6.3.5    Clinical evidence

The studies considered in this review looked at predictors of treatment response from a variety of perspectives (see Table 34). For the purposes of this review, the evidence was assessed with regard to factors predicting: (a) response/remission, (b) risk of recurrence and (c) non-adherence to treatment. Due to the nature of the studies, they have been narratively reviewed.

*Factors predicting response/remission*
Numerous treatments exist for depression, and research exists assessing the extent to which certain factors predict response to treatment. In general, it has been found that an initial good response to treatment predicts good outcome for recovery (FEKADU2009).

Predictors of response to antidepressant treatment can be broken down into biological and non-biological predictors, and medical predictors, as well as predictors for specific treatment. Each of these will now be considered in turn.

DODD2004 outlined a number of biological predictors that influence response to antidepressant treatment. Most of the biological predictors, although important, are not applicable to primary care (the primary focus of this guideline) and will only be discussed briefly. Using the dexamethasone suppression test, it was found that post-treatment dexamethasone predicts the course of treatment. Blunted thyrotropin response at admission is indicative of recovery at 9 weeks. Treatment non-response has also been associated with lower levels of [$^3$H] imipramine recognition-site densities (measured prior to treatment), and low rapid eye movement density and sleep onset difficulty (DODD2004).

There are some biological factors that, rather than predicting treatment response in general, predict response to specific treatment agents. 3-methoxy-4-hydroxy-phenylglycol levels prior to treatment predicted response to imipramine. Monoamine oxidase activity has been found to have varying effects, depending on the drug in question. Decreased monoamine oxidase activity following sleep deprivation can lead to response to clomipramine treatment, but non-response to maprotiline. Conversely, increased monoamine oxidase activity following sleep deprivation has been associated with non-response to clomipramine treatment and response to maprotiline (DODD2004).

Biological predictors are not the only predictors available to clinicians when deciding on the appropriateness of antidepressant treatment. In fact, many of the non-biological predictors may actually be of more benefit to primary care practitioners because they do not require complex biological tests.

Other clinical predictors include a range of factors specific to the disorder. For example, according to DODD2004, an initially more severe depression was associated with a reduced response to therapy. Similarly, endogenous-type depression may be more responsive to antidepressant treatment than reactive depression. However, depression with comorbid disorders (particularly panic disorder and alcohol misuse) is associated with a reduced response rate (DODD2004). Interestingly, early age of onset is not directly related to treatment response. Instead early age of onset appears to be related to a more malignant course of depression (DODD2004).

Clinical factors can have effects on specific antidepressant treatments. Several studies cited in DODD2004 suggest that atypical depression responds better to monoamine oxidase inhibitors than to other first-generation antidepressants. However, results are mixed, with other studies failing to find a depression subtype that significantly influences treatment response. Atypical depression may be associated with better response to phenelzine than to imipramine in a 6-week double-blinded trial, although, when depression is associated with an absence of a life event, better outcomes are seen for imipramine. Response to moclobemide and phenelzine in comparison with second-generation antidepressants does not appear to be influenced by depression type (DODD2004).

A number of personality factors may also impact on the chance of recovery following antidepressant treatment. DODD2004 found that having any of the

162

following reduced the likelihood of recovery following antidepressant treatment: passive/aggressive personality, antisocial personality traits, mild depression (Hamilton Rating Scale for Depression score <20) with personality dysfunction, high harm avoidance and high reward dependence, high harm avoidance and low reward dependence, and low harm avoidance and high reward dependence.

Conversely, some personality factors have been found to increase the chance of recovery following antidepressant treatment. These include having an obsessive-compulsive personality, high levels of cooperativeness and self-directedness and low levels of novelty seeking, harm avoidance and reward dependence (DODD2004).

Service user factors not directly related to personality have been highlighted as important in predicting response to treatment (DODD2004). Rumination, poor occupational functioning, psychosocial vulnerabilities (including physical, emotional and sexual abuse, and physical and emotional neglect), current stress, lack of social support, and length of interval between the onset of depressive symptoms and commencement of treatment have all been found to reduce the response to antidepressant treatment (DODD2004).

Just as personality factors have the potential to influence treatment response in general, they have also been found to influence response to specific antidepressant treatment. Presence of anxiety symptoms has been associated with a positive response to lofepramine, whereas non-response is associated with observed sadness, psychomotor retardation and subjective lassitude (DODD2004). Surprisingly, despite being a common treatment for anxiety disorders, non-response to fluoxetine has been associated with presence of anxiety symptoms (DODD2004). However, NELSON2009 has contradicted this finding, showing similar response rates to both drug and placebo conditions in non-anxious and anxious depressed participants (OR = 1.57, 95% CI, 1.15 to 2.14 and OR = 1.44, 95% CI, 1.15 to 1.80, respectively; $\chi^2$ = 0.88, p = 0.35). According to one meta-analysis, the pooled response rates to drug and placebo respectively were 49.4% versus 37.4% in anxious patients and 44.2% versus 35.5% in non-anxious patients. Response rates to drug treatment were similar for both groups (OR = 1.21, 95% CI, 0.93 to 1.57).

Demographic factors may also influence response to treatment. Age in particular appears to have an association with treatment response. Although older populations have a higher mortality rate, younger patients seem to have reduced treatment response, and experience persistent residual symptoms (MITCHELL2009). However, younger participants in these studies often have a significantly greater number of previous episodes in this study, making interpretation difficult. In light of problems associated with poor control, results are often mixed with some studies finding significantly lower rates of remission in participants over the age of 60 years (MITCHELL2009) and others finding no effect of age (DODD2004).

MITCHELL2009 also examined age as a prognostic indicator for treatment success in ECT. Service users aged 65 years and over have been found to have a better rate of recovery than younger participants (67% and 40% at 4-year follow-up, respectively). However, the exact effect is masked by problems of control for confounding factors such as past episode characteristics, and illness comorbidity. Furthermore, ECT is often used for different reasons in older and younger populations. For younger service users, ECT tends to be used less frequently, and for treatment-resistant disorders. It is more likely to be used as first-line treatment in older populations. As a result, findings are often mixed, with some studies reporting no effect of age on treatment response.

Finally, it is important to consider some of the therapeutic factors that can improve treatment response. DODD2004 report that the greater the therapist–patient alliance, the better the pharmacological outcome, especially when the alliance is rated positively by the therapist. Optimism, from the psychiatrist or the patient, is also an important predictor and research suggests that optimism correlates positively with improved response (DODD2004).

*Factors predicting risk of recurrence*

Neither gender, age, socioeconomic status or marital status were found to be associated with the risk of recurrence (FEKADU2009, HARDEVELD2010). However, older age may be associated with more previous episodes and greater medical comorbidity, which in turn increases rates of relapse (MITCHELL2009).

With regard to personal factors, service users who, after achieving remission, experience impaired functioning (be it in work, relationship or leisure domains) appear to have a higher risk for recurrence of major depression. Similarly, use of moderate coping skills and having low self-efficacy can also result in higher risk of recurrence of major depression. Finally, although the evidence is mixed, having a personality disorder can also be a predictor for recurrence (HARDEVELD2010). Interestingly, experiencing a severe life event and having low social support did not appear to relate to recurrence.

A large number of clinical factors have been found to predict rates of recurrence. Age of onset of first depressive episode in particular is an important factor, with each additional year of age at onset lowering the risk by 0.96 (95% CI, 0.93 to 0.99). However, this finding has not always been successfully replicated (FEKADU2009). Similarly, shorter duration of illness at intake, lower illness severity during follow-up and fewer previous episodes are often cited as reducing the rate of recurrence (HARDEVELD2010). Risk of relapse has been found to increase from 55.3% after Step 2 of treatment to 64.6% after Step 3 and 71.1% after Step 4 (FEKADU2009).

The presence of both subclinical symptoms and comorbid axis I disorders also appear to increase the rate of recurrence. With regard to comorbid symptoms, dysthymia and social phobia (HARDEVELD2010), and delusions and agitation (FEKADU2009) have all been associated with an increase in the risk of recurrence. Research indicates that service users with subclinical symptoms after recovery from major depression relapse around three times faster than those without such symptoms (HARDEVELD2010). The rate of relapse for those entering follow-up with residual symptoms has been estimated at around 58.6%, compared with 47.4% for those without residual symptoms ($\chi^2 = 6.4$; p = 0.01; FEKADU2009). However, the time frame in which to measure relapse is important, because at 8 to 10 years' follow-up this difference is no longer significant (HARDEVELD2010). Residual symptoms affect not only remission but also global functioning. According to FEKADU2009, participants with residual symptoms were more likely than participants without residual symptoms to have a longer period of impaired occupational functioning when they had reached remission.

*Factors predicting non-adherence to treatment*
One of the key factors associated with treatment response is rate of adherence to treatment. POMPILI2009 conducted a systematic review of the factors that can influence likelihood of treatment non-adherence. Reported rates of non-adherence increase weekly, starting at 16% in week one and increasing to 41% in week two, 59% in week three and 68% in week four. Approximately 30% of people on antidepressants will stop taking them within 1 month of commencing treatment, with as many as 60% stopping by 3 months.

Many factors predict non-adherence. These include medication-specific issues, service user factors and physician factors. Looking first at medication-specific issues, problems of non-adherence have been associated with treatment-related adverse events, delayed onset of action, complicated dosage, titration schedule and sub-therapeutic dosing, hyperstimulation due to antidepressants, non-cooperation from the service users' family, fear of the drug and a lack of an adequate long-term treatment regimen (POMPILI2009).

Looking next at patient factors, POMPILI2009 also identified a number of variables that could influence adherence. Poor motivation, failure to perceive a benefit, education, age of first episode, presence of melancholia or anxiety, psychiatric morbidity or clinical setting and concerns about the cost have all been found to influence non-adherence.

Finally, with regard to physician factors, it has been found that the patient–doctor relationship is vital in determining adherence. According to POMPILI2009, having a good alliance can enhance long-term treatment adherence, reduce drop-out rates to less than 10% and increase adherence rates to more than 85%. The alliance has been found to be especially important during the early stages of treatment, particularly when the short-term benefits are often outweighed by adverse events.

### 6.3.6 Clinical evidence summary

Response to antidepressant treatment is influenced by an array of factors. Initially, more severe depression, reactive depression and comorbid depression may all be associated with reduced response to treatment. The GDG considered these factors and felt many were already taken into account in the existing guidelines and recommendations. Specific personality factors have also been identified in the reviews as having a potentially important role, with passive/aggressive personality, antisocial personality traits, mild depression with personality dysfunction, high harm avoidance and high reward dependence, high harm avoidance and low reward dependence, and low harm avoidance and high reward dependence all being identified as possible causes of a reduced likelihood of recovery with antidepressant treatment. Similarly, rumination, poor occupational functioning, psychosocial vulnerabilities and length of interval between the onset of depressive symptoms and commencement of treatment may also

**Table 34: Summary of findings for systematic reviews of factors that predict treatment response/recurrence of depression/non-adherence**

| Study ID | Outcome | Summary of findings |
|---|---|---|
| DODD2004 | Treatment response | The following non-biological factors predicted better response:<br>• moderate depression (compared with severe depression)<br>• endogenous depression (compared with situational/reactive depression)<br>• high autonomy and low sociotropy<br>• high co-operativeness and self-directedness<br>• high reward dependence and novelty seeking and low harm avoidance<br>• greater non-verbal attunement between patient and interviewer<br>• psychiatrist's initial optimism<br>• strong alliance between therapist and service user<br>• strongly held religious beliefs and activities.<br><br>The following non-biological factors predicted poor response:<br>• comorbidity of GAD<br>• comorbidity of panic disorder<br>• bipolarity<br>• alcohol misuse and dependance<br>• poor occupational functioning.<br><br>Biological predictive factors included neuro-endocrine factors, platelet markers, electroen-cephalographic markers and magnetic resonance markers, but the review authors suggest that while these are useful in research they are of only limited use to the treating clinican. |
| FEKADU2009 | Depression recovery | The following factors predicted good outcome and recovery:<br>• initial responsiveness to lithium<br>• absence of previous history of admission<br>• shorter duration of illness at intake<br>• less severe illness during follow-up.<br>The following factors predicted poorer outcome and readmission:<br>• prior history of treatment with lithium<br>• presence of delusions and agitation.<br><br>Age, sex and history of dysthymia were not predictive of recovery. |
| HARDEVELD2010 | Recurrence of MDD | The following factors predicted recurrence of MDD:<br>• the number of previous episodes<br>• subclinical residual symptoms after recovery for the last episode. |

## Table 34:  (*Continued*)

|  |  | Demographic factors such as gender, civil status and socioeconomic status were not related to the recurrence of MDD. |
|---|---|---|
|  |  | The percentage of recurrence of MDD in specialised mental healthcare settings is high (85% after 15 years) and may be similar in primary care. In the general population, recurrence of MDD is lower (35% after 15 years). |
| MITCHELL2005 | Response rates/remission rates | Response and remission rates to pharmacotherapy and ECT are not significantly different in depression in older and middle-aged people. |
|  |  | The evidence suggests that older patients have a higher risk of further episodes, short intervals to recurrence and experience more confounding factors, for example medical comorbidity, than younger patients. Therefore, it is important to look at age-related factors rather than just age when assessing risk factors for recurrence. |
|  |  | Although rates of response are not substantially different between groups, systematic differences in treatment of depression by age exist. In general, the evidence overall supports the notion that depression in the elderly is equally responsive to initial treatment but has a more adverse longitudinal trajectory than depression in middle age. |
| NELSON2009 | Response to second-generation antidepressant treatment | There was no evidence that anxiety affected response to second-generation antidepressant treatment in placebo-controlled trials of major depression in older adults. |
| POMPILI2009 | Non-adherence | Factors that predict medication non-adherence specific to unipolar/bipolar depression can be categorised as:<br>• variables unique to the disorder (early onset, high number of hospitalisations)<br>• treatment issues (complex treatment regimen, medication side effects, delayed onset of action, cost of medication, inadequate medication dosage and inadequate therapy duration)<br>• patient factors (gender, age, marital status, educational level and social support, ethnicity, cognitive dysfunction, higher level of personality pathology, lack of insight, substance misuse, mood-incongruent psychotic features)<br>• physician factors (poor physician–patient communication).<br><br>Comorbid symptoms had no effect on adherence. |

be associated with a reduced response to antidepressant treatment. Presence of anxiety symptoms, on the other hand, may not influence response to antidepressant treatment. The GDG were of the view that a number of these factors had already been reviewed in existing guidelines and that the uncertainty surrounding much of this evidence did not support the development of additional recommendations.

The impact of age on treatment response has produced mixed findings. Younger patients seem to have reduced antidepressant and ECT treatment response, and experience persistent residual symptoms. However, studies are often associated with poor control, making findings difficult to interpret.

Optimism in treatment has also been identified as an important factor. The greater the therapist–patient alliance, the better the pharmacological outcome, especially when the alliance was rated positively by the therapist or service user. This area was also well covered in existing NICE guidelines, although it was not considered to be a patient-specific factor that might guide choice of treatment.

Studies have found that factors related to the individual can influence the rate of recurrence. These factors include impaired functioning following remission, poor coping skills, low self-efficacy and the presence of a personality disorder. Clinical factors including age of onset of first depressive episode, duration of illness, illness severity, the number of previous episodes, subclinical symptoms and comorbid disorders have also all been found to influence rates of relapse. Again, the GDG felt that these areas had also been adequately addressed in existing NICE guidelines.

One of the key factors associated with treatment response is the rate of adherence, which is influenced by a number of factors. Treatment-related factors that reduce adherence include treatment-related adverse events, delayed onset of action, complicated dosage, titration schedule and sub-therapeutic dosing, hyper-stimulation due to antidepressants, non-cooperation from the service users' family, fear of the drug and a lack of an adequate long-term treatment regimen. Factors related to the individual include poor motivation, failure to perceive a benefit, education, age of first episode, presence of melancholia or anxiety, psychiatric morbidity or clinical setting and concerns about the cost. Finally, physician factors include poor therapeutic alliance, especially in the initial stages of treatment. Again, the GDG felt that these areas had also been well covered in existing NICE guidelines on depressive and anxiety disorders, and also in the NICE *Medicines Adherence* guideline (NICE, 2009c).

### 6.3.7    From evidence to recommendations

As can be seen from the clinical review, the GDG drew on two sources of evidence in developing the recommendations in this section. First, the existing recommendations from NICE clinical guidelines relevant to people with common mental health disorders, which provided advice on appropriate treatment for individuals, depending on a number of clinical and demographic factors. Second, the search of the evidence identified a number of systematic reviews that pointed to factors potentially associated with treatment response, including the nature of the disorder (for example,

168

chronicity and severity, and previous response to treatment). In addition, the systematic reviews included some biological markers that had not been identified in previous clinical guidelines (for example, the dexamethasone suppression test). These biological markers were not considered for recommendations as the guideline is focused on primary care and the routine use of such markers in primary care was not felt to be feasible by the GDG.

An important concern of the GDG was to develop recommendations that would support the referral of people from primary care into appropriate treatment interventions in primary or secondary care. This meant that the recommendations were revised and developed in a way that was focused on primary care. The GDG took the view that the recommendations developed by the existing NICE guidelines had taken into account and, indeed, had been developed in light of evidence reviewed by a number of systematic reviews identified in the searches for this guideline. This meant that the systematic reviews identified generally provided additional support for the recommendations developed for the previous NICE guidelines and at times provided evidence that led to some minor changes in the wording, structure and/or content of recommendations, but did not alter the meaning of the original recommendations. The GDG also determined that as far as possible it was sensible and appropriate to try to integrate recommendations from existing guidelines (for recommendations from within the same guideline and from different guidelines) into a clear, coherent and comprehensible format to facilitate understanding and uptake, particularly in primary care settings. However, in doing this the GDG took great care not to alter the meaning or intent of each recommendation because the evidence base for these recommendations was not reviewed by the GDG. Because it was outside of the scope of this guideline to review the evidence for the treatment recommendations, the primary impact of any further evidence (from the systematic review) or from expert opinion (of GDG members) was to shape and adjust the presentation of the recommendations rather than change the meaning or intent of any recommendation.

All of the guidelines on depressive and anxiety disorders so far developed by NICE have adopted a stepped-care framework in which to present their recommendations. This approach was also adopted for this guideline, and the recommendations are organised around the steps that cover primary care identification, assessment and treatment (that is, Steps 1 to 3 in most NICE guidelines). A summary of the recommendations from the original NICE guidelines are organised in a stepped-care framework in Figure 11. Given the breadth of disorders covered by this guideline, the stepped-care model should be seen as an organising principle to guide the development of locally developed care pathways.

### 6.3.8    Recommendations

The recommendations in this section regarding treatment and referral for common mental health disorders are also presented in the form of tables organised by disorder (see Table 35 and Table 36).

# Figure 11: Stepped-care model: a combined summary for common mental health disorders

**Focus of the intervention**

**Step 3:** Persistent subthreshold depressive symptoms or mild to moderate depression that has not responded to a low-intensity intervention; initial presentation of moderate or severe depression; GAD with marked functional impairment or that has not responded to a low-intensity intervention; moderate to severe panic disorder; OCD with moderate or severe functional impairment; PTSD.

**Step 2:** Persistent subthreshold depressive symptoms or mild to moderate depression; GAD; mild to moderate panic disorder; mild to moderate OCD; PTSD (including people with mild to moderate PTSD).

**Step 1:** All disorders – known and suspected presentations of common mental health disorders.

**Nature of the intervention**

**Depression:** CBT, IPT, behavioural activation, behavioural couples therapy, counselling\*, short-term psychodynamic psychotherapy\*, antidepressants, combined interventions, collaborative care\*\*, self-help groups.
**GAD:** CBT, applied relaxation, drug treatment, combined interventions, self-help groups.
**Panic disorder:** CBT, antidepressants, self-help groups.
**OCD:** CBT (including ERP), antidepressants, combined interventions and case management, self-help groups.
**PTSD:** Trauma-focused CBT, EMDR, drug treatment.
**All disorders:** Support groups, befriending, rehabilitation programmes, educational and employment support services; referral for further assessment and interventions.

**Depression:** Individual facilitated self-help, computerised CBT, structured physical activity, group-based peer support (self-help) programmes\*\*, non-directive counselling delivered at home†, antidepressants, self-help groups.
**GAD and panic disorder:** Individual non-facilitated and facilitated self-help, psychoeducational groups, self-help groups.
**OCD:** Individual or group CBT (including ERP), self-help groups.
**PTSD:** Trauma-focused CBT or EMDR.
**All disorders:** Support groups, educational and employment support services; referral for further assessment and interventions.

**All disorders:** Identification, assessment, psychoeducation, active monitoring; referral for further assessment and interventions.

\* Discuss with the person the uncertainty of the effectiveness of counselling and psychodynamic psychotherapy in treating depression.
\*\* For people with depression and a chronic physical health problem.
† For women during pregnancy or the postnatal period.

**Table 35: Step 2 treatment and referral advice**

| Disorder | Psychological interventions | Pharmacological interventions | Psychosocial interventions |
|---|---|---|---|
| **Depression** – persistent subthreshold symptoms or mild to moderate depression | Offer or refer for one or more of the following low-intensity interventions:<br>• individual facilitated self-help based on the principles of CBT<br>• CCBT<br>• a structured group physical activity programme<br>• a group-based peer support (self-help) programme (for those who also have a chronic physical health problem)<br>• non-directive counselling delivered at home (listening visits) (for women during pregnancy or the postnatal period)[a,b,c] | Do not offer antidepressants routinely but consider them for; or refer for an assessment, people with:<br>• initial presentation of subthreshold depressive symptoms that have been present for a long period (typically at least 2 years) **or**<br>• subthreshold depressive symptoms or mild depression that persist(s) after other interventions **or**<br>• a past history of moderate or severe depression **or**<br>• mild depression that complicates the care of a physical health problem[a,b]. | Consider:<br>• informing people about self-help groups, support groups and other local and national resources<br>• educational and employ-ment support services[a]. |
| **GAD** – that has not improved after psychoeducation and active monitoring in Step 1 | Offer or refer for one of the following low-intensity interventions:<br>• individual non-facilitated self-help<br>• individual facilitated self-help<br>• psychoeducational groups[d]. | N/A | |
| **Panic disorder** – mild to moderate | Offer or refer for one of the following low-intensity interventions:<br>• individual non-facilitated self-help<br>• individual facilitated self-help. | N/A | |
| **OCD** – mild to moderate | Offer or refer for individual CBT including ERP of limited duration (typically up to 10 hours), which could be provided using self-help materials or by telephone **or**<br>Refer for group CBT (including ERP)[e,f]. | N/A | |

*Continued*

171

**Table 35:** *(Continued)*

| Disorder | Psychological interventions | Pharmacological interventions | Psychosocial interventions |
|---|---|---|---|
| **PTSD** – including mild to moderate PTSD | Refer for a formal psychological intervention (trauma-focused CBT or EMDR)[g]. | N/A | Consider:<br>• informing people about support groups and other local and national resources<br>• educational and employment support services[a]. |
| **All disorders** – women planning a pregnancy, during pregnancy or following pregnancy who have subthreshold symptoms that significantly interfere with personal and social functioning | For women who have had a previous episode of depression or anxiety, consider providing or referring for individual brief psychological treatment (four to six sessions), such as IPT or CBT[c].<br><br>Women requiring psychological interventions during pregnancy or the postnatal period should be seen for treatment within 1 month of (and no longer than 3 months from) initial assessment[c]. | When considering drug treatments for women who are pregnant, breastfeeding or planning a pregnancy, consult *Antenatal and Postnatal Mental Health* (NICE, 2007a) for advice on prescribing. | For women who have not had a previous episode of depression or anxiety, consider providing or referring for social support during pregnancy and the postnatal period; such support may consist of regular informal individual or group-based support[c]. |

[a]Adapted from *Depression* (NICE, 2009a).
[b]Adapted from *Depression in Adults with a Chronic Physical Health Problem* (NICE, 2009b).
[c]Adapted from *Antenatal and Postnatal Mental Health* (NICE, 2007a).
[d]Adapted from *Generalised Anxiety Disorder and Panic Disorder (with or without Agoraphobia) in Adults* (NICE, 2011a).
[e]Adapted from *Obsessive-compulsive Disorder* (NICE, 2005a).
[f]Group formats may deliver more than 10 hours of therapy.
[g]Adapted from *Post-traumatic Stress Disorder* (NICE, 2005b).

**Table 36: Step 3 treatment and referral**

| Disorder | Psychological or pharmacological interventions | Combined and complex interventions | Psychosocial interventions |
|---|---|---|---|
| **Depression** – persistent subthreshold depressive symptoms or mild to moderate depression that has not responded to a low-intensity intervention | Offer or refer for: <br>• antidepressant medication **or** <br>• a psychological intervention (CBT, IPT, behavioural activation or behavioural couples therapy)[a]. <br><br>For people who decline the interventions above, consider providing or referring for: <br>• counselling for people with persistent subthreshold depressive symptoms or mild to moderate depression <br>• short-term psychodynamic psychotherapy for people with mild to moderate depression[a]. <br><br>Discuss with the person the uncertainty of the effectiveness of counselling and psychodynamic psychotherapy in treating depression[a]. | N/A | Consider: <br>• informing people about self-help groups, support groups and other local and national resources <br>• befriending or a rehabilitation programme for people with long-standing moderate or severe disorders <br>• educational and employment support services[a]. |
| **Depression** – moderate or severe (first presentation) | See combined and complex interventions column | Offer or refer for a psychological intervention (CBT or IPT) in combination with an antidepressant[a]. | |
| **Depression** – moderate to severe depression and a chronic physical health problem | See combined and complex interventions column | For people with no, or only a limited, response to psychological or drug treatment alone or combined in the current or in a past episode, consider referral to collaborative care[b]. | |
| **GAD** – with marked functional impairment or non-response to a low-intensity intervention | Offer or refer for one of the following: <br>• CBT **or** <br>• applied relaxation **or** <br>• if the person prefers, drug treatment[c]. | N/A | |

*Continued*

173

**Table 36:** *(Continued)*

| Disorder | Psychological or pharmacological interventions | Combined and complex interventions | Psychosocial interventions |
|---|---|---|---|
| **Panic disorder** – moderate to severe (with or without agoraphobia) | Consider referral for:<br>• CBT **or**<br>• an antidepressant if the disorder is long-standing or the person has not benefitted from or has declined psychological interventions[c]. | N/A | Consider:<br>• informing people about self-help groups, support groups and other local and national resources<br>• befriending or a rehabilitation programme for people with long-standing moderate or severe disorders<br>• educational and employment support services[a]. |
| **OCD** – moderate or severe functional impairment, and in particular where there is significant comorbidity with other common mental health disorders[d] | For moderate impairment, offer or refer for:<br>• CBT (including ERP) or antidepressant medication[e].<br><br>Offer home-based treatment where the person is unable or reluctant to attend a clinic or has specific problems (for example, hoarding)[e]. | For severe impairment, offer or refer for:<br>• CBT (including ERP) combined with antidepressant medication and case management[e,f]. | |
| **PTSD** | Offer or refer for a psychological intervention (trauma-focused CBT or EMDR). Do not delay the intervention or referral, particularly for people with severe and escalating symptoms in the first month after the traumatic event[g].<br><br>Offer or refer for drug treatment only if a person declines an offer of a psychological intervention or expresses a preference for drug treatment[g]. | N/A | Consider:<br>• informing people about support groups and other local and national resources<br>• befriending or a rehabilitation programme for people with long-standing moderate or severe disorders<br>• educational and employment support services[a]. |

[a]Adapted from *Depression* (NICE, 2009a).
[b]Adapted from *Depression in Adults with a Chronic Physical Health Problem* (NICE, 2009b).
[c]Adapted from *Generalised Anxiety Disorder and Panic Disorder (with or without Agoraphobia) in Adults* (NICE, 2001a).
[d]For people with long-standing OCD or with symptoms that are severely disabling and restrict their life, consider referral to a specialist mental health service.
[e]Adapted from *Obsessive-compulsive Disorder* (NICE, 2005a).
[f]For people with OCD who have not benefitted from two courses of CBT (including ERP) combined with antidepressant medication, refer to a service with specialist expertise in OCD.
[g]Adapted from *Post-traumatic Stress Disorder* (NICE, 2005b).

*All steps: Treatment and referral for treatment*

**Identifying the correct treatment options**

6.3.8.1    When discussing treatment options with a person with a common mental health disorder, consider:
- their past experience of the disorder
- their experience of, and response to, previous treatment
- the trajectory of symptoms
- the diagnosis or problem specification, severity and duration of the problem
- the extent of any associated functional impairment arising from the disorder itself or any chronic physical health problem
- the presence of any social or personal factors that may have a role in the development or maintenance of the disorder
- the presence of any comorbid disorders.

6.3.8.2    When discussing treatment options with a person with a common mental health disorder, provide information about:
- the nature, content and duration of any proposed intervention
- the acceptability and tolerability of any proposed intervention
- possible interactions with any current interventions
- the implications for the continuing provision of any current interventions.

6.3.8.3    When making a referral for the treatment of a common mental health disorder, take account of patient preference when choosing from a range of evidence-based treatments.

6.3.8.4    When offering treatment for a common mental health disorder or making a referral, follow the stepped-care approach, usually offering or referring for the least intrusive, most effective intervention first (see Figure 11).

6.3.8.5    When a person presents with symptoms of anxiety and depression, assess the nature and extent of the symptoms, and if the person has:
- depression that is accompanied by symptoms of anxiety, the first priority should usually be to treat the depressive disorder, in line with the NICE guideline on depression
- an anxiety disorder and comorbid depression or depressive symptoms, consult the NICE guidelines for the relevant anxiety disorder and consider treating the anxiety disorder first
- both anxiety and depressive symptoms, with no formal diagnosis, that are associated with functional impairment, discuss with the person the symptoms to treat first and the choice of intervention[27].

6.3.8.6    When a person presents with a common mental health disorder and harmful drinking or alcohol dependence, refer them for treatment of the alcohol misuse first as this may lead to significant improvement in depressive or anxiety symptoms[28].

---

[27]Adapted from *Depression* (NICE, 2009a).

[28]Adapted from *Alcohol-use Disorders: Diagnosis, Assessment and Management of Harmful Drinking and Alcohol Dependence* (NICE, 2011b).

6.3.8.7   When a person presents with a common mental health disorder and a mild
          learning disability or mild cognitive impairment:
          ● where possible provide or refer for the same interventions as for other
            people with the same common mental health disorder
          ● if providing interventions, adjust the method of delivery or duration of
            the assessment or intervention to take account of the disability or
            impairment[29].

6.3.8.8   When a person presents with a common mental health disorder and has a
          moderate to severe learning disability or a moderate to severe cognitive
          impairment, consult a specialist concerning appropriate referral and treat-
          ment options.

6.3.8.9   Do not routinely vary the treatment strategies and referral practice for
          common mental health disorders described in this guideline either by
          personal characteristics (for example, sex or ethnicity) or by depression
          subtype (for example, atypical depression or seasonal depression) as there
          is no convincing evidence to support such action[29].

6.3.8.10  If a person with a common mental health disorder needs social, educational
          or vocational support, consider:
          ● informing them about self-help groups (but not for people with PTSD),
            support groups and other local and national resources
          ● befriending or a rehabilitation programme for people with long-standing
            moderate or severe disorders
          ● educational and employment support services[29].

*Step 2: Treatment and referral advice for subthreshold symptoms and mild to
moderate common mental health disorders*

6.3.8.11  For people with persistent subthreshold depressive symptoms or mild to
          moderate depression, offer or refer for one or more of the following low-
          intensity interventions:
          ● individual facilitated self-help based on the principles of cognitive
            behavioural therapy (CBT)
          ● computerised CBT
          ● a structured group physical activity programme
          ● a group-based peer support (self-help) programme (for those who also
            have a chronic physical health problem)
          ● non-directive counselling delivered at home (listening visits) (for
            women during pregnancy or the postnatal period)[30].

---

[29]Adapted from *Depression* (NICE, 2009a).
[30]Adapted from *Depression* (NICE, 2009a), *Depression in Adults with a Chronic Physical Health Problem*
(NICE, 2009b) and *Antenatal and Postnatal Mental Health* (NICE, 2007a).

6.3.8.12 For pregnant women who have subthreshold symptoms of depression and/or anxiety that significantly interfere with personal and social functioning, consider providing or referring for:

- individual brief psychological treatment (four to six sessions), such as interpersonal therapy (IPT) or CBT for women who have had a previous episode of depression or anxiety
- social support during pregnancy and the postnatal period for women who have not had a previous episode of depression or anxiety; such support may consist of regular informal individual or group-based support[31].

6.3.8.13 Do not offer antidepressants routinely for people with persistent subthreshold depressive symptoms or mild depression, but consider them for, or refer for an assessment, people with:

- initial presentation of subthreshold depressive symptoms that have been present for a long period (typically at least 2 years) or
- subthreshold depressive symptoms or mild depression that persist(s) after other interventions or
- a past history of moderate or severe depression or
- mild depression that complicates the care of a physical health problem[32].

6.3.8.14 For people with generalised anxiety disorder that has not improved after psychoeducation and active monitoring, offer or refer for one of the following low-intensity interventions:

- individual non-facilitated self-help
- individual facilitated self-help
- psychoeducational groups[33].

6.3.8.15 For people with mild to moderate panic disorder, offer or refer for one of the following low-intensity interventions:

- individual non-facilitated self-help
- individual facilitated self-help.

6.3.8.16 For people with mild to moderate OCD:

- offer or refer for individual CBT including exposure and response prevention (ERP) of limited duration (typically up to 10 hours), which could be provided using self-help materials or by telephone **or**
- refer for group CBT (including ERP) (note, group formats may deliver more than 10 hours of therapy)[34].

6.3.8.17 For people with PTSD, including those with mild to moderate PTSD, refer for a formal psychological intervention (trauma-focused CBT or eye movement desensitisation and reprocessing [EMDR])[35].

---

[31]Adapted from *Antenatal and Postnatal Mental Health* (NICE, 2007a).

[32]Adapted from *Depression* (NICE, 2009a) and *Depression in Adults with a Chronic Physical Health Problem* (NICE, 2009b).

[33]Adapted from *Generalised Anxiety Disorder and Panic Disorder (with or without Agoraphobia) in Adults* (NICE, 2011a).

[34]Adapted from *Obsessive-compulsive Disorder* (NICE, 2005a).

[35]Adapted from *Post-traumatic Stress Disorder* (NICE, 2005b).

*Step 3: Treatment and referral advice for persistent subthreshold depressive symptoms or mild to moderate common mental health disorders with inadequate response to initial interventions, or moderate to severe common mental health disorders*

If there has been an inadequate response following the delivery of a first-line treatment for persistent subthreshold depressive symptoms or mild to moderate common mental health disorders, a range of psychological, pharmacological or combined interventions may be considered. This section also recommends interventions or provides referral advice for first presentation of moderate to severe common mental health disorders.

6.3.8.18 For people with persistent subthreshold depressive symptoms or mild to moderate depression that has not responded to a low-intensity intervention, offer or refer for:
- antidepressant medication **or**
- a psychological intervention (CBT, IPT, behavioural activation or behavioural couples therapy)[36].

6.3.8.19 For people with an initial presentation of moderate or severe depression, offer or refer for a psychological intervention (CBT or IPT) in combination with an antidepressant[36].

6.3.8.20 For people with moderate to severe depression and a chronic physical health problem consider referral to collaborative care if there has been no, or only a limited, response to psychological or drug treatment alone or combined in the current or in a past episode[37].

6.3.8.21 For people with depression who decline an antidepressant, CBT, IPT, behavioural activation and behavioural couples therapy, consider providing or referring for:
- counselling for people with persistent subthreshold depressive symptoms or mild to moderate depression
- short-term psychodynamic psychotherapy for people with mild to moderate depression.

Discuss with the person the uncertainty of the effectiveness of counselling and psychodynamic psychotherapy in treating depression[36].

6.3.8.22 For people with generalised anxiety disorder who have marked functional impairment or have not responded to a low-intensity intervention, offer or refer for one of the following:
- CBT **or**
- applied relaxation **or**
- if the person prefers, drug treatment[38].

---

[36]Adapted from *Depression* (NICE, 2009a).
[37]Adapted from *Depression in Adults with a Chronic Physical Health Problem* (NICE, 2009b).
[38]Adapted from *Generalised Anxiety Disorder and Panic Disorder (with or without Agoraphobia) in Adults* (NICE, 2011a).

6.3.8.23   For people with moderate to severe panic disorder (with or without agoraphobia), consider referral for:
- CBT **or**
- an antidepressant if the disorder is long-standing or the person has not benefitted from or has declined psychological interventions[39].

6.3.8.24   For people with OCD and moderate or severe functional impairment, and in particular where there is significant comorbidity with other common mental health disorders, offer or refer for:
- CBT (including ERP) or antidepressant medication for moderate impairment
- CBT (including ERP) combined with antidepressant medication and case management for severe impairment.

Offer home-based treatment where the person is unable or reluctant to attend a clinic or has specific problems (for example, hoarding)[40].

6.3.8.25   For people with long-standing OCD or with symptoms that are severely disabling and restrict their life, consider referral to a specialist mental health service[40].

6.3.8.26   For people with OCD who have not benefitted from two courses of CBT (including ERP) combined with antidepressant medication, refer to a service with specialist expertise in OCD[40].

6.3.8.27   For people with PTSD, offer or refer for a psychological intervention (trauma-focused CBT or EMDR). Do not delay the intervention or referral, particularly for people with severe and escalating symptoms in the first month after the traumatic event[41].

6.3.8.28   For people with PTSD, offer or refer for drug treatment only if a person declines an offer of a psychological intervention or expresses a preference for drug treatment[41].

*Treatment and referral advice to help prevent relapse*

6.3.8.29   For people with a common mental health disorder who are at significant risk of relapse or have a history of recurrent problems, discuss with the person the treatments that might reduce the risk of recurrence. The choice of treatment or referral for treatment should be informed by the response to previous treatment, including residual symptoms, the consequences of relapse, any discontinuation symptoms when stopping medication, and the person's preference.

---

[39]Adapted from *Generalised Anxiety Disorder and Panic Disorder (with or without Agoraphobia) in Adults* (NICE, 2011a).

[40]Adapted from *Obsessive-compulsive Disorder* (NICE, 2005a).

[41]Adapted from *Post-traumatic Stress Disorder* (NICE, 2005b).

6.3.8.30   For people with a previous history of depression who are currently well and who are considered at risk of relapse despite taking antidepressant medication, or those who are unable to continue or choose not to continue antidepressant medication, offer or refer for one of the following:
- individual CBT
- mindfulness-based cognitive therapy (for those who have had three or more episodes)[42].

6.3.8.31   For people who have had previous treatment for depression but continue to have residual depressive symptoms, offer or refer for one of the following:
- individual CBT
- mindfulness-based cognitive therapy (for those who have had three or more episodes)[42].

### 6.3.9   Research recommendations

6.3.9.1   For people with a common mental health disorder, is the use of a simple algorithm (based on factors associated with treatment response), when compared with a standard clinical assessment, more clinically and cost effective? (See Appendix 11 for further details.)

6.3.9.2   For people with both anxiety and depression, which disorder should be treated first to improve their outcomes? (See Appendix 11 for further details.)

## 6.4   ROUTINE OUTCOME MONITORING

### 6.4.1   Introduction

ROM has increasingly become a part of mental healthcare. Within the field of psychological therapies, recent developments in the IAPT programme led by the Department of Health (CSIP [Care Services Improvement Partnership] Choice and Access Team, 2007) have placed considerable emphasis on ROM. In a report emerging from the IAPT programme, Clark and colleagues (2009) describe the benefits associated with ROM. From an individual service user perspective, it can lead to an increased focus on outcomes and provide feedback for both psychological therapist and client on the benefits of any intervention. In turn this may lead to changes in the delivery of any intervention. At the service level there is evidence (see Clark *et al.*, 2009) that the use of outcome measurement can provide a more accurate picture of the overall success of a service. For example, the two IAPT programme pilot programmes had ROM

---

[42]Adapted from *Depression* (NICE, 2009a).

returns of over 90%. This was based on sessional outcome monitoring and can be contrasted with outcome monitoring at designated times, for example at the beginning and end of treatment. It is clear from this comparison that session-by-session monitoring can lead to a more accurate (and realistic) assessment of treatment outcome. Elsewhere in mental health, others have shown that there is considerable concern about and poor uptake of outcome monitoring among many mental healthcare professionals (for example, Gilbody *et al.*, 2002). There are a number of reasons for this, including the design, content and feasibility of the measures used, with significant concerns that the process will be burdensome on both patients and staff, but with little of value emerging for either group. This supports the view that brief measures are more likely to be used routinely. More recent developments in mental health services in the NHS (see for example, the Health of the Nation Outcome Scales, Payment by Results [HoNOS-PbR][43]) that focus on developing outcome-related clustering and costing tools have also focused on the use of ROM. In addition, Department of Health developments to promote the development of National Quality Standards from NICE[44] will lead to an increased focus on outcome monitoring. Taken together these various developments suggest that outcome monitoring will become standard practice in the NHS and, therefore, it is important to consider its feasibility and applicability to routine care. The benefits of ROM are summarised in Table 37 below.

*Current practice*
Current practice regarding ROM is limited. As mentioned above, healthcare professionals often have doubts about the value of routine monitoring, and there is a lack of appropriate and effective electronic systems to support them and the potential costs implications thereof. The IAPT programme's (Clark *et al.*, 2009) success or otherwise in meeting targets for data completion is in significant part related to the availability of effective information system to support routine data collection.

### 6.4.2     Clinical review protocol

The aim of this review was to perform a narrative synthesis of existing NICE guidelines and published systematic reviews addressing ROM for people with a common mental health disorder. The review protocol including the review question, information about databases searched and the eligibility criteria used in this section of the guideline can be found in Table 38. Although the search was conducted for the period 1995 to 2010, the focus was on systematic reviews published since 2003. Further information about the rationale for the method employed here can be found in Chapter 3 and the search strategy can be found in Appendix 6.

---

[43]http://webarchive.nationalarchives.gov.uk/+/www.dh.gov.uk/en/Managingyourorganisation/
Financeandplanning/NHSFinancialReforms/DH_4137762
[44]http://www.nice.org.uk/guidance/qualitystandards/qualitystandards.jsp

**Table 37:  Principles and benefits of outcome measurement (IAPT, 2010)**

| Principles |
| --- |
| • The primary purpose of outcome measurement is to improve people's experience and benefits from the service and is part of ongoing, collaborative service evaluation, with feedback from patients at its heart.<br>• Outcomes feedback to clinicians helps improve the quality of their interventions.<br>• Outcomes feedback to supervisors supports case reviews and collaborative treatment planning.<br>• Routinely collected outcomes data helps managers and commissioners of services to respond to diverse needs, and monitor and improve overall service performance.<br>• Intelligent use of aggregate outcomes data aims to define best practice models of service delivery.<br>• The requirement for data collection should be proportionate to the treatment being offered, and integrated with clinical priorities. |
| **Benefits** |
| • People chart their progress towards recovery and see at what point their psychometric score falls within the normal range.<br>• Therapists and supervisors, and the clinical team, can chart progress and adjust treatment plans, if the feedback indicates the current plan is not working.<br>• Clinicians can check performance against their peers to keep their skills up to date.<br>• Service managers can use an outcomes framework to manage performance and improve quality, helping commissioners ensure contracts are providing good value for money.<br>• Local, regional and national leads will benefit from having accurate, comprehensive outcomes data being fed in to the policy-making system, helping drive up standards by setting benchmarks as well as improving whole system care pathways and future resource planning. |

### 6.4.3    Studies considered

The literature search for systematic reviews and RCTs yielded 9,323 papers. Scanning titles/abstracts identified 34 potentially relevant reviews[45]; however, further inspection found only one systematic review, KNAUP2009 (Knaup *et al.*, 2009), and one meta-analysis of three studies, LAMBERT2003 (Lambert *et al.*, 2003), that met the eligibility criteria for inclusion in this narrative synthesis. During consultation, an update to the LAMBERT2003 review that included six studies was identified

---

[45]This includes reviews potentially relevant to the assessment topics covered in Chapter 5.

182

**Table 38: Clinical review protocol for the review of ROM**

| Component | Description |
|---|---|
| Review question | In adults (18 years and older) identified with depression (including subthreshold disorders) or an anxiety disorder*, should ROM be used, and if so, what systems are effective for the delivery of ROM and use within clinical decision making? |
| Objectives | To perform a narrative synthesis of systematic reviews addressing the use of ROM for people with a common mental health disorder |
| Population | Adults (18 years and older) identified with depression (including subthreshold disorders) or an anxiety disorder* |
| Intervention(s) | ROM, systems for the delivery of ROM |
| Comparison | Standard management strategy |
| Critical outcomes | Common mental health disorder symptoms, duration of treatment |
| Electronic databases | Systematic reviews: CDSR, CINAHL, DARE, EMBASE, MEDLINE, PsycINFO<br>RCTs: CENTRAL |
| Date searched | Systematic reviews: 1 January 1995 to 10 September 2010<br>RCTs: 1 January 2008 up to 10 September 2010 |
| Study design | Systematic review and RCTs |
| *Including GAD, panic disorder, social anxiety disorder, OCD, specific phobias and PTSD. | |

(SHIMOKAWA2010 [Shimokawa *et al.*, 2010]). Therefore, only the more recent review was included in this chapter. KNAUP2009 assessed the impact of routine feedback to both healthcare professionals and service users on mental health outcomes in specialist mental health services. SHIMOKAWA2010 focused specifically on ROM for service users who showed a poor initial response to treatment. Given that KNAUP2009 conducted their search in 2008, the search for this guideline was conducted for RCTs published between January 2008 and September 2010. The search resulted in 2,402 articles. Scanning titles/abstracts identified no potentially relevant trials that were not already included in the existing reviews.

The characteristics of the reviews included in this section can be found in Table 39. Further information about both included and excluded studies can be found in Appendix 14.

**Table 39: Study information table for systematic reviews of ROM**

| Study ID | KNAUP2009 | SHIMOKAWA2010 |
|---|---|---|
| Type of ROM | General | Therapist signal alarm feedback |
| Outcome of ROM | Mental health outcome | Improvement/worsening of symptoms |
| Method used to synthesise evidence | Meta-analysis | Meta-analysis |
| Design of included studies | Controlled trials using outcome management | RCT and quasi-experimental |
| Dates searched | Inception to 2008 | Not applicable |
| Diagnosis | Common mental health disorder (some studies included people with personality disorders, eating disorders or schizophrenia) | Common mental health disorder |
| No. of included studies | 12 | 6 |
| Review quality | Moderate risk of bias (quality of included studies not assessed/reported) | Moderate risk of bias (this study did not claim to be a systematic review, but rather was a meta-analysis of six major studies using the Outcome Questionnaire-45) |

### 6.4.4    Clinical evidence

KNAUP2009 reviewed a total of 12 studies to assess the effectiveness of ROM. The review focused on ROM methods, the effect of ROM on short-term mental health outcomes, long-term mental health outcomes and length of treatment, and finally on moderator variables influencing the effect of ROM on short-term mental health outcomes. SHIMOKAWA2010 meta-analysed six controlled studies to investigate the effects of ROM, specifically signal-alarm feedback, on treatment outcome and attendance rates. It is important to note that this study was a meta-analysis of studies previously conducted by the same research group and is not a systematic review. It has been included here due to lack of available evidence in the area. The results of the two reviews are discussed in more detail below.

## Methods of routine outcome monitoring

ROM can be given at regular intervals, often at every session, at 1- or 2-week intervals throughout therapy or at set time-points to restrict the number of data collection points. The results from standardised assessments of psychological functioning usually focus on current treatment status and changes in symptomatology over time. The easiest way to report this data was found to be using graphs and charts, with accompanying verbal explanations, and sometimes treatment recommendations (KNAUP2009).

## Efficacy of routine outcome monitoring

To evaluate the effectiveness of ROM, a number of outcomes have been measured, including mental health, met and unmet needs, physical impairment, social functioning, quality of life, patient satisfaction, acceptance or appraisal of feedback, rate of significant clinical change, rate of treatment response and saved cost.

KNAUP2009 conducted a meta-analysis of the short- and long-term outcomes and the length of treatment for service users receiving ROM in comparison with those not receiving ROM. With regard to short-term outcomes, KNAUP2009 reported that despite moderate between-study heterogeneity ($I^2 = 31\%$, p $= 0.16$), there was a small but statistically significant effect favouring the feedback intervention in ten studies including a total of 4,009 participants (SMD $= 0.10$, 95% CI, 0.01 to 0.19). For long-term effects of ROM, meta-analysis of five studies (N $= 573$) demonstrated a very small, unexpected and non-significant trend in favour of the no feedback group (SMD $= -0.06$, 95% CI, $-0.22$ to 0.11; $I^2 = 0\%$, p $= 0.69$).

SHIMOKAWA2010 performed both a traditional meta-analysis and an individual patient data meta-analysis of studies using a feedback model based on the routine administration of the Outcome Questionnaire-45 (Lambert *et al.*, 2004). Based on the traditional meta-analysis of intent-to-treat data, they report that following a signal alarm, individuals who were responding poorly to treatment and whose therapist received feedback showed an improvement in functioning compared with those receiving standard care (four studies, N $= 587$, SMD $= -0.28$, 95% CI, $-0.47$ to $-0.10$). The individual patient data meta-analysis confirmed this finding. For those participants whose therapists received treatment feedback, the proportion that had a clinically significant worsening/deterioration (13.6%) was lower than in the standard-care group (20.1%). This difference was statistically significant (OR $= 0.62$, 95% CI, 0.40 to 0.98). The individual patient data meta-analysis confirmed this finding.

ROM was not found to significantly change the length of treatment in the meta-analysis by KNAUP2009 (SMD $= 0.05$, 95% CI, $-0.05$ to 0.15) or SHIMOKAWA2010 (SMD $= 0.27$, 95% CI, $-0.16$ to 0.70). However, SHIMOKAWA2010 reported that their individual patient data meta-analysis demonstrated attendance of more sessions by those in the feedback group.

## Moderator analysis

According to KNAUP2009, a number of factors might act as moderators but none were statistically significant.

### 6.4.5 Clinical evidence summary

The evidence shows that across a range of methods used to monitor outcomes, frequent ROM can have benefits (albeit of a limited size) on the short-term mental health outcomes for service users. There is, however, limited evidence on the long-term impact on mental health outcomes. There was also evidence that feedback could not only improve a mental health outcome for individual service users but also might do so through an impact on healthcare professional behaviour. This is in line with emerging evidence from the IAPT programme (Clark *et al.*, 2009).

### 6.4.6 Health economic evidence

No studies were identified in the systematic literature review that considered the cost effectiveness of ROM for people with a common mental health disorder.

### 6.4.7 From evidence to recommendations

The primary aim of the use of ROM in healthcare is to improve outcomes for service users. The studies reviewed in this section clearly demonstrated that ROM and feedback to clinicians resulted in improved outcomes for services users in both RCTs and high-quality observational studies. In addition, ROM can provide information about the overall functioning and effectiveness of services, and so provides information about and can be used to improve the effective use of health resources through audit and benchmarking systems. This evidence review supports the outlook that ROM can have a positive impact on the capacity of a healthcare system to provide effective feedback both for individual patients and for services. There is also some evidence to suggest that the benefits that accrue from ROM are mediated by the impact of healthcare professional behaviour.

Two other factors were also considered important by the GDG, drawing on their expert knowledge. These were that, first, brief self-completed measures have increased feasibility and utility, and therefore are more likely to be used, and second, that the use of electronic systems that can collect, analyse and report on data are central to the success of ROM. The GDG in developing its recommendations was also mindful of current developments in the NHS, for example in the QOF (British Medical Association and NHS Employers, 2006) and the National Quality Standards[46] that are in development for secondary care for mental health services. Both of these programmes promote the use of measures, such as the PHQ-9, HADS and GAD-7, which by their structure and design lend themselves to ROM. These measures also have the advantage of reasonable psychometric properties, are free to use and are feasible for everyday use. With this in mind, and also taking into consideration the

---

[46]http://www.nice.org.uk/guidance/qualitystandards/qualitystandards.jsp

impact of routine feedback, the GDG decided to support ROM, for the benefits it may bring both to the individual patients and to the information it may supply about the overall effectiveness of local care pathways. Therefore, the GDG recommended the adoption of sessional ROM using measures already in place in the NHS, but with flexibility for individual practitioners to draw on a range of other formal assessment measures that have good psychometric properties and are feasible for routine use. The GDG was aware that such a recommendation has, essentially, a service focus and so developed the recommendation with the intent of ensuring that it formed an important element of any local care pathway for people with a common mental health disorder.

### 6.4.8    Recommendations

6.4.8.1    Primary and secondary care clinicians, managers and commissioners should work together to design local care pathways that have robust systems for outcome measurement in place, which should be used to inform all involved in a pathway about its effectiveness. This should include providing:
- individual routine outcome measurement systems
- effective electronic systems for the routine reporting and aggregation of outcome measures
- effective systems for the audit and review of the overall clinical and cost effectiveness of the pathway.

### 6.4.9    Research recommendations

6.4.9.1    In people with a common mental health disorder, what is the clinical utility of routine outcome measurement and is it cost effective compared with standard care? (See Appendix 11 for further details.)

# 7    SYSTEMS FOR ORGANISING AND DEVELOPING LOCAL CARE PATHWAYS

## 7.1    INTRODUCTION

It has long been argued that the effective and efficient organisation of healthcare systems is associated with better outcomes, and much of the effort of managers and funders of healthcare is focused on the re-organisation of healthcare systems. Unfortunately, few of these re-organisations have been subject to formal evaluation so the benefits that may have followed from this process have been difficult to quantify and, in the absence of accurate description, difficult to replicate. Although this has led to considerable uncertainty about the best methods by which to organise healthcare systems, in recent years a consensus has emerged to support the development of clinical care pathways as one model for doing this (Vanhaecht *et al.*, 2007; Whittle & Hewison, 2007), including interest in the field of mental health (Evans-Lacko *et al.*, 2008).

Recent developments in the NHS have supported the development of clinical care pathways for the organisation of care, and discussions are currently underway as to whether these may also form the basis for the future funding of mental healthcare (see HoNOS-PbR[47]). While there is general agreement about the potential advantages for clinical care, there is less evidence for benefits such as changes in professional practice, more efficient care, and more informed and empowered patients (Dy *et al.*, 2005; Emmerson *et al.*, 2006). Within specific areas of mental health there is emerging evidence, for example in the area of collaborative care for depression (Bower *et al.*, 2006; Gilbody *et al.*, 2006), but precise methods for the organisation of care across the whole range of mental healthcare have not been well developed. An additional problem, particularly with common mental health disorders, is that most care is delivered in a primary care setting. Historically, the development of care pathways has tended to focus more on the provision of specialist services, and so uncertainty remains about the best way of structuring mental healthcare in primary care (the major focus on this guideline) and the links between primary and secondary/specialist services. In addition, as has been noted elsewhere in guidelines developed by NICE (NICE, 2009b), many people, particularly as they get older, develop comorbid physical health problems, and pathways therefore potential need to take into account not only the links with secondary and specialist mental health services but also with secondary care and specialist physical health services. Again, there is some emerging evidence (NICE, 2009b) demonstrating that integration (for example, the integration for physical and mental healthcare for people with depression) can bring real benefits.

---

[47]http://webarchive.nationalarchives.gov.uk/+/www.dh.gov.uk/en/Managingyourorganisation/Financeandplanning/NHSFinancialReforms/DH_4137762

The purpose of this chapter is to examine the evidence for clinical pathways, to try and identify key characteristics of these pathways that are associated with positive outcomes. In addition, the GDG aimed to provide advice on the principles by which local care pathways should be established. In any national guidance it is extremely difficult to prescribe specific care pathways. Therefore the approach taken in this guideline was to develop some overall principles to guide the development of local care pathways, drawing on the evidence to underpin and support these principles.

### 7.1.1    Defining clinical care pathways

Clinical care pathways (also referred to as 'critical pathways', 'integrated care pathways', or simply 'care pathways') are defined for the purpose of this guideline as systems designed to improve the overall quality of healthcare by standardising the care process. In doing so, they seek to promote organised, efficient patient care, based on best evidence, which is intended to optimise patient outcomes. Usually they draw on clinical guidance (for example, technology appraisals and clinical guidelines) as sources of evidence. Clinical care pathways are usually multidisciplinary in structure and, importantly, are focused on a specific group of service users. These service users have a broadly predictable clinical course in which different interventions provided are defined, optimised and sequenced in a manner appropriate to the needs of the service users and the setting in which they are provided.

A number of recent developments in the NHS in the UK have supported the development of clinical care pathways. Of particular note is the development of integrated care pathways in NHS Scotland (which has seen the development of locally agreed multidisciplinary and multiagency practice, including pathways for mental health services[48]). In a recently proposed reorganisation of the NHS by Lord Darzi ('High quality care for all: NHS Next Stage Review final report'[49]), considerable emphasis was also placed on care pathways as a means to improve healthcare.

However, the evidence for the effectiveness of care pathways remains uncertain (Dy *et al.*, 2005; Emmerson *et al.*, 2006). This may be a particular problem in mental health where comorbidities (including mental and physical health problems), and considerable difference in severity and uncertainty about treatment options, mean that specifying interventions for defined patient groups can be challenging and with consequent uncertainty about the benefits (Panella *et al.*, 2006; Wilson *et al.*, 1997).

### 7.1.2    Current practice in the National Health Service

With the possible exception of the developments in Scotland (described above) there has been little systematic development of care pathways in the NHS, although it could

---

[48]http://www.healthcareimprovementscotland.org/home.aspx
[49]http://www.dh.gov.uk/en/Publicationsandstatistics/Publications/PublicationsPolicyAndGuidance/DH_085825

be argued that the IAPT[50] (CSIP, 2007) stepped-care model, with its clear focus on evidence-based psychological interventions, is a form of care pathway, albeit without an explicit claim to such. Outside of common mental health disorders, the work of the National Treatment Agency on models of care for alcohol users has something in common with the care pathway model (Department of Health, 2006). More recently, the development of care clusters in mental health, with the intention that such clusters form future funding schemes through Payment by Results, suggest that care pathways will be an increasing aspect of care in the NHS (HoNOS-PbR[51]).

## 7.2    CLINICAL EVIDENCE REVIEW

### 7.2.1    Clinical review protocol

The aim of this review was to perform a narrative synthesis of existing systematic reviews of clinical care pathways for people with common mental health disorders. The review protocol, including the review question, information about databases searched and the eligibility criteria used in this section of the guideline, can be found in Table 40. Although the search was conducted for the period 1995 to 2010, the focus was on systematic reviews published since 2003. Further information about the rationale for the method employed here can be found in Chapter 3 and the search strategy can be found in Appendix 6.

### 7.2.2    Studies considered[52]

The literature search for systematic reviews yielded 3,641 papers. Scanning titles/abstracts identified 28 potentially relevant reviews, but further inspection revealed that only 21 met eligibility criteria.

ADLI2006 (Adli *et al.*, 2006), BUTLER2007 (Butler *et al.*, 2007) and VANHERCK2004 (Vanherck *et al.*, 2004) investigated the utility of general algorithms and care pathways in healthcare. Twelve studies looked at models of treatment delivery. Two of these studies, CHRISTENSEN2008 (Christensen *et al.*, 2008) and GRIF-FITHS2008 (Griffiths & Christensen, 2008), looked at models of delivery for depression treatment in general. Ten studies, BADAMGARAV2003 (Badamgarav *et al.*, 2003), BOWER2006 (Bower *et al.*, 2006), CHANGQUAN2009 (Chang-Quan *et al.*, 2009), CRAVEN2006 (Craven & Bland, 2006), FOY2010 (Foy *et al.*, 2010), FREDER-ICK2007 (Frederick *et al.*, 2007), GENSICHEN2005 (Gensichen *et al.*, 2005),

---

[50]http://www.iapt.nhs.uk/

[51]http://webarchive.nationalarchives.gov.uk/+/www.dh.gov.uk/en/Managingyourorganisation/ FinanceandplanningyNHSFinancialReforms/DH_4137762

[52]Here and elsewhere in the guideline, each study considered for review is referred to by a study ID in capital letters (primary author and date of study publication, except where a study is in press or only submitted for publication, then a date is not used).

**Table 40: Clinical review protocol for the review of care pathways**

| Component | Description |
|---|---|
| Review question | In adults (18 years and older) with depression (including subthreshold disorders) or an anxiety disorder*, what are the aspects of a clinical care pathway that are associated with better individual or organisations outcomes? |
| Objectives | To perform a narrative synthesis of systematic reviews addressing care pathways |
| Population | Adults (18 years and older) identified with depression (including subthreshold disorders) or an anxiety disorder* |
| Intervention(s) | Care pathways |
| Comparison | Standard management strategy |
| Critical outcomes | Any |
| Electronic databases | CINAHL, DARE, EMBASE, MEDLINE, PsycINFO, |
| Date searched | 1 January 1995 to 14 June 2010 |
| Study design | Systematic review |
| *Including GAD, panic disorder, social anxiety disorder, OCD, specific phobias and PTSD. | |

GILBODY2006 (Gilbody *et al.*, 2006), GUNN2006 (Gunn *et al.*, 2006), NEUMEYER-GROMEN2004 (Neumeyer-Gromen *et al.*, 2004) and SMOLDERS2008 (Smolders *et al.*, 2008) looked at collaborative care and case management as specific models of care. One further study, CALLAGHAN2003 (Callaghan *et al.*, 2003), looked at liaison mental health services as a model of care. Two studies, HEIDEMAN2005 (Heideman *et al.*, 2005) and AGARWAL2008 (Agarwal & Crooks, 2008), also investigated continuity of care, but for anxiety disorders rather than depression. One study, ADLER2010 (Adler *et al.*, 2010), looked at continuity of care; the aforementioned AGARWAL2008 (Agarwal *et al.*, 2008) looked ways of improving informational continuity and GILBODY2003 (Gilbody *et al.*, 2003) investigated the effect of educational interventions on depression outcomes.

The characteristics of the studies included in this review can be found in Table 41. Further information about both included and excluded studies can be found in Appendix 14.

### 7.2.3 Clinical evidence

On the basis of an initial review of the references identified by the literature search, the GDG was able to group the included studies under a number of headings. These

**Table 41: Study information table for systematic reviews of care pathways**

| Study ID | ADLER2010 | ADLI2006 | AGARWAL2008 | BADAMGARAV2003 | BOWER2006 |
|---|---|---|---|---|---|
| Method used to synthesise evidence | Narrative and meta-regression | Narrative | Narrative | Meta-analysis | Meta-analysis |
| Design of included studies | Various | Various | Various | RCTs | RCTs |
| Search strategy | CINAHL and MEDLINE were searched to 2007 | MEDLINE (no dates given) | CINAHL, EMBASE, MEDLINE, PsycINFO and Web of Science were searched to 2006 | Cochrane Library, HealthSTAR, MEDLINE were searched to 2001 | CINAHL, the Cochrane Library, DARE, EMBASE, MEDLINE and PsycINFO were searched to 2005 |
| No. of included studies | 12 | Not given | 34 | 19 | 72 |
| Review quality | Adequate | Poor | Adequate | Adequate | Adequate |
| Interventions | Continuity of care | Algorithms | Informational continuity | Disease management | Collaborative care |
| Outcomes | Patient satisfaction | Recovery, quality of life, patient satisfaction, remission or response to treatment, treatment adherence, symptom reduction, suicidal ideation, side-effect burden and functional impairment | Accuracy | Improvements in symptoms, physical functioning, social and health status and patient satisfaction, impact on healthcare utilisation, hospitalisations, healthcare costs, depression detection, referral rates, prescribing adequacy and adherence | Antidepressant use and symptom improvement |
| Participant diagnoses | Various medical concerns | Depression | Various mental and non-mental health conditions | Depression | Depression or depressive symptoms |

| Study ID | BUTLER2007 | CALLAGHAN2003 | CHANGQUAN2009 | CHRISTENSEN2008 | CRAVEN2006 |
|---|---|---|---|---|---|
| Method used to synthesise evidence | Narrative | Narrative | Meta-analysis | Statistical (based on counting number of significant findings in primary studies) | Narrative |
| Design of included studies | Systematic reviews and RCTs | Reviews, descriptive studies and evaluative studies | RCTs | RCT and controlled trials | RCTs and intervention studies with outcome measures |
| Search strategy | Cochrane, EMBASE, HTA, MEDLINE, NHS Centre of Reviews and Disseminations, NHS Centre for Database of Abstracts of Reviews of Effects, NICE guidance PsycINFO and Turning Research Into Practice were searched to 2006 | ASSIA, Best Evidence, British Nursing Index, CINAHL, the Cochrane Library, DARE, EMBASE, MEDLINE, National Research Register, Nursing collection, PsycINFO and Royal College of Nursing Library were searched to 2001 | Cochrane Library, EMBASE and MEDLINE were searched to 2007 | Cochrane Library, The National Library of Medicine's collection database (PubMed) and PsycINFO were searched from inception to October 2005 | CINAHL, Cochrane Library, Education Resources Information Center, EMBASE, Google, MEDLINE, PsycINFO, PubMed and Social Science Abstracts were searched to 2005 |
| No. of included studies | 10 systematic reviews and 4 RCTs | 48 | 3 | 55 | 38 |
| Review quality | Adequate | Adequate | Adequate | Poor | Adequate |
| Interventions | Care pathways using befriending, cognitive therapy, combining antidepressant drugs and psychological treatments, interpersonal | Liaison mental health services | Collaborative care | Training and feedback, care management, enhancements of extensions to general practice, self-help, teams external to the practice, | Collaborative care |

*(Continued)*

**Table 41: (*Continued*)**

| Study ID | BUTLER2007 | CALLAGHAN2003 | CHANGQUAN2009 | CHRISTENSEN2008 | CRAVEN2006 |
|---|---|---|---|---|---|
| | psychotherapy, non-directive counselling, problem-solving therapy or relapse prevention programmes | | | community-based mental health professionals, health maintenance organisation-based interventions and broad community-based interventions | |
| Outcomes | Effectiveness and safety | Symptom reduction, physician skill improvements, referral rates, acceptability and appointment compliance | Depression symptoms, response rates, remission, suicidal ideation and treatment seeking | Significant improvement on the key depression measure | Improved patient response |
| Participant diagnoses | Mild, moderate and severe depression | Various mental health problems | Depression in older people | Depression | Various |

| Study ID | FOY2010 | FREDERICK2007 | GENSICHEN2005 | GILBODY2003 | GILBODY2006 |
|---|---|---|---|---|---|
| Method used to synthesise evidence | Meta-analysis | Narrative | Meta-analysis | Narrative | Meta-analysis |
| Design of included studies | RCT | Various | RCTs | RCTs, controlled before-and-after studies, interrupted time series analyses | RCTs |
| Search strategy | CDSR, CINAHL, DARE, EMBASE, PsycINFO, | To 2005 (no further details given) | Cochrane Library (2003, 2nd edition), EMBASE | CINAHL, Cochrane, Cochrane Controlled | CINAHL (from the beginning of 1980), |

| | PubMed and Web of Science to 2008 | | (1980 to May 2003) and MEDLINE (1966 to May 2003) | Trials Register, Cochrane Depression Anxiety and Neurosis Group Register, EMBASE, MEDLINE, PsycLIT and UK NHS EED were searched to 2003 | Cochrane Library (from the beginning of 1966), DARE (from the beginning of 1980), EMBASE (from the beginning of 1980), MEDLINE (from the beginning of 1966) and PsycINFO (from the beginning of 1980) |
|---|---|---|---|---|---|
| No. of included studies | 38 | 121 | 13 | 36 | 37 |
| Review quality | Adequate | Adequate | Adequate | Adequate | Adequate |
| Interventions | Collaborative care | Community-based interventions for depression in older adults | Case management | Educational and organisational methods to improve depression management | Collaborative care |
| Outcomes | Depression symptoms | Depression symptoms | Symptom reduction, relative risk (RR) reduction, treatment response rate and medication adherence | Medication concordance and adherence, depression outcomes, rate of recovery, persistent depression benefits, recognition rates, management effectiveness | Symptom outcomes (6 months and longer term) |
| Participant diagnoses | Depression | Depression in older adults | Depression | Depression | Depression |

*(Continued)*

195

**Table 41: (Continued)**

| Study ID | GRIFFITHS2008 | GUNN2006 | HEIDEMAN2005 | NEUMEYERG-ROMEN2004 | SMOLDERS2008 | VANHERCK2004 |
|---|---|---|---|---|---|---|
| Method used to synthesise evidence | Narrative | Narrative | Meta-analysis | Meta-analysis | Meta-analysis and narrative | Narrative |
| Design of included studies | Systematic reviews | RCTs and cluster RCTs | RCTs and controlled before-and-after studies | RCTs | RCTs and controlled before-and-after studies | Experimental, quasi-experimental observational, systematic reviews, subjective opinion and unclear |
| Search strategy | Discussion of six systematic reviews | Cochrane Library MEDLINE and PubMed were searched to 2004 | Cochrane Library, EMBASE, MEDLINE and PsycINFO searched to 2003 | BMJ Clinical Trials, CINAHL, Cochrane Library, EMBASE, HTA databases, MEDLINE, NHS EED, PsyINDEX and PsycLIT were searched to 2002 | CINAHL, Cochrane Library, EMBASE, MEDLINE and PsycINFO were searched to 2003, and then again to 2006 | MEDLINE was searched from 2000 to 2002 |
| No. of included studies | 6 | 11 | 7 | 10 | 24 | 200 |
| Review quality | Poor | Adequate | Adequate | Adequate | Adequate | Poor |
| Interventions | Depression management | System-level interventions to improve recovery | Audit and feedback, brief education and educational outreach | Disease-management programs | Audit and feedback, education and educational outreach | Care pathways (not mental health-specific) |
| Outcomes | Depression symptoms | Recovery rates | Symptom improvement, rates of recognition, correct diagnoses, levels of recovery and appropriate prescriptions | Depression severity, quality of life, employment status, patient satisfaction, adherence and cost | Prescription rates, referrals, physician knowledge, anxiety symptom improvement, satisfaction and cost-effectiveness | Clinical outcome and team, process and financial effects |
| Participant diagnoses | Depression | Depression | Anxiety | Depressive disorders | Anxiety | Medical and psychiatric conditions |

included two broad categories; the first concerned the overall design and structure of a care pathway, and the second concerned various aspects or components of the care pathway that were associated with positive outcomes including case management, care coordination, liaison and communication. In this review the GDG also drew on existing reviews that were not restricted to mental health (although non-mental reviews were in the minority). Of those reviews that focused on mental health, and common mental health disorders in particular, the majority were focused on depression. The outcomes reported by the reviews varied considerably and included patients' satisfaction with care, engagement, and clinical outcomes such as remission and symptom reduction. Very little health economic evidence was identified. Wherever possible, the GDG considered the implications of the review for all common mental health disorders.

*The design and structure of care pathways*

Three reviews were identified in this area (ADLI2006, BUTLER2007, VANHERCK2004). ADLI2006 conducted a systematic narrative review of studies (exact number not provided) that investigated the effectiveness of algorithms and collaborative care systems for depression. The review provided helpful information on the use of objective 'critical decision points' that were associated with the use of objective formal measurement scales on pre-defined response criteria, and appropriate scheduling of their use. They concluded that such characteristics of a care pathway were effective in reducing overall symptomatology and improving function, but questions remained about the cost effectiveness of these approaches.

BUTLER2007 conducted a systematic, narrative review of ten systematic reviews and four RCTs to investigate the outcomes associated with integrated care pathways (broadly defined) as part of a wider review of psychological and combined psychological and pharmacology treatments for depression. They suggested that care pathways, including collaborative care models, and community mental health teams could all contribute to patient-centred outcomes. Although they were confident of the benefit of care pathways, they were unable to identify which specific elements contributed to the overall effectiveness of the pathways. They concluded that all elements of multidisciplinary care pathway should be introduced routinely into the care of people with depression.

VANHERCK2004 conducted a systematic narrative review of 200 studies, including experimental, quasi-experimental and observational studies, and systematic reviews. Only eight of these studies were directly related to clinical pathways in mental health. Commonly identified characteristics of successful pathways included the use of both process and outcome measures. They concluded that the overall effect of pathways was positive, with a stronger impact on the process of delivery of care than individual clinical targets or service style changes.

*Components of the care pathway*
**Care coordination and collaborative care**
Eleven reviews were identified in this area: BADAMGARAV2003, BOWER2006, CHANGQUAN2009, CHRISTENSEN2008, CRAVEN2006, FREDERICK2007, GENSICHEN2005, GILBODY2003, GILBODY2006, NEUMEYERGROMEN2004,

SMOLDERS2008. A large number of these studies focused on some aspect of collaborative care or case management. The majority of these reviews were on the care and management of depression. The reviews often identified common themes, but many reported on different aspects of the delivery and coordination of care, and, as a whole, provide for a substantial review of the effectiveness or otherwise of various aspects of the care pathway. Care coordination in this review was broadly defined, with a number of the reviews adopting broader definitions than have been used in other NICE guidelines (for example, NICE, 2009a and 2009b). Because the focus of this review was on the potential contribution of the aspects of the care provided and not collaborative care or case management *per se*, the GDG took the view that it was appropriate to except the definition developed by the authors and not use these as eligibility criteria on which to base a decision to include or exclude a study.

BADAMGARAV2003 conducted a meta-analysis of 19 RCTs of case management approaches for treatment of depression. These studies showed case management approaches to be associated with improved outcomes but with little impact on physical functioning, social status or hospital costs for admission rates.

GILBODY2003 conducted a systematic narrative review of 36 RCTs, controlled before-and-after studies and interrupted time-series analyses, to investigate the educational and organisational interventions designed to improve both the care and management of depression in primary care. The authors concluded that educational interventions, guideline implementations, patient reminders and less intensive forms of continuous quality management alone were less effective, and that an integrated approach to the improvement of care for people with depression was required. Such a programme would likely be a population-based intensive intervention incorporating shared care and decision making and organisational interventions to support delivery, such as education, patient-specific reminders, case management and enhanced integration of all aspects of a patient's care.

BOWER2006 conducted a meta-regression of 72 RCTs, based on the initial GILBODY2003 dataset, to identify the mutative components of collaborative care of depression. The authors identified the systematic identification of depression, the mental health background of staff and the provision of specialist supervision of case managers as being associated with improved process focused outcomes. In a review from the same group, GILBODY2006 conducted a meta-analysis of 37 RCTs to provide further evidence for the effectiveness of collaborative care. Medication compliance and case manager background were also important, but brief psychological interventions had limited impact on outcomes. CHANGQUAN2009 conducted another meta-analysis of collaborative care focused on older people with depression, based on three RCTs. Again, they found that collaborative care improved outcomes for people with depression.

A number of reviews that looked at collaborative care examined the monitoring system associated with case management or collaborative care. NEUMEYER-GROMEN2004 conducted a meta-analysis of ten RCTs to identify the importance of self-management systems, and the use of outcome monitoring and reminder systems with improved outcomes. FREDERICK2007 conducted a narrative systematic review of various study types (number of studies included not reported). The authors state that case-management approaches based either in the home or the clinic were effective in producing positive outcomes for older people with depression who were also in receipt of individual CBT.

CHRISTENSEN2008 conducted a meta-analysis of 55 RCTs and case-control trials to review models for depression treatment in primary care. They concluded that case management systems were associated with better outcomes when the monitoring of treatment was delivered by a mental health professional practice, but training and clinical guidelines were not associated with better outcomes.

CRAVEN2006 conducted a systematic narrative review of 208 studies. The authors took a broader view of the definition of collaborative care, and focused on communication, personal contact between professional, sharing clinical information and joint educational programmes. They noted that such systems took time to establish and that patient involvement was crucial. They also noted that the extent and degree of collaboration did not seem to predict outcomes, with limited collaboration still involved in producing good outcomes. Systematic follow up was again identified as one of the most powerful factors predictive of clinical outcome. Patient choice about modality may also be an important factor in treatment.

GENSICHEN2005 reviewed 13 RCTs of case management in a meta-analysis. In line with the findings of CRAVEN2006, the authors showed an impact on depression outcomes, but the complexity of the case management did not appear to impact on the nature of the overall outcomes.

SMOLDERS2008 was one of the few studies that looked at anxiety disorders. They reviewed a total of 24 RCTs in their systematic review. In common with the reviews of depression, the authors found that audit and educational strategies had limited impact when focused on professionals only improving process of care, but did improve the outcome of care when imbedded in organisational-level interventions. They concluded that collaborative care interventions may prove effective for treatment of anxiety.

**Satisfaction**

ADLER2010 conducted a systematic narrative review of 12 studies, focusing on the relationship between continuity of care and patients satisfaction. The review found that continuity of care was associated with overall increased satisfaction, but some variations existed and consequently there was uncertainty due to differences in the measures of continuity that were used by the included studies.

**Liaison**

CALLAGAHAN2003 conducted a systematic narrative review of 41 reviews, and descriptive and evaluative studies. This review included a large number of UK-based studies and looked at the impact of liaison between multidisciplinary teams and non-specialist teams. The study focused on the relationship between acute and chronic physical health services, but also included mental health services. The overall conclusion was that the liaison between the mental health services improved access to these services and reduced readmission rates for people with mental health problems. FOY2010 conducted a meta-analysis of 38 RCTs to investigate the effective interactive components between primary care physicians and specialists. Their conclusion was that interaction and communication between primary and secondary care leads to significant improvement of outcomes for people with depression. In contrast, needs assessment and joint care of planning had relatively little impact on overall outcome.

**System-level interventions**

GRIFFITHS2008 conducted a narrative review of six previous systematic reviews to evaluate a number of models for the delivery of effective treatments of depression in primary care. These included care management extended/enhanced care, facilitated self-help, systematic tracking by non-medical professionals, and revised professional roles that incorporated patient preference into care, all of which were associated with positive outcomes. In contrast, GP training with feedback, pharmacist-led interventions, community context, telephone support and the use of the internet were not associated with positive outcomes.

GUNN2006 conducted a systematic narrative review of 11 RCTs and cluster RCTs to review system-level interventions. These were defined as having a multi-professional element with a structured management plan, scheduled patient follow-ups and enhanced inter-professional communication. They concluded that these approaches could potentially produce benefits for moderate to severely depressed patients, but were unsure about the potential benefits for patients with milder forms of depression. They also raised some questions about the generalisability of these studies beyond the US, where all but one of the studies reviewed was undertaken.

HEIDEMAN2005 conducted a meta-analysis of seven RCTs and controlled before-and-after studies to investigate the efficacy of interventions in primary care focused on improving outcomes for patients with anxiety disorders. The authors examined a number of organisational interventions including audit and feedback, professional replacement models and education. Audit and feedback did little in terms of improving outcomes, but brought about some improved recognition. A brief psychoeducational group intervention brought some improvement, as did a nurse substitution intervention and collaborative care.

AGARWAL2008 conducted a systematic narrative review of 34 studies of information provided through primary care settings. They identified a number of systems, including formal electronic records and patient involvement in what should be in their records, which were associated with improved emotional continuity.

### 7.2.4    Clinical evidence summary

The majority of the studies identified in this review concentrated on the treatment of depression and a large number were systematic reviews of collaborative care (see Table 42). The original intention of this review was to identify important components of local care pathways for common mental health disorders. The review identified a number of aspects of care pathways relating to their design and structure. The use of clear and objective entry and response criteria, where possible, based on formal measures, were associated with positive outcomes.

**Table 42: Summary of findings for systematic reviews of pathways**

| Study ID | Outcomes | Results |
|---|---|---|
| ADLER2010 | Patient satisfaction | In general, continuity of care was associated with overall satisfaction of care. However, results were not always consistent and varied depending on measures of continuity. Duration of doctor-patient relationship showed no significant effect on satisfaction, whereas subjective measures did. |
| ADLI2006 | Recovery, quality of life, patient satisfaction, remission or response to treatment, treatment adherence, symptom reduction, suicidal ideation, side-effect burden and functional impairment | In clinical practice, treatment algorithms should be embedded in a multi-faceted disease management or collaborative care program. They must be understandable and acceptable, and be capable of overcoming administrative and clinician-related hurdles.

Critical decision points can be useful for algorithm implementation, provided that they use objective symptom scales, are based on pre-defined response criteria, include a rigorous assessment of side-effects, are scheduled at appropriate time points and are adaptable to various clinical circumstances.

In comparison with treatment as usual, algorithms can help to improve the likelihood of recovery, quality of life and patient satisfaction, to achieve remission or response to treatment, to maintain treatment adherence and to reduce depressive symptoms, suicidal ideation, side-effect burden and functional impairment. |

*(Continued)*

**Table 42:** (*Continued*)

| Study ID | Outcomes | Results |
|---|---|---|
| AGARWAL2008 | Accuracy | Duration and depth of the patient–doctor relationship is important because accurate histories often require a good knowledge base.<br><br>Doctors were found to rarely ask about social/lifestyle and medical histories, preferring to rely on memory.<br><br>Around 30% of patients report enjoying discussing what should be entered in their records. However, they can be selective and often prioritise biomedical issues over socio-contextual or personal ones. |
| BADAMGARAV2003 | Improvements in symptoms, physical functioning, social and health status and patient satisfaction, impact on healthcare utilisation, hospitalisations, healthcare costs, depression detection, referral rates, prescribing adequacy and adherence | In comparison with standard care, disease management was significantly better at:<br>• Reducing symptoms of depression (effect size = 0.33, 95% CI, 0.16 to 0.49)<br>• Improving patient satisfaction (effect size = 0.51, 95% CI, 0.33 to 0.68)<br>• Increasing primary care visits (effect size = −0.1, 95% CI, −0.18 to −0.02)<br>• Detecting depression, but only when programs contained an explicit screening component (effect size = 0.18, 95% CI, −0.11 to 0.18)<br>• Improving treatment adequacy (effect size = 0.44, 95% CI, 0.30 to 0.59) |

| | | |
|---|---|---|
| | | • Improving patient adherence to treatment (effect 95% CI, 0.17 to 0.54). |
| | | In comparison with standard care, disease management had no effect on: |
| | | • Physical functioning (effect size = −0.05, 95% CI, −0.72 to 0.62) |
| | | • Social and health status (effect size = 0.06, 95% CI, −0.51 to 0.62) |
| | | • Hospitalisation rates (effect size = −0.2, 95% CI, −0.35 to 0.04) |
| | | • Healthcare costs (effect size = −1.03, 95% CI, −2.62 to 0.54). |
| | | Outcomes affected by patient and provider adherence to treatment (effect size = 0.57, 95% CI, −0.11 to 1.26). |
| | | Referral to specialist care (effect size = 0.13, 95% CI, −0.32 toĨ 0.57). |
| BOWER2006 | Antidepressant use and symptom improvement | Collaborative care had a positive effect on depressive symptom outcomes (SMD = 0.24, 95% CI, 0.17 to 0.32). |
| | | No intervention content variables predicted antidepressant use. |
| | | Intervention content variables that predicted depressive symptom improvement were: |
| | | • Recruitment by systematic identification |
| | | • Case managers with specific mental health backgrounds |
| | | • Provision of regular supervision for case managers |

*(Continued)*

**Table 42:** (*Continued*)

| Study ID | Outcomes | Results |
|---|---|---|
| BUTLER2007 | Effectiveness and safety | Compared with standard care:<br>• Care pathways were more effective at improving symptoms and response rates<br>• Recurrence prevention programmes were equally effective at improving relapse rates at 6 months, regardless of specific treatment components<br>• It is unclear what effect care pathways have in the very long term (2+ years).<br><br>However, much of the evidence was considered to be of low quality. |
| CALLAGHAN2003 | Symptom reduction, physician skill improvements, referral rates, acceptability and appointment compliance | Liaison mental health services were found to:<br>• Reduce levels of psychological morbidity, cardiac mortality and healthcare costs<br>• Increase rates of referral for follow up appointments<br>• Be acceptable to clients in terms of the information they received, and overall satisfaction<br>• Have little effect on compliance with psychiatric appointments. |
| CHANGQUAN2009 | Depression symptoms, response rates, remission, suicidal ideation and treatment seeking | At 18 and 24 months, collaborative care interventions were superior to usual care in improving depression scores (mean difference [MD] = −0.44, 95% CI, −0.55 to −0.33 and MD = −0.35, 95% CI, −0.46 to −0.24, respectively), response |

| | | rates (OR = 2.38, 95% CI, 1.88 to 3.02 and OR = 1.67, 95% CI, 1.63 to 2.12, respectively) and remission rates (OR = 2.29, 95% CI, 1.42 to 3.10 and OR = 1.83, 95% CI, 1.34 to 1.98, respectively). |
|---|---|---|
| CHRISTENSEN2008 | Quality of life, depression symptoms | Treatment monitoring and delivery was best done by a professional with a mental health background ($\chi^2$ [2, 22] = 7.558, p = 0.021). |
| | | GP training and clinical practice guideline provision alone were not associated with improved outcomes. |
| | | There was no association between number of treatment components and outcome. |
| CRAVEN2006 | Improved patient response | Degree of collaboration does not in itself appear to predict clinical outcome. |
| | | Systematic follow-up strongly predicts clinical outcome. |
| | | Enhanced patient education often improved patient outcomes. |
| | | Collaborative interventions took time to establish and are hard to maintain outside of the study environment. |
| | | Patient choice is an important factor in treatment engagement in collaborative care. |
| FOY2010 | Depression symptoms | GP and psychiatrist collaboration led to a significant improvement in depression outcomes (effect size = −0.48, 95% CI, −0.67 to −0.30). |

*(Continued)*

**Table 42:** (*Continued*)

| Study ID | Outcomes | Results |
|---|---|---|
| | | Interventions that improved the quality of information exchange had significantly better outcomes than those with no such focus on information exchange (effect size = –0.84, 95% CI, –1.14 to –0.55 and –0.27, 95% CI, –0.49 to –0.05, respectively).<br><br>Needs assessment and joint care planning had little effect on outcome. |
| FREDERICK2007 | Depression symptoms | Depression care management, home or primary care clinics and individual CBT can be strongly recommended. |
| GENSICHEN2005 | Symptom reduction, relative risk reduction, treatment response rate and medication adherence | Case management was associated with a significant reduction in depression severity and the relative risk of long-lasting depression, and an increase in response rate and medication adherence at 6 to 12 months in comparison with usual care.<br><br>Simple and complex case management did not differ from each other. |
| GILBODY2003 | Patient outcomes | Effective strategies included collaborative care, stepped collaborative care, quality improvement, case management, for the pharmacist to provide prescribing information and patient education (medication outcomes only), and guideline implementation strategies when embedded in complex interventions. |

| | | Ineffective strategies included guidelines and educational strategies when not accompanied by organisational support, chronic care clinics and computer-based decision support systems. |
| --- | --- | --- |
| GILBODY2006 | Depression symptoms at 6 months | Collaborative care had a positive effect on depression outcomes at 6 months compared with standard care (SMD = 0.25, 95% CI, 0.18–0.32), which were maintained at 12 months (SMD = 0.31; 95% CI, 0.01 to 0.53), 18 months (SMD = 0.25; 95% CI, 0.03 to 0.46) and 5 years (SMD = 0.15; 95% CI, 0.001 to 0.30). |
| | | Regular supervision and the mental health background of case managers were significantly related to study effect size (β = 0.15; 95% CI, –0.02 to –0.31 and β = 0.18; 95% CI, 0.04 to 0.32, respectively). |
| | | The addition of psychotherapy to medication management in collaborative care was not associated with any significantly increased effect size (β = 0.10, 95% CI, –0.05 to 0.25). |
| | | The number of case management sessions had no impact on effect size (β = 0.02; 95% CI, –0.008 to 0.04). |
| GRIFFITHS2008 | Depression symptoms | The following were associated with an improvement in depression outcomes relative to treatment-as-usual or control condition: <br>• Care management <br>• Enhanced/extended care <br>• Guided self-help in general practice |

*(Continued)*

**Table 42:** (*Continued*)

| Study ID | Outcomes | Results |
|---|---|---|
| | | • Systematic tracking by a non-doctor<br>• Revision of professional roles<br>• Incorporation of patient preferences into care.<br><br>The following were associated with no improvement in depression outcomes relative to treatment-as-usual or control condition:<br>• GP training and feedback<br>• Pharmacist interventions<br>• Community context.<br><br>Telephone interventions, internet support groups and passive education did not have enough evidence for evaluation of their effectiveness. |
| GUNN2006 | Recovery rates | Studies generally favoured the multi-professional intervention groups in comparison with the control groups at various follow-up points for depression outcomes. |
| HEIDEMAN2005 | Symptom improvement, rates of recognition, correct diagnoses, levels of recovery and appropriate prescriptions | Audit and feedback had no effect on the majority of anxiety outcomes, but did lead to significantly higher rates of recognition (RR = 1.71, 95% CI, 1.27 to 2.29), treatment, chart notation (RR = 1.66, 95% CI, 1.23 to 2.30) and referral in comparison with the control group (RR = 2.94, 95% CI, 1.33 to 6.51). |

| | | |
|---|---|---|
| | | Brief education intervention led to significantly higher rates of correct agoraphobia, panic, GAD and adjustment disorder diagnoses than the control group (RR = 1.32, 95% CI, 1.24 to 1.42, RR = 1.14, 95% CI, 1.07 to 1.21, RR = 1.53, 95% CI, 1.38 to 1.69 and RR = 1.12, 95% CI, 1.04 to 1.21, respectively)<br><br>Nurse substitution intervention led to significantly greater improvements in symptoms than the control group<br><br>Collaborative care led to significantly greater levels of recovery (RR = 2.29, 95% CI, 1.29 to 4.06) and more anxiety free days per patient than the control group. |
| NEUMEYERGROMEN2004 | Depression severity, quality of life, employment status, patient satisfaction, adherence and cost | In comparison with usual care, disease management programs significantly improved HRQoL scales at 12 and 24 months (MD = 11.83, 95% CI, 7.38 to 16.28 and MD = 24.42, 95% CI, 17.92 to 30.92, respectively), significantly higher rates of patient satisfaction (RR = 0.57, 95% CI, 0.37 to 0.87; p = 0.009) and significantly reduced depression severity in comparison with usual care (RR = 0.75, 95% CI, 0.70 to 0.81), although 2-year follow-up showed inconsistent results. |
| SMOLDERS2008 | Prescription rates, referrals, physician knowledge, anxiety symptom improvement, satisfaction and cost effectiveness | Intensive programs that incorporated education and shared care were associated with increased anxiety-free days and better employment status. |

*(Continued)*

**Table 42:** (*Continued*)

| Study ID | Outcomes | Results |
|---|---|---|
| | | Education and audit and feedback strategies alone were not successful at increasing anxiety outcomes. Brief education was successful at influencing treatment recommendations for panic disorder only and CBT training sessions increased the use of CBT techniques. Studies that used guideline concordant treatment and medication adherence strategies were associated with short-term effects only. |
| | | Collaborative care improved receipt of adequate medication and medication adherence over 6 months, but not 12 months. |
| | | Interventions had a high probability of being cost effective. |
| VANHERCK2004 | Clinical outcome and team, process and financial effects | Most studies agreed that pathways had positive effects, and all domains were associated with positive effects more than they were with negative effects. |
| | | Pathways had stronger positive influence on process, team and financial effects than clinical outcome and service effects. |
| | | Negative effects were consistently low. |

With regard to the specific components of care pathways, reliance on single approaches to develop or improve care pathways, such as educational interventions or guideline intervention, were not associated with positive outcomes. Although a focus on outcomes, to monitor and measure effectiveness, is clearly desirable there is also evidence that process measures could be of benefit. With regard to the specific components of care pathways, interventions or systems that focus on the coordination and/or organisation of individual care were associated with positive outcomes. Identified case managers (particularly those with a mental health background) and the active engagement of the patient in the planning, delivery and monitoring of their own care, were associated with positive outcomes. Effective communication about patient care, both with the patient and between professionals, was also associated with positive outcomes. Interestingly, the extent of communication did not need to be great, but was enhanced by direct contact between professionals. Improved communication was also associated with improved patient satisfaction.

The majority of the evidence, as noted above, was focused on people with depression. There was some suggestion that substantial organisational interventions may be of more benefit for moderately to severely depressed people. There was less evidence for people with anxiety disorders, but nevertheless the reviews that focused on anxiety disorders reported much the same findings as those that focused on depression. Flexibility in the provision of services was both valued and associated with better outcomes, for example, having multiple points of access to the care pathway and the ability to progress within the care pathway were associated with better outcomes.

## 7.3 HEALTH ECONOMIC EVIDENCE

The systematic search of the economic literature undertaken for the guideline identified one eligible study on different care pathways for people with common mental health disorders (Hakkart-van Roijen *et al.*, 2006). The study compared CBT with brief therapy (more accurately described as a form of stepped care) and care as usual for the treatment of people with depression and anxiety from a societal perspective in the Netherlands. Care as usual was defined as a mixture of therapeutic strategies based on professional experience, while the number of sessions depended on the therapy provided to the patient. Brief therapy was described as a formalised 'stepped- care' approach; a stepped-care approach was adopted in the case of CBT as well. Namely, patients initially received a first-line treatment and were switched to an alternative treatment if the first proved insufficient. Patients were offered a maximum of 15 sessions. The study population consisted of adult patients (aged between 18 and 65 years) with DSM-IV diagnoses of major depressive disorder (MDD; single episode or recurrent), dysthymic disorder, panic disorder (with or without agoraphobia), social phobia and GAD who were referred to Dutch outpatient mental healthcare centres by GPs. The measure of outcome for the economic analysis was the number of QALYs gained. The source of clinical effectiveness data was a multicentre randomised trial conducted in seven mental healthcare centres in the Netherlands. Resource-use estimates were based on actual data collected prospectively on the same sample of patients as were used in the effectiveness study using the Trimbos/iMTA Questionnaire on Costs Associated with Psychiatric Illness (TiC-P). Costs were derived from published sources. The TiC-P questionnaire was also used to estimate productivity losses due to absenteeism from work. The analysis estimated that use of CBT was the dominant strategy compared with care as usual because CBT resulted in a higher number of QALYs at lower cost. The incremental cost of providing brief therapy rather than CBT was €222,956 per QALY gained (2002 prices). Although the study was based on an RCT, it was considered to be non-applicable to the UK setting for the following reasons: it was conducted in the Netherlands; care as usual was not described in sufficient depth and was likely to differ significantly from standard care in the NHS context; and the utility weightings were based on Dutch and not UK preferences. Therefore the study was not considered further during the guideline development process.

Details on the methods used for the systematic review of the economic literature are described in Chapter 3; the evidence table providing details of the study is presented in Appendix 10. The completed methodology checklist of the study is provided in Appendix 12.


### 7.4　　FROM EVIDENCE TO RECOMMENDATIONS

In developing these recommendations for local care pathways for common mental health disorders, the GDG was mindful that a considerable amount of evidence reviewed was drawn from non-UK studies. In addition, the majority of reviews that were mental health-specific focused on depression alone. This led to some caution in the development of the recommendations and the GDG took the view that, as far as possible, the recommendations should identify the principles or functions underlying local care pathways rather than attempt to specify in detail the nature and structure of it. A further factor that influenced the GDG's approach was the requirement to develop recommendations that would be appropriate for both depression and the anxiety disorders.

A number of clear principles emerged from the evidence review that were associated with positive outcomes and these are reflected in the recommendations below. They focus on the provision of information, the active involvement of the patient in the process of care, clarity about the pathways through care and the processes by which this is assessed, the provision of effective follow-up, the need for inter-professional communication and an overarching principle that all of these approaches should be delivered in an integrated manner. It was also clear that having staff with specific responsibility to assist in coordination and organisation of care was important, particularly with those patients with more severe disorders.

In delivering the recommendations for local care pathways, the GDG drew on the evidence base and also considered the recommendations developed or reproduced from other NICE guidelines in the other chapters of this guideline. The GDG also considered the principles of the stepped-care models developed and the evidence for them summarised in other NICE guidelines (for example, NICE, 2009a) and the need for the local care pathway recommendations to support and integrate with existing

NICE guidelines, for example in the location of care pathways within a broad stepped-care framework, which underpins the organisation of care in most NICE guidelines for common mental health disorders.

## 7.5    RECOMMENDATIONS

7.5.1.1    Local care pathways should be developed to promote implementation of key principles of good care. Pathways should be:
  ● negotiable, workable and understandable for people with common mental health disorders, their families and carers, and professionals
  ● accessible and acceptable to all people in need of the services served by the pathway
  ● responsive to the needs of people with common mental health disorders and their families and carers
  ● integrated so that there are no barriers to movement between different levels of the pathway
  ● outcomes focused (including measures of quality, service-user experience and harm).

7.5.1.2    Responsibility for the development, management and evaluation of local care pathways should lie with a designated leadership team, which should include primary and secondary care clinicians, managers and commissioners. The leadership team should have particular responsibility for:
  ● developing clear policy and protocols for the operation of the pathway
  ● providing training and support on the operation of the pathway
  ● auditing and reviewing the performance of the pathway.

7.5.1.3    Primary and secondary care clinicians, managers and commissioners should work together to design local care pathways that promote a stepped-care model of service delivery that:
  ● provides the least intrusive, most effective intervention first
  ● has clear and explicit criteria for the thresholds determining access to and movement between the different levels of the pathway
  ● does not use single criteria such as symptom severity to determine movement between steps
  ● monitors progress and outcomes to ensure the most effective interventions are delivered and the person moves to a higher step if needed.

7.5.1.4    Primary and secondary care clinicians, managers and commissioners should work together to design local care pathways that promote a range of evidence-based interventions at each step in the pathway and support people with common mental health disorders in their choice of interventions.

7.5.1.5    All staff should ensure effective engagement with families and carers, where appropriate, to:
  ● inform and improve the care of the person with a common mental health disorder
  ● meet the identified needs of the families and carers.

7.5.1.6 Primary and secondary care clinicians, managers and commissioners should work together to design local care pathways that promote the active engagement of all populations served by the pathway. Pathways should:
- offer prompt assessments and interventions that are appropriately adapted to the cultural, gender, age and communication needs of people with common mental health disorders
- keep to a minimum the number of assessments needed to access interventions.

7.5.1.7 Primary and secondary care clinicians, managers and commissioners should work together to design local care pathways that respond promptly and effectively to the changing needs of all populations served by the pathways. Pathways should have in place:
- clear and agreed goals for the services offered to a person with a common mental health disorder
- robust and effective means for measuring and evaluating the outcomes associated with the agreed goals
- clear and agreed mechanisms for responding promptly to identified changes to the person's needs.

7.5.1.8 Primary and secondary care clinicians, managers and commissioners should work together to design local care pathways that provide an integrated programme of care across both primary and secondary care services. Pathways should:
- minimise the need for transition between different services or providers
- allow services to be built around the pathway and not the pathway around the services
- establish clear links (including access and entry points) to other care pathways (including those for physical healthcare needs)
- have designated staff who are responsible for the coordination of people's engagement with the pathway.

7.5.1.9 Primary and secondary care clinicians, managers and commissioners should work together to ensure effective communication about the functioning of the local care pathway. There should be protocols for:
- sharing and communicating information with people with common mental health disorders, and where appropriate families and carers, about their care
- sharing and communicating information about the care of service users with other professionals (including GPs)
- communicating information between the services provided within the pathway
- communicating information to services outside the pathway.

# 8 SUMMARY OF RECOMMENDATIONS

## 8.1 IMPROVING ACCESS TO SERVICES

8.1.1.1 Primary and secondary care clinicians, managers and commissioners should collaborate to develop local care pathways (see also Section 8.5) that promote access to services for people with common mental health disorders by:
- supporting the integrated delivery of services across primary and secondary care
- having clear and explicit criteria for entry to the service
- focusing on entry and not exclusion criteria
- having multiple means (including self-referral) to access the service
- providing multiple points of access that facilitate links with the wider healthcare system and community in which the service is located.

8.1.1.2 Provide information about the services and interventions that constitute the local care pathway, including the:
- range and nature of the interventions provided
- settings in which services are delivered
- processes by which a person moves through the pathway
- means by which progress and outcomes are assessed
- delivery of care in related health and social care services.

8.1.1.3 When providing information about local care pathways to people with common mental health disorders and their families and carers, all healthcare professionals should:
- take into account the person's knowledge and understanding of mental health disorders and their treatment
- ensure that such information is appropriate to the communities using the pathway.

8.1.1.4 Provide all information about services in a range of languages and formats (visual, verbal and aural) and ensure that it is available from a range of settings throughout the whole community to which the service is responsible.

8.1.1.5 Primary and secondary care clinicians, managers and commissioners should collaborate to develop local care pathways (see also Section 8.5) that promote access to services for people with common mental health disorders from a range of socially excluded groups including:
- black and minority ethnic groups
- older people
- those in prison or in contact with the criminal justice system
- ex-service personnel.

8.1.1.6    Support access to services and increase the uptake of interventions by:
- ensuring systems are in place to provide for the overall coordination and continuity of care of people with common mental health disorders
- designating a healthcare professional to oversee the whole period of care (usually a GP in primary care settings).

8.1.1.7    Support access to services and increase the uptake of interventions by providing services for people with common mental health disorders in a variety of settings. Use an assessment of local needs as a basis for the structure and distribution of services, which should typically include delivery of:
- assessment and interventions outside normal working hours
- interventions in the person's home or other residential settings
- specialist assessment and interventions in non-traditional community-based settings (for example, community centres and social centres) and where appropriate, in conjunction with staff from those settings
- both generalist and specialist assessment and intervention services in primary care settings.

8.1.1.8    Primary and secondary care clinicians, managers and commissioners should consider a range of support services to facilitate access and uptake of services. These may include providing:
- crèche facilities
- assistance with travel
- advocacy services.

8.1.1.9    Consider modifications to the method and mode of delivery of assessment and treatment interventions and outcome monitoring (based on an assessment of local needs), which may typically include using:
- technology (for example, text messages, email, telephone and computers) for people who may find it difficult to, or choose not to, attend a specific service
- bilingual therapists or independent translators.

8.1.1.10   Be respectful of, and sensitive to, diverse cultural, ethnic and religious backgrounds when working with people with common mental health disorders, and be aware of the possible variations in the presentation of these conditions. Ensure competence in:
- culturally sensitive assessment
- using different explanatory models of common mental health disorders
- addressing cultural and ethnic differences when developing and implementing treatment plans
- working with families from diverse ethnic and cultural backgrounds[53].

---

[53]Adapted from *Depression* (NICE, 2009a).

8.1.1.11 Do not significantly vary the content and structure of assessments or interventions to address specific cultural or ethnic factors (beyond language and the cultural competence of staff), except as part of a formal evaluation of such modifications to an established intervention, as there is little evidence to support significant variations to the content and structure of assessments or interventions.

## 8.2 STEPPED CARE

A stepped-care model (shown below in Figure 12) is used to organise the provision of services and to help people with common mental health disorders, their families, carers and healthcare professionals to choose the most effective interventions. The model presents an integrated overview of the key assessment and treatment interventions from this guideline.

Recommendations focused solely on specialist mental health services are not included (these can be found in related guidance). Recommendation 8.5.1.3 sets out the components of a stepped-care model of service delivery, which should be included in the design of local care pathways for people with common mental health disorders.

## 8.3 STEP 1: IDENTIFICATION AND ASSESSMENT

### 8.3.1 Identification

8.3.1.1 Be alert to possible depression (particularly in people with a past history of depression, possible somatic symptoms of depression or a chronic physical health problem with associated functional impairment) and consider asking people who may have depression two questions, specifically:
- During the last month, have you often been bothered by feeling down, depressed or hopeless?
- During the last month, have you often been bothered by having little interest or pleasure in doing things?
If a person answers 'yes' to either of the above questions consider depression and follow the recommendations for assessment (see Section 8.3.2)[54].

8.3.1.2 Be alert to possible anxiety disorders (particularly in people with a past history of an anxiety disorder, possible somatic symptoms of an anxiety disorder or in those who have experienced a recent traumatic event). Consider asking the person about their feelings of anxiety and their ability to stop or control worry, using the 2-item Generalized Anxiety Disorder scale (GAD-2; see Appendix 13).

---

[54]Adapted from *Depression* (NICE, 2009a).

# Figure 12: Stepped-care model: a combined summary for common mental health disorders

**Focus of the intervention**

**Nature of the intervention**

**Step 3:** Persistent subthreshold depressive symptoms or mild to moderate depression that has not responded to a low-intensity intervention; initial presentation of moderate or severe depression; GAD with marked functional impairment or that has not responded to a low-intensity intervention; moderate to severe panic disorder; OCD with moderate or severe functional impairment; PTSD.

**Depression:** CBT, IPT, behavioural activation, behavioural couples therapy, counselling*, short-term psychodynamic psychotherapy*, antidepressants, combined interventions, collaborative care**, self-help groups.
**GAD:** CBT, applied relaxation, drug treatment, combined interventions, self-help groups.
**Panic disorder:** CBT, antidepressants, self-help groups.
**OCD:** CBT (including ERP), antidepressants, combined interventions and case management, self-help groups.
**PTSD:** Trauma-focused CBT, EMDR, drug treatment.
**All disorders:** Support groups, befriending, rehabilitation programmes, educational and employment support services; referral for further assessment and interventions.

**Step 2:** Persistent subthreshold depressive symptoms or mild to moderate depression; GAD; mild to moderate panic disorder; mild to moderate OCD; PTSD (including people with mild to moderate PTSD).

**Depression:** Individual facilitated self-help, computerised CBT, structured physical activity, group-based peer support (self-help) programmes**, non-directive counselling delivered at home†, antidepressants, self-help groups.
**GAD and panic disorder:** Individual non-facilitated and facilitated self-help, psychoeducational groups, self-help groups.
**OCD:** Individual or group CBT (including ERP), self-help groups.
**PTSD:** Trauma-focused CBT or EMDR.
**All disorders:** Support groups, educational and employment support services; referral for further assessment and interventions.

**Step 1:** All disorders – known and suspected presentations of common mental health disorders.

**All disorders:** Identification, assessment, psychoeducation, active monitoring; referral for further assessment and interventions

* Discuss with the person the uncertainty of the effectiveness of counselling and psychodynamic psychotherapy in treating depression.
** For people with depression and a chronic physical health problem.
† For women during pregnancy or the postnatal period.

- If the person scores three or more on the GAD-2 scale, consider an anxiety disorder and follow the recommendations for assessment (see Section 8.3.2).
- If the person scores less than three on the GAD-2 scale, but you are still concerned they may have an anxiety disorder, ask the following: 'Do you find yourself avoiding places or activities and does this cause you problems?'. If the person answers 'yes' to this question consider an anxiety disorder and follow the recommendations for assessment (see Section 8.3.2).

8.3.1.3    For people with significant language or communication difficulties, for example people with sensory impairments or a learning disability, consider using the Distress Thermometer[55] and/or asking a family member or carer about the person's symptoms to identify a possible common mental health disorder. If a significant level of distress is identified, offer further assessment or seek the advice of a specialist[56].

## 8.3.2    Assessment

8.3.2.1    If the identification questions (see Section 8.3.1) indicate a possible common mental health disorder, but the practitioner is not competent to perform a mental health assessment, refer the person to an appropriate healthcare professional. If this professional is not the person's GP, inform the GP of the referral[56].

8.3.2.2    If the identification questions (see Section 8.3.1) indicate a possible common mental health disorder, a practitioner who is competent to perform a mental health assessment should review the person's mental state and associated functional, interpersonal and social difficulties[56].

8.3.2.3    When assessing a person with a suspected common mental health disorder, consider using:

- a diagnostic or problem identification tool or algorithm, for example, the Improving Access to Psychological Therapies (IAPT) screening prompts tool[57]
- a validated measure relevant to the disorder or problem being assessed, for example, the 9-item Patient Health Questionnaire (PHQ-9), the Hospital Anxiety and Depression Scale (HADS) or the 7-item

---

[55]The Distress Thermometer is a single-item question screen that will identify distress coming from any source. The person places a mark on the scale answering: 'How distressed have you been during the past week on a scale of 0 to 10?' Scores of 4 or more indicate a significant level of distress that should be investigated further. (Roth *et al.*, 1998).

[56]Adapted from *Depression* (NICE, 2009a).

[57]For further information see *The IAPT Data Handbook* (IAPT, 2010; Appendix C, 'IAPT Provisional Diagnosis Screening Prompts', available from www.iapt.nhs.uk/services/measuring-outcomes).

Generalized Anxiety Disorder scale (GAD-7) to inform the assessment and support the evaluation of any intervention.

8.3.2.4  All staff carrying out the assessment of suspected common mental health disorders should be competent to perform an assessment of the presenting problem in line with the service setting in which they work, and be able to:

● determine the nature, duration and severity of the presenting disorder

● take into account not only symptom severity but also the associated functional impairment

● identify appropriate treatment and referral options in line with relevant NICE guidance.

8.3.2.5  All staff carrying out the assessment of common mental health disorders should be competent in:

● relevant verbal and non-verbal communication skills, including the ability to elicit problems, the perception of the problem(s) and their impact, tailoring information, supporting participation in decision-making and discussing treatment options

● the use of formal assessment measures and routine outcome measures in a variety of settings and environments.

8.3.2.6  In addition to assessing symptoms and associated functional impairment, consider how the following factors may have affected the development, course and severity of a person's presenting problem:

● a history of any mental health disorder

● a history of a chronic physical health problem

● any past experience of, and response to, treatments

● the quality of interpersonal relationships

● living conditions and social isolation

● a family history of mental illness

● a history of domestic violence or sexual abuse

● employment and immigration status.

If appropriate, the impact of the presenting problem on the care of children and young people should also be assessed, and if necessary local safeguarding procedures followed[58].

8.3.2.7  When assessing a person with a suspected common mental health disorder, be aware of any learning disabilities or acquired cognitive impairments, and if necessary consider consulting with a relevant specialist when developing treatment plans and strategies[58].

8.3.2.8  If the presentation and history of a common mental health disorder suggest that it may be mild and self-limiting (that is, symptoms are improving) and the disorder is of recent onset, consider providing psychoeducation and active monitoring before offering or referring for further assessment or treatment. These approaches may improve less severe presentations and avoid the need for further interventions.

---

[58]Adapted from *Depression* (NICE, 2009a).

8.3.2.9    Always ask people with a common mental health disorder directly about suicidal ideation and intent. If there is a risk of self-harm or suicide:
- assess whether the person has adequate social support and is aware of sources of help
- arrange help appropriate to the level of risk (see Section 8.3.3)
- advise the person to seek further help if the situation deteriorates[59].

### Antenatal and postnatal mental health

8.3.2.10   During pregnancy or the postnatal period, women requiring psychological interventions should be seen for treatment normally within 1 month of initial assessment, and no longer than 3 months afterwards. This is because of the lower threshold for access to psychological interventions during pregnancy and the postnatal period arising from the changing risk–benefit ratio for psychotropic medication at this time[60].

8.3.2.11   When considering drug treatments for common mental health disorders in women who are pregnant, breastfeeding or planning a pregnancy, consult *Antenatal and Postnatal Mental Health* (NICE, 2007a) for advice on prescribing.

### 8.3.3    Risk assessment and monitoring

8.3.3.1    If a person with a common mental health disorder presents a high risk of suicide or potential harm to others, a risk of significant self-neglect, or severe functional impairment, assess and manage the immediate problem first and then refer to specialist services. Where appropriate inform families and carers.

8.3.3.2    If a person with a common mental health disorder presents considerable and immediate risk to themselves or others, refer them urgently to the emergency services or specialist mental health services[59].

8.3.3.3    If a person with a common mental health disorder, in particular depression, is assessed to be at risk of suicide:
- take into account toxicity in overdose, if a drug is prescribed, and potential interaction with other prescribed medication; if necessary, limit the amount of drug(s) available
- consider increasing the level of support, such as more frequent direct or telephone contacts
- consider referral to specialist mental health services[59].

---

[59]Adapted from *Depression* (NICE, 2009a).
[60]Adapted from *Antenatal and Postnatal Mental Health* (NICE, 2007a).

**8.4      STEPS 2 AND 3: TREATMENT AND REFERRAL FOR TREATMENT**

**8.4.1      Identifying the correct treatment options**

8.4.1.1      When discussing treatment options with a person with a common mental health disorder, consider:
- their past experience of the disorder
- their experience of, and response to, previous treatment
- the trajectory of symptoms
- the diagnosis or problem specification, severity and duration of the problem
- the extent of any associated functional impairment arising from the disorder itself or any chronic physical health problem
- the presence of any social or personal factors that may have a role in the development or maintenance of the disorder
- the presence of any comorbid disorders.

8.4.1.2      When discussing treatment options with a person with a common mental health disorder, provide information about:
- the nature, content and duration of any proposed intervention
- the acceptability and tolerability of any proposed intervention
- possible interactions with any current interventions
- the implications for the continuing provision of any current interventions.

8.4.1.3      When making a referral for the treatment of a common mental health disorder, take account of patient preference when choosing from a range of evidence-based treatments.

8.4.1.4      When offering treatment for a common mental health disorder or making a referral, follow the stepped-care approach, usually offering or referring for the least intrusive, most effective intervention first (see Figure 12).

8.4.1.5      When a person presents with symptoms of anxiety and depression, assess the nature and extent of the symptoms, and if the person has:
- depression that is accompanied by symptoms of anxiety, the first priority should usually be to treat the depressive disorder, in line with the NICE guideline on depression
- an anxiety disorder and comorbid depression or depressive symptoms, consult the NICE guidelines for the relevant anxiety disorder and consider treating the anxiety disorder first
- both anxiety and depressive symptoms, with no formal diagnosis, that are associated with functional impairment, discuss with the person the symptoms to treat first and the choice of intervention[61].

---

[61]Adapted from *Depression* (NICE, 2009a).

8.4.1.6    When a person presents with a common mental health disorder and harmful drinking or alcohol dependence, refer them for treatment of the alcohol misuse first as this may lead to significant improvement in depressive or anxiety symptoms[62].

8.4.1.7    When a person presents with a common mental health disorder and a mild learning disability or mild cognitive impairment:

● where possible provide or refer for the same interventions as for other people with the same common mental health disorder

● if providing interventions, adjust the method of delivery or duration of the assessment or intervention to take account of the disability or impairment[63].

8.4.1.8    When a person presents with a common mental health disorder and has a moderate to severe learning disability or a moderate to severe cognitive impairment, consult a specialist concerning appropriate referral and treatment options.

8.4.1.9    Do not routinely vary the treatment strategies and referral practice for common mental health disorders described in this guideline either by personal characteristics (for example, sex or ethnicity) or by depression subtype (for example, atypical depression or seasonal depression) as there is no convincing evidence to support such action[63].

8.4.1.10   If a person with a common mental health disorder needs social, educational or vocational support, consider:

● informing them about self-help groups (but not for people with PTSD), support groups and other local and national resources

● befriending or a rehabilitation programme for people with long-standing moderate or severe disorders

● educational and employment support services[63].

**8.4.2    Step 2: Treatment and referral advice for subthreshold symptoms and mild to moderate common mental health disorders**

8.4.2.1    For people with persistent subthreshold depressive symptoms or mild to moderate depression, offer or refer for one or more of the following low-intensity interventions:

● individual facilitated self-help based on the principles of cognitive behavioural therapy (CBT)

● computerised CBT

● a structured group physical activity programme

---

[62]Adapted from *Alcohol-use Disorders* (NICE, 2011b).
[63]Adapted from *Depression* (NICE, 2009a).

- a group-based peer support (self-help) programme (for those who also have a chronic physical health problem)
- non-directive counselling delivered at home (listening visits) (for women during pregnancy or the postnatal period)[64].

8.4.2.2 For pregnant women who have subthreshold symptoms of depression and/or anxiety that significantly interfere with personal and social functioning, consider providing or referring for:

- individual brief psychological treatment (four to six sessions), such as interpersonal therapy (IPT) or CBT for women who have had a previous episode of depression or anxiety
- social support during pregnancy and the postnatal period for women who have not had a previous episode of depression or anxiety; such support may consist of regular informal individual or group-based support[65].

8.4.2.3 Do not offer antidepressants routinely for people with persistent subthreshold depressive symptoms or mild depression, but consider them for, or refer for an assessment, people with:

- initial presentation of subthreshold depressive symptoms that have been present for a long period (typically at least 2 years) or
- subthreshold depressive symptoms or mild depression that persist(s) after other interventions or
- a past history of moderate or severe depression or
- mild depression that complicates the care of a physical health problem[66].

8.4.2.4 For people with generalised anxiety disorder that has not improved after psychoeducation and active monitoring, offer or refer for one of the following low-intensity interventions:

- individual non-facilitated self-help
- individual facilitated self-help
- psychoeducational groups[67].

8.4.2.5 For people with mild to moderate panic disorder, offer or refer for one of the following low-intensity interventions:

- individual non-facilitated self-help
- individual facilitated self-help.

8.4.2.6 For people with mild to moderate OCD:

- offer or refer for individual CBT including exposure and response prevention (ERP) of limited duration (typically up to 10 hours), which could be provided using self-help materials or by telephone or

---

[64]Adapted from *Depression* (NICE, 2009a), *Depression in Adults with a Chronic Physical Health Problem* (NICE, 2009b) and *Antenatal and Postnatal Mental Health* (NICE, 2007a).

[65]Adapted from *Antenatal and Postnatal Mental Health* (NICE, 2007a).

[66]Adapted from *Depression* (NICE, 2009a) and *Depression in Adults with a Chronic Physical Health Problem* (NICE, 2009b).

[67]Adapted from *Generalised Anxiety Disorder and Panic Disorder (With or Without Agoraphobia) in Adults* (NICE, 2011a).

- refer for group CBT (including ERP) (note, group formats may deliver more than 10 hours of therapy)[68].

8.4.2.7   For people with PTSD, including those with mild to moderate PTSD, refer for a formal psychological intervention (trauma-focused CBT or eye movement desensitisation and reprocessing [EMDR])[69].

### 8.4.3   Step 3: Treatment and referral advice for persistent subthreshold depressive symptoms or mild to moderate common mental health disorders with inadequate response to initial interventions, or moderate to severe common mental health disorders

If there has been an inadequate response following the delivery of a first-line treatment for persistent subthreshold depressive symptoms or mild to moderate common mental health disorders, a range of psychological, pharmacological or combined interventions may be considered. This section also recommends interventions or provides referral advice for first presentation of moderate to severe common mental health disorders.

8.4.3.1   For people with persistent subthreshold depressive symptoms or mild to moderate depression that has not responded to a low-intensity intervention, offer or refer for:
- antidepressant medication or
- a psychological intervention (CBT, IPT, behavioural activation or behavioural couples therapy)[70].

8.4.3.2   For people with an initial presentation of moderate or severe depression, offer or refer for a psychological intervention (CBT or IPT) in combination with an antidepressant[70].

8.4.3.3   For people with moderate to severe depression and a chronic physical health problem consider referral to collaborative care if there has been no, or only a limited, response to psychological or drug treatment alone or combined in the current or in a past episode[71].

8.4.3.4   For people with depression who decline an antidepressant, CBT, IPT, behavioural activation and behavioural couples therapy, consider providing or referring for:
- counselling for people with persistent subthreshold depressive symptoms or mild to moderate depression
- short-term psychodynamic psychotherapy for people with mild to moderate depression.

---

[68]Adapted from *Obsessive-compulsive Disorder* (NICE, 2005a).
[69]Adapted from *Post-traumatic Stress Disorder* (NICE, 2005b).
[70]Adapted from *Depression* (NICE, 2009a).
[71]Adapted from *Depression in Adults with a Chronic Physical Health Problem* (NICE, 2009b).

Discuss with the person the uncertainty of the effectiveness of counselling and psychodynamic psychotherapy in treating depression[72].

8.4.3.5 For people with generalised anxiety disorder who have marked functional impairment or have not responded to a low-intensity intervention, offer or refer for one of the following:

- CBT or
- applied relaxation or
- if the person prefers, drug treatment[73].

8.4.3.6 For people with moderate to severe panic disorder (with or without agoraphobia), consider referral for:

- CBT or
- an antidepressant if the disorder is long-standing or the person has not benefitted from or has declined psychological interventions[73].

8.4.3.7 For people with OCD and moderate or severe functional impairment, and in particular where there is significant comorbidity with other common mental health disorders, offer or refer for:

- CBT (including ERP) or antidepressant medication for moderate impairment
- CBT (including ERP) combined with antidepressant medication and case management for severe impairment.

Offer home-based treatment where the person is unable or reluctant to attend a clinic or has specific problems (for example, hoarding)[74].

8.4.3.8 For people with long-standing OCD or with symptoms that are severely disabling and restrict their life, consider referral to a specialist mental health service[74].

8.4.3.9 For people with OCD who have not benefitted from two courses of CBT (including ERP) combined with antidepressant medication, refer to a service with specialist expertise in OCD[74].

8.4.3.10 For people with PTSD, offer or refer for a psychological intervention (trauma-focused CBT or EMDR). Do not delay the intervention or referral, particularly for people with severe and escalating symptoms in the first month after the traumatic event[75].

8.4.3.11 For people with PTSD, offer or refer for drug treatment only if a person declines an offer of a psychological intervention or expresses a preference for drug treatment[75].

---

[72]Adapted from *Depression* (NICE, 2009a).

[73]Adapted from *Generalised Anxiety Disorder and Panic Disorder (With or Without Agoraphobia) in Adults* (NICE, 2011a).

[74]Adapted from *Obsessive-compulsive Disorder* (NICE, 2005a).

[75]Adapted from *Post-traumatic Stress Disorder* (NICE, 2006b).

**8.4.4      Treatment and referral advice to help prevent relapse**

8.4.4.1    For people with a common mental health disorder who are at significant risk of relapse or have a history of recurrent problems, discuss with the person the treatments that might reduce the risk of recurrence. The choice of treatment or referral for treatment should be informed by the response to previous treatment, including residual symptoms, the consequences of relapse, any discontinuation symptoms when stopping medication, and the person's preference.

8.4.4.2    For people with a previous history of depression who are currently well and who are considered at risk of relapse despite taking antidepressant medication, or those who are unable to continue or choose not to continue antidepressant medication, offer or refer for one of the following:
- individual CBT
- mindfulness-based cognitive therapy (for those who have had three or more episodes)[76].

8.4.4.3    For people who have had previous treatment for depression but continue to have residual depressive symptoms, offer or refer for one of the following:
- individual CBT
- mindfulness-based cognitive therapy (for those who have had three or more episodes)[76].

**8.5       DEVELOPING LOCAL CARE PATHWAYS**

8.5.1.1    Local care pathways should be developed to promote implementation of key principles of good care. Pathways should be:
- negotiable, workable and understandable for people with common mental health disorders, their families and carers, and professionals
- accessible and acceptable to all people in need of the services served by the pathway
- responsive to the needs of people with common mental health disorders and their families and carers
- integrated so that there are no barriers to movement between different levels of the pathway
- outcomes focused (including measures of quality, service-user experience and harm).

8.5.1.2    Responsibility for the development, management and evaluation of local care pathways should lie with a designated leadership team, which should

---

[76]Adapted from *Depression* (NICE, 2009a).

include primary and secondary care clinicians, managers and commissioners. The leadership team should have particular responsibility for:

- developing clear policy and protocols for the operation of the pathway
- providing training and support on the operation of the pathway
- auditing and reviewing the performance of the pathway.

8.5.1.3     Primary and secondary care clinicians, managers and commissioners should work together to design local care pathways that promote a stepped-care model of service delivery that:

- provides the least intrusive, most effective intervention first
- has clear and explicit criteria for the thresholds determining access to and movement between the different levels of the pathway
- does not use single criteria such as symptom severity to determine movement between steps
- monitors progress and outcomes to ensure the most effective interventions are delivered and the person moves to a higher step if needed.

8.5.1.4     Primary and secondary care clinicians, managers and commissioners should work together to design local care pathways that promote a range of evidence-based interventions at each step in the pathway and support people with common mental health disorders in their choice of interventions.

8.5.1.5     All staff should ensure effective engagement with families and carers, where appropriate, to:

- inform and improve the care of the person with a common mental health disorder
- meet the identified needs of the families and carers.

8.5.1.6     Primary and secondary care clinicians, managers and commissioners should work together to design local care pathways that promote the active engagement of all populations served by the pathway. Pathways should:

- offer prompt assessments and interventions that are appropriately adapted to the cultural, gender, age and communication needs of people with common mental health disorders
- keep to a minimum the number of assessments needed to access interventions.

8.5.1.7     Primary and secondary care clinicians, managers and commissioners should work together to design local care pathways that respond promptly and effectively to the changing needs of all populations served by the pathways. Pathways should have in place:

- clear and agreed goals for the services offered to a person with a common mental health disorder
- robust and effective means for measuring and evaluating the outcomes associated with the agreed goals
- clear and agreed mechanisms for responding promptly to identified changes to the person's needs.

8.5.1.8     Primary and secondary care clinicians, managers and commissioners should work together to design local care pathways that provide an integrated programme of care across both primary and secondary care services. Pathways should:

- minimise the need for transition between different services or providers
- allow services to be built around the pathway and not the pathway around the services
- establish clear links (including access and entry points) to other care pathways (including those for physical healthcare needs)
- have designated staff who are responsible for the coordination of people's engagement with the pathway.

8.5.1.9 Primary and secondary care clinicians, managers and commissioners should work together to ensure effective communication about the functioning of the local care pathway. There should be protocols for:

- sharing and communicating information with people with common mental health disorders, and where appropriate families and carers, about their care
- sharing and communicating information about the care of service users with other professionals (including GPs)
- communicating information between the services provided within the pathway
- communicating information to services outside the pathway.

8.5.1.10 Primary and secondary care clinicians, managers and commissioners should work together to design local care pathways that have robust systems for outcome measurement in place, which should be used to inform all involved in a pathway about its effectiveness. This should include providing:

- individual routine outcome measurement systems
- effective electronic systems for the routine reporting and aggregation of outcome measures
- effective systems for the audit and review of the overall clinical and cost-effectiveness of the pathway.

# 9    APPENDICES

Appendix 1: Scope for the development of the clinical guideline          231

Appendix 2: Declarations of interests by Guideline Development
Group members                                                           236

Appendix 3: Stakeholders and experts who submitted comments in
response to the consultation draft of the guideline                     246

Appendix 4: Analytic framework and review questions                     247

Appendix 5: Review protocols                                            On CD

Appendix 6: Search strategies for the identification of clinical studies  On CD

Appendix 7: Methodology checklists for clinical studies and reviews     On CD

Appendix 8: Search strategies for the identification of health
economics evidence                                                      On CD

Appendix 9: Methodology checklists for economic studies                 256

Appendix 10: Evidence tables for economic studies                       270

Appendix 11: High priority research recommendations                     272

Appendix 12: Completed methodology checklists for economic studies      On CD

Appendix 13: GAD-2 questionnaire                                        276

Appendix 14: Clinical study characteristics tables                      On CD

# APPENDIX 1:

# SCOPE FOR THE DEVELOPMENT OF THE

# CLINICAL GUIDELINE

*Final version*
December 2009

## 1 GUIDELINE TITLE

Common mental health disorders: identification and pathways to care

### 1.1 SHORT TITLE

Common mental health disorders.

## 2 THE REMIT

Following the decision to update NICE clinical guideline 22, 'Anxiety', and NICE clinical guideline 23, 'Depression' NICE has asked the National Collaborating Centre for Mental Health to develop a guideline on the identification and recognition of, and referral advice for, depression and anxiety in primary care.

## 3 CLINICAL NEED FOR THE GUIDELINE

### 3.1 EPIDEMIOLOGY

a)  Depression and anxiety disorders are common and may affect up to 15% of the UK population over the course of a year. Depression and anxiety disorders (panic disorder, generalised anxiety disorder, obsessive-compulsive disorder, social phobia, post-traumatic stress disorder) vary considerably in their severity but all conditions may be associated with significant long-term disability and have significant impact on a person's social and personal functioning. For example, the World Health Organization estimates that depression will be the second greatest contributor to disability-adjusted life years throughout the world by the year 2020. Depression is also associated with high levels of morbidity and also with high mortality, and is the most common disorder contributing to suicide. The presence of a depressive disorder is also associated with a higher incidence of morbidity and mortality in a range of physical disorders including cardiovascular disease.

b) The prevalence of individual disorders varies considerably. In the 2007 UK Psychiatric Morbidity Survey, the 1-week prevalence was 4.4% for generalised anxiety disorder, 3.0% for PTSD, 2.3% for depression, 1.4% for phobia, 1.1% for panic disorder and 1.1% for obsessive compulsive disorder.

c) For many people the onset of these disorders occurs in adolescence or early adult life, but the disorders can affect people at any point in their life (for example in PTSD the onset of the disorder relates to specific traumatic events). Earlier onset is generally associated with poorer outcomes.

d) Depressive disorders often have a relapsing and remitting course, which may be lifelong. Many anxiety disorders have a chronic course. This chronic course may be associated with a considerable delay in presenting to services, with consequent significant personal, occupational and social impairment and possible negative consequences for their physical health.

e) Depressive and anxiety disorders are common in both men and women but tend to have a higher prevalence in women. Some ethnic groups also have a higher incidence of common mental disorders and depression is more common in those with chronic physical health problems. Common mental disorders may present in combination. For example, up to 50% of depressive disorders will be accompanied with comorbid anxiety disorders or significant anxiety symptoms.

## 3.2    CURRENT PRACTICE

a) The vast majority of depression and anxiety disorders (up to 90%) are treated in primary care. Relatively few (typically the more severe depressive and anxiety disorders) go forward to treatment in secondary care.

b) Many people do not seek treatment, and both anxiety and depression are often undiagnosed. Recognition of anxiety disorders by GPs is often poor, and only a small minority of people who experience anxiety disorders actually receive treatment. For example, it is likely only 30% of people presenting with depressive disorder are diagnosed and offered treatment. This is a source of concern, although it is probably more the case for mild rather than more severe disorders. The problem of under-recognition for anxiety disorders has recently been highlighted by evidence that the prevalence of PTSD is significantly under-recognised in primary care. In part this may stem from GPs not recognising the disorder, and the lack of clearly defined care pathways. But from a patient's perspective, stigma and avoidance may also contribute to under-recognition. Pessimism about possible treatment outcomes may further contribute to this.

c) In primary care these disorders are mainly treated with psychotropic medication. Psychological interventions are generally preferred by patients but there is limited availability of these interventions in primary care. However, recent developments in the Improving Access to Psychological Therapies programme have begun to address this issue.

## 4 THE GUIDELINE

The guideline development process is described in detail on the NICE website (see Section 6, 'Further information').

This scope defines what the guideline will (and will not) examine, and what the guideline developers will consider.

The areas that will be addressed by the guideline are described in the following sections.

### 4.1 POPULATION

#### 4.1.1 Groups that will be covered

a) Adults (18 years and older) with common mental health disorders, that is:
  - depression (including subthreshold disorders)
  - anxiety disorders (including generalised anxiety disorder, panic disorder, social anxiety, obsessive compulsive disorder and post-traumatic stress disorder)
  - Comorbid presentations of anxiety and depression will be covered, but subthreshold mixed anxiety and depression will not.

#### 4.1.2 Groups that will not be covered

a) Adults with:
  - psychotic and related disorders (including schizophrenia and bipolar disorder)
  - those for whom drug and alcohol misuse are the primary problem
  - those for whom eating disorders are the primary problem
b) Children and young people (17 years and younger).

### 4.2 HEALTHCARE SETTING

a) The guideline will focus on identification and assessment in primary care settings, but will also be applicable to community services funded and provided by the NHS and secondary care acute medical settings.
b) The guideline will not provide specific recommendations for prison medical services but it will be relevant to their work.

### 4.3 CLINICAL MANAGEMENT

#### 4.3.1 Key clinical issues that will be covered

a) Identification and recognition of the full range of depression and anxiety disorders (including the tools used in this area).

b) Assessment of anxiety and depressive disorders, including assessment systems that have been tested and validated for the relevant disorders.
c) Systems for improving access to and uptake of mental health services for common mental disorders.
d) Systems (such as stepped care and triage) for organising and developing care pathways.

### 4.3.2    Clinical issues that will not be covered

a) Population based screening for common mental health disorders.
b) Evidence for the efficacy of treatment interventions.

### 4.4    MAIN OUTCOMES

a) Diagnostic accuracy (sensitivity, specificity, positive predictive. value, negative predictive value, area under the curve) of identification tools.
b) Percentage of people receiving appropriate treatment.
c) The proportion of people from groups identified as having a greater incidence of unidentified disorders (for example, people from ethnic minorities) is in line with epidemiological data for the prevalence of the disorder in those groups.
d) Measures of efficiency (for example, reduced waiting times for appropriate treatment) and cost-effectiveness.

### 4.5    ECONOMIC ASPECTS

Developers will take into account cost effectiveness when making recommendations involving a choice between alternative interventions. A review of the economic evidence will be conducted and analyses will be carried out as appropriate. The preferred unit of effectiveness is the quality-adjusted life year (QALY), and the costs considered will usually be only from an NHS and personal social services (PSS) perspective. Further details on the methods can be found in 'The guidelines manual' (see section 6).

### 4.6    STATUS

### 4.6.1    Scope

This is the final scope

### 4.6.2    Timing

The development of the guideline recommendations will begin in December 2009.

# 5 RELATED NICE GUIDANCE

## 5.1 PUBLISHED GUIDANCE

### 5.1.1 NICE guidance to be incorporated

- *Post-traumatic Stress Disorder* (PTSD). NICE Clinical Guideline 26 (2005). Available at: www.nice.org.uk/CG26.
- *Obsessive-compulsive Disorder.* NICE Clinical Guideline 31 (2005). Available at: www.nice.org.uk/CG31.
- *Depression.* NICE Clinical Guideline 90 (2009). Available at: www.nice.org.uk/ CG90.
- *Depression in Adults with a Chronic Physical Health Problem.* NICE Clinical Guideline 91 (2009). Available at: www.nice.org.uk/CG91.

## 5.2 GUIDANCE UNDER DEVELOPMENT

NICE is currently developing the following guidance, which will be incorporated into this guideline (details available from the NICE website).
- *Anxiety* (partial update of NICE Clinical Guideline 22). NICE Clinical Guideline. Publication expected January 2011.[77]

# 6 FURTHER INFORMATION

Information on the guideline development process is provided in:
- 'How NICE clinical guidelines are developed: an overview for stakeholders, the public and the NHS' (Appendix O, *The Guidelines Manual*)
- *The Guidelines Manual.*
  These are available from the NICE website (www.nice.org.uk/guidelinesmanual). Information on the progress of the guideline will also be available from the NICE website (www.nice.org.uk).

---

[77]This guideline was subsequently published as *Generalised Anxiety Disorder and Panic Disorder (With or Without Agoraphobia) in Adults* (NICE, 2011a).

# APPENDIX 2:

# DECLARATIONS OF INTERESTS BY GUIDELINE DEVELOPMENT GROUP MEMBERS

With a range of practical experience relevant to common mental health disorders in the GDG, members were appointed because of their understanding and expertise in healthcare for people with common mental health disorders and support for their families and carers, including: scientific issues; health research; the delivery and receipt of healthcare, along with the work of the healthcare industry; and the role of professional organisations and organisations for people with common mental health disorders and their families and carers.

To minimise and manage any potential conflicts of interest, and to avoid any public concern that commercial or other financial interests have affected the work of the GDG and influenced guidance, members of the GDG must declare as a matter of public record any interests held by themselves or their families which fall under specified categories (see below). These categories include any relationships they have with the healthcare industries, professional organisations and organisations for people with common mental health disorders and their families and carers.

Individuals invited to join the GDG were asked to declare their interests before being appointed. To allow the management of any potential conflicts of interest that might arise during the development of the guideline, GDG members were also asked to declare their interests at each GDG meeting throughout the guideline development process. The interests of all the members of the GDG are listed below, including interests declared prior to appointment and during the guideline development process.

## CATEGORIES OF INTEREST

- Paid employment
- Personal pecuniary interest: financial payments or other benefits from either the manufacturer or the owner of a product or service under consideration in this guideline, or the industry or sector from which the product or service comes. This includes: holding a directorship, or other paid position; carrying out consultancy or fee paid work; having shareholdings or other beneficial interests; receiving expenses and hospitality over and above what would be reasonably expected to attend meetings and conferences.
- Personal family interest: financial payments or other benefits from the healthcare industry that were received by a member of the GDG member's family.
- Non-personal pecuniary interest: financial payments or other benefits received by the GDG member's organisation or department, but where the GDG member has not personally received payment, including fellowships and other support

236

provided by the healthcare industry. This includes a grant or fellowship or other payment to sponsor a post, or contribute to the running costs of the department; commissioning of research or other work; contracts with, or grants from, NICE.

Personal non-pecuniary interest: these include, but are not limited to, clear opinions or public statements you have made about common mental health disorders, holding office in a professional organisation or advocacy group with a direct interest in common mental health disorders, other reputational risks relevant to common mental health disorders.

| Declarations of interest - GDG | |
|---|---|
| **Professor Tony Kendrick - Chair, Guideline Development Group** | |
| Employment | Professor of Primary Care and Dean, York Medical School, University of Hull (from September 2010). Associate Dean for Clinical Research Professor of Primary Medical Care University of Southampton (until August 2010). |
| Personal pecuniary interest | None |
| Personal family interest | None |
| Non-personal pecuniary interest | In receipt of a grant to look at patient and practitioner views of depression questionnaires and a grant to look at prediction of response to low intensity interventions. Has had some involvement with a trial of stepped and matched care. |
| Personal non-pecuniary interest | GP whose practice may be affected by the guideline. Chaired an expert advisory group which recommended screening for depression in diabetes and heart disease, and the use of severity questionnaire measures, in the GP contract QOF. GP and researcher in the field of common mental health disorders in primary care. Guideline recommendations will apply to his practice and may apply to his research. Co-editor of *British Journal of Psychiatry* article on a review of the Depression guideline. |
| Actions taken | None |

| Mr Mike Bessant | |
|---|---|
| Employment | Mental Health Nurse, Regional Mental Health Lead, Bristol |
| Personal pecuniary interest | None |
| Personal family interest | None |
| Non-personal pecuniary interest | None |
| Personal non-pecuniary interest | None |
| Actions taken | None |
| **Ms Mary Burd** | |
| Employment | Head of Psychology and Counselling, Tower Hamlets Primary Care Trust |
| Personal pecuniary interest | None |
| Personal family interest | None |
| Non-personal pecuniary interest | None |
| Personal non-pecuniary interest | Work in primary care. |
| Actions taken | None |
| **Dr Alan Cohen** | |
| Employment | Director of Primary Care, West London Mental Health Trust; National Primary Care Advisor, IAPT, Department of Health |
| Personal pecuniary interest | None |
| Personal family interest | None |
| Non-personal pecuniary interest | None |
| Personal non-pecuniary interest | None |
| Actions taken | None |
| **Dr Barbara Compitus** | |
| Employment | General Practitioner, Southville |
| Personal pecuniary interest | None |
| Personal family interest | None |
| Non-personal pecuniary interest | None |

| Personal non-pecuniary interest | None |
|---|---|
| Actions taken | None |

| **Ms Lillian Dimas** | |
|---|---|
| Employment | Service User/Carer Representative. |
| Personal pecuniary interest | None |
| Personal family interest | None |
| Non-personal pecuniary interest | None |
| Personal non-pecuniary interest | None |
| Actions taken | None |

| **Mr David Ekers** | |
|---|---|
| Employment | Nurse Consultant, Primary Care Mental Health, Tees, Esk and Wear Valleys NHS Foundation Trust; Honorary Clinical Lecturer, Centre for Mental Health Research, Durham University |
| Personal pecuniary interest | None |
| Personal family interest | None |
| Non-personal pecuniary interest | None |
| Personal non-pecuniary interest | Working at Tees, Esk and Wear Valleys NHS Foundation Trust and will be looking at implementation of findings.<br>Member of Mental Health Research Centre at Durham University – may link to potential research applications. |
| Actions taken | None |

| **Professor Linda Gask** | |
|---|---|
| Employment | Professor of Primary Care Psychiatry, University of Manchester; Honorary Consultant Psychiatrist, Salford Primary Care Trust |
| Personal pecuniary interest | None |
| Personal family interest | None |
| Non-personal pecuniary interest | Has had some involvement with a trial of stepped and matched care |

| Personal non-pecuniary interest | Has carried out research relating to, and expressed opinions in writing about, the topic of this guideline.<br>Carrying out work on classification of disorders for ICD-11, in primary care.<br>Carrying out work on responses to low-intensity interventions in primary care, for ICD-11. |
|---|---|
| Actions taken | None |
| **Professor Simon Gilbody** | |
| Employment | Professor of Psychological Medicine and Health Services, University of York |
| Personal pecuniary interest | None |
| Personal family interest | None |
| Non-personal pecuniary interest | Undertaking research into stepped, matched and stratified care. |
| Personal non-pecuniary interest | None |
| Actions taken | None |
| **Mr Terence Lewis** | |
| Employment | Service User/Carer Representative |
| Personal pecuniary interest | None |
| Personal family interest | None |
| Non-personal pecuniary interest | None |
| Personal non-pecuniary interest | None |
| Actions taken | None |
| **Mr Francesco Palma** | |
| Employment | Service User/Carer Representative |
| Personal pecuniary interest | None |
| Personal family interest | None |
| Non-personal pecuniary interest | None |
| Personal non-pecuniary interest | None |
| Actions taken | None |
| | None |

| Dr Matthew Ridd | |
|---|---|
| Employment | General Practitioner, Portishead; Clinical Lecturer, National Institute for Health Research, Bristol |
| Personal pecuniary interest | None |
| Personal family interest | None |
| Non-personal pecuniary interest | None |
| Personal non-pecuniary interest | GP clinical practice mat be affected by the outcomes of the GDG. As a researcher, may wish to take up some of the research areas identified by the GDG. |
| Actions taken | None |
| **Professor Roz Shafran** | |
| Employment | Professor of Psychology, School of Psychology and Clinical Language Sciences, University of Reading |
| Personal pecuniary interest | None |
| Personal family interest | None |
| Non-personal pecuniary interest | Has been commissioned by South Central Strategic Health Authority to develop five modular training sessions to be delivered by IAPT workers to primary care staff, which include modules on the detection of anxiety and depression in primary care, and the application of 'guided' self-help and behavioural activation. |
| Personal non-pecuniary interest | An interest in training clinicians to deliver NICE guidelines via the Charlie Waller Institute of Evidence-based Psychological treatment. Conducts research in mental health problems, especially OCD. Has been commissioned by South Central Strategic Health Authority to develop five modular training sessions to be delivered by IAPT workers to primary care staff, which include modules on the detection of anxiety |

| | |
|---|---|
| | and depression in primary care, and the application of 'guided' self-help and behavioural activation. (January 2011) |
| Actions taken | None |
| **Mr Rupert Suckling** | |
| Employment | Deputy Director of Public Health; Consultant in Public Health Medicine, Doncaster Primary Care Trust |
| Personal pecuniary interest | None |
| Personal family interest | None |
| Non-personal pecuniary interest | None |
| Personal non-pecuniary interest | Employee of NHS Doncaster and a member of the Faculty of Public Health's Mental Health Committee. Was involved and led the local evaluation of the Doncaster IAPT National Demonstration site. Has published research on Doncaster IAPT programme. Future research interests may coincide. |
| Actions taken | None |

*NCCMH staff*

| **Professor Stephen Pilling – Facilitator, Guideline Development Group** | |
|---|---|
| Employment | Director, NCCMH. Professor of Clinical Psychology and Clinical Effectiveness, University College London Director, Centre for Outcomes Research and Effectiveness, University College London |
| Personal pecuniary interest | Funding of £1,200,000 per annum from NICE to develop clinical guidelines. Funding from British Psychological Society (2005–2011) £6,100,000 to establish the Clinical Effectiveness Programme at Centre for Outcomes Research and Effectiveness, University College London; with Professor P. Fonagy and Professor S. Michie. |

| Personal family interest | None |
|---|---|
| Non-personal pecuniary interest | RCT to evaluate multi-systemic therapy with Professor Peter Fonagy; Department of Health funding of £1,000,000 (2008 to 2012).<br>RCT to evaluate collaborative care for depression; with Professor D Richards; Medical Research Council Funding of £2,200,000 (2008 to 2012).<br>Developing a UK Evidence Base for Contingency Management in Addiction with Professor J. Strang;<br>National Institute of Health Research Grant of £2,035,042 (2009 to 2013). |
| Personal non-pecuniary interest | None |
| Actions taken | None |
| **Ms Beth Dumonteil** | |
| Employment | Project Manager and Centre Administrator, NCCMH (September 2009 to February 2010) |
| Personal pecuniary interest | None |
| Personal family interest | None |
| Non-personal pecuniary interest | None |
| Personal non-pecuniary interest | None |
| Actions taken | None |
| **Ms Laura Gibbon** | |
| Employment | Project Manager, NCCMH (from September 2010) |
| Personal pecuniary interest | None |
| Personal family interest | None |
| Non-personal pecuniary interest | None |
| Personal non-pecuniary interest | None |
| Actions taken | None |
| **Ms Flora Kaminski** | |
| Employment | Research Assistant, NCCMH |
| Personal pecuniary interest | None |

| Personal family interest | None |
|---|---|
| Non-personal pecuniary interest | None |
| Personal non-pecuniary interest | None |
| Actions taken | None |
| **Dr Dimitra Lambrelli** | |
| Employment | Health Economist, NCCMH |
| Personal pecuniary interest | None |
| Personal family interest | None |
| Non-personal pecuniary interest | None |
| Personal non-pecuniary interest | None |
| Actions taken | None |
| **Ms Caroline Salter** | |
| Employment | Research Assistant, NCCMH |
| Personal pecuniary interest | None |
| Personal family interest | None |
| Non-personal pecuniary interest | None |
| Personal non-pecuniary interest | None |
| Actions taken | None |
| **Ms Christine Sealey** | |
| Employment | Head of NCCMH |
| Personal pecuniary interest | None |
| Personal family interest | None |
| Non-personal pecuniary interest | None |
| Personal non-pecuniary interest | None |
| Actions taken | None |
| **Ms Melinda Smith** | |
| Employment | Research Assistant, NCCMH |
| Personal pecuniary interest | None |
| Personal family interest | None |
| Non-personal pecuniary interest | None |

| Personal non-pecuniary interest | None |
|---|---|
| Actions taken | None |

| **Ms Sarah Stockton** | |
|---|---|
| Employment | Senior Information Scientist, NCCMH |
| Personal pecuniary interest | None |
| Personal family interest | None |
| Non-personal pecuniary interest | None |
| Personal non-pecuniary intercst | None |
| Actions taken | None |

| **Dr Clare Taylor** | |
|---|---|
| Employment | Senior Editor, NCCMH |
| Personal pecuniary interest | None |
| Personal family interest | None |
| Non-personal pecuniary interest | None |
| Personal non-pecuniary interest | None |
| Actions taken | None |

| **Dr Amina Yesufu-Udechuku** | |
|---|---|
| Employment | Systematic Reviewer, NCCMH |
| Personal pecuniary interest | None |
| Personal family interest | None |
| Non-personal pecuniary interest | None |
| Personal non-pecuniary interest | None |
| Actions taken | None |

| **Dr Craig Whittington** | |
|---|---|
| Employment | Senior Systematic Reviewer, NCCMH |
| Personal pecuniary interest | None |
| Personal family interest | None |
| Non-personal pecuniary interest | None |
| Personal non-pecuniary interest | None |
| Actions taken | None |

# APPENDIX 3:

# STAKEHOLDERS AND EXPERTS WHO SUBMITTED COMMENTS IN RESPONSE TO THE CONSULTATION DRAFT OF THE GUIDELINE

Anxiety UK
Association for Family Therapy and Systemic Practice in the UK (AFT)
British Association for Counselling and Psychotherapy
British Association for Psychopharmacology
British Psychological Society, The
Connecting for Health
Department for Education
Department for Work and Pensions
Department of Health
Humber NHS Foundation Trust
Lilly UK
Ministry of Defence (MoD)
National Treatment Agency for Substance Misuse
NIHR (National Institute for Health Research) Evaluation, Trials and Studies Coordinating Centre
NHS Direct
Pfizer Limited
Princess Royal Trust for Carers, The
Ridgeway Partnership
Royal College of General Practitioners
Royal College of Nursing
Royal College of Psychiatrists
Royal Pharmaceutical Society of Great Britain
Ultrasis Ltd
United Kingdom Council of Psychotherapists
Whitstone Head Educational (Charitable) Trust Ltd

# APPENDIX 4:
# ANALYTIC FRAMEWORK AND
# REVIEW QUESTIONS

## INTRODUCTION

Review questions typically fall into one of three main areas:
1. Intervention
2. Diagnosis
   a. Test accuracy
   b. Clinical value
3. Prognosis

Patient experience is a component of each of these and should inform the development of a structured review question. In addition, review questions that focus on a specific element of patient experience may merit consideration in their own right.

An analytic framework (to frame the questions, rather than the clinical pathway) and associated review questions should be developed for each topic area. For most review questions, we use the PICO format (see below).

## PICO format

| Patients/population: | Which patients or populations of patients are we interested in? How can they be best described? Are there subgroups that need to be considered? Can diagnosis be refined? |
|---|---|
| Intervention: | Which intervention, treatment or approach should be used? |
| Comparison: | What is/are the main alternative/s to compare with the intervention being considered? |
| Outcome: | What is really important for the patient? Which outcomes should be considered? |

**Access/identification/assessment/systems for organising and developing local care pathways**

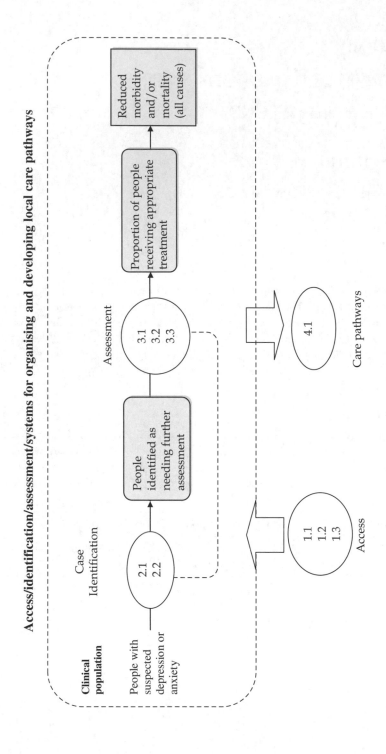

**Access to healthcare**

| No. | Primary review questions |
|---|---|
| 1.1 | In adults (18 years and older) at risk of depression or anxiety disorders* (in particular BME groups and older people), what factors prevent people accessing mental healthcare services? |
| Subquestions | • What factors, or attributes of the individual who requires mental healthcare, can inhibit access to services?<br>• What practitioner-level factors or attributes can inhibit an individual from accessing healthcare?<br>• Do systems and processes utilised in mental healthcare services inhibit access to healthcare?<br>• What practical or resource-based factors inhibit access to mental healthcare services? |
| 1.2 | In adults (18 years and older) at risk of depression or anxiety disorders* (in particular older people and people from ethnic minorities), do changes to specific models of service delivery (that is, community based outreach clinics, clinics or services in non-health settings), increase the proportion of people from the target group who access treatment, when compared with standard care? |
| Subquestions | • Do adaptations to existing services improve access to mental healthcare for all individuals?<br>• Do adaptations improve access to mental healthcare for vulnerable groups (for example, older people, BME groups)? |
| 1.3 | In adults (18 years and older) at risk of depression or anxiety disorders* (in particular, older people and people from ethnic minorities), do service developments which are specifically designed to promote access, increase the proportion of people from the target group who access treatment, when compared with standard care? |
| Subquestions | • Do new service developments targeted at changing the behaviour of the individual or the practitioner improve access to healthcare services?<br>• Do service developments targeted at the healthcare system improve access to healthcare services?<br>• Do specific treatments or interventions developed for vulnerable groups improve access to healthcare services? |
| *Including GAD, panic disorder, social anxiety disorder, OCD, specific phobias and PTSD. | |

**Case identification**

| No. | Primary review questions |
|-----|--------------------------|
| 2.1 | In adults (18 years and older) with suspected depression (including subthreshold disorders) at first point of contact, what identification tools when compared with a gold standard diagnosis (based on DSM or ICD criteria) improve identification (that is, sensitivity, specificity, positive likelihood ratio, negative likelihood ratio, diagnostic OR) of people with depression (including subthreshold disorders)? |
| 2.2 | In adults (18 years and older) with a suspected anxiety disorder at first point of contact, what ultra-brief identification tools (one to three items) when compared with a gold standard diagnosis (based on DSM or ICD criteria) improve identification (that is, sensitivity, specificity, positive likelihood ratio, negative likelihood ratio, diagnostic OR) of people with an anxiety disorder? |
| 2.3 | In adults (18 years and older) with a suspected anxiety disorder at first point of contact, what longer identification tools (four to 12 items) when compared with a gold standard diagnosis (based on DSM or ICD criteria) improve identification (that is, sensitivity, specificity, positive likelihood ratio, negative likelihood ratio, diagnostic OR) of people with an anxiety disorder? |

**Assessment**

| No. | Primary review questions |
|-----|--------------------------|
| 3.1 | In adults (18 years and older) identified with depression (including subthreshold disorders) or an anxiety disorder*, what is the clinical utility of more formal assessments of the nature and severity of the common mental health disorder (including problem specification or diagnosis) when compared another management strategy? |
| 3.2 | In adults (18 years and older) identified with depression (including subthreshold disorders) or an anxiety disorder*, what is the definition, delivery and value (or otherwise) of risk assessment? |
| 3.3 | In adults (18 years and older) identified with depression (including subthreshold disorders) or an anxiety disorder*, what factors predict treatment response and/or treatment failure? |
| 3.4 | In adults (18 years and older) identified with depression (including subthreshold disorders) or an anxiety disorder*, should ROM be used, and if so, what systems are effective for the delivery of ROM and use within clinical decision making? |
| *Including GAD, panic disorder, social anxiety disorder, OCD, specific phobias and PTSD. | |

**Systems for organising and developing local care pathways**

| No. | Primary review questions |
| --- | --- |
| 4.1 | In adults (18 years and older) with depression (including subthreshold disorders) or an anxiety disorder*, what are the specific components of a good care pathway? |
| *Including GAD, panic disorder, social anxiety disorder, OCD, specific phobias and PTSD. | |

# APPENDIX 5:
# REVIEW PROTOCOLS

The completed forms can be found on the CD accompanying this guideline.

# APPENDIX 6:
# SEARCH STRATEGIES FOR THE IDENTIFICATION
# OF CLINICAL STUDIES

The completed forms can be found on the CD accompanying this guideline.

# APPENDIX 7:
# METHODOLOGY CHECKLISTS FOR CLINICAL STUDIES AND REVIEWS

The completed forms can be found on the CD accompanying this guideline.

# APPENDIX 8:
# SEARCH STRATEGIES FOR THE IDENTIFICATION
# OF HEALTH ECONOMICS EVIDENCE

The completed forms can be found on the CD accompanying this guideline.

# APPENDIX 9:
# METHODOLOGY CHECKLISTS FOR
# ECONOMIC STUDIES

| Study identification |
|---|
| **Study identification**<br>*Including author, title, reference, year of publication* |

| | | |
|---|---|---|
| **Guideline topic:** | | **Question no:** |
| **Checklist completed by:** | | |

| **Section 1: Applicability (relevance to specific guideline review question(s) and the NICE reference case). This checklist should be used first to filter out irrelevant studies.** | **Yes/Partly/ No/Unclear/ NA** | **Comments** |
|---|---|---|
| 1.1 | Is the study population appropriate for the guideline? | | |
| 1.2 | Are the interventions appropriate for the guideline? | | |
| 1.3 | Is the healthcare system in which the study was conducted sufficiently similar to the current UK NHS context? | | |
| 1.4 | Are costs measured from the NHS and personal social services (PSS) perspective? | | |
| 1.5 | Are all direct health effects on individuals included? | | |
| 1.6 | Are both costs and health effects discounted at an annual rate of 3.5%? | | |
| 1.7 | Is the value of health effects expressed in terms of quality-adjusted life years (QALYs)? | | |
| 1.8 | Are changes in health-related quality of life (HRQoL) reported directly from patients and/or carers? | | |

| 1.9 | Is the valuation of changes in HRQoL (utilities) obtained from a representative sample of the general public? | |
|---|---|---|
| 1.10 | Overall judgement: Directly applicable/Partially applicable/Not applicable<br>There is no need to use section 2 of the checklist if the study is considered 'not applicable'. | |
| Other comments: | | |

| Section 2: Study limitations (the level of methodological quality) This checklist should be used once it has been decided that the study is sufficiently applicable to the context of the clinical guideline. | | Yes/ Partly/ No/ Unclear/ NA | Comments |
|---|---|---|---|
| 2.1 | Does the model structure adequately reflect the nature of the health condition under evaluation? | | |
| 2.2 | Is the time horizon sufficiently long to reflect all important differences in costs and outcomes? | | |
| 2.3 | Are all important and relevant health outcomes included? | | |
| 2.4 | Are the estimates of baseline health outcomes from the best available source? | | |
| 2.5 | Are the estimates of relative treatment effects from the best available source? | | |
| 2.6 | Are all important and relevant costs included? | | |
| 2.7 | Are the estimates of resource use from the best available source? | | |
| 2.8 | Are the unit costs of resources from the best available source? | | |
| 2.9 | Is an appropriate incremental analysis presented or can it be calculated from the data? | | |

| 2.10 | Are all important parameters whose values are uncertain subjected to appropriate sensitivity analysis? | | |
|------|----------------------------------------------------|---|---|
| 2.11 | Is there no potential conflict of interest? | | |
| 2.12 | Overall assessment: Minor limitations/ Potentially serious limitations/Very serious limitations | | |
| Other comments: | | | |

**Notes on use of methodology checklist: economic evaluations**

For all questions:

● answer 'yes' if the study fully meets the criterion

● answer 'partly' if the study largely meets the criterion but differs in some important respect

● answer 'no' if the study deviates substantively from the criterion

● answer 'unclear' if the report provides insufficient information to judge whether the study complies with the criterion

● answer 'NA (not applicable)' if the criterion is not relevant in a particular instance.

For 'partly' or 'no' responses, use the comments column to explain how the study deviates from the criterion.

## SECTION 1: APPLICABILITY

### 1.1     IS THE STUDY POPULATION APPROPRIATE FOR THE GUIDELINE?

The study population should be defined as precisely as possible and should be in line with that specified in the guideline scope and any related review protocols. This includes consideration of appropriate subgroups that require special attention. For many interventions, the capacity to benefit will differ for participants with differing characteristics. This should be explored separately for each relevant subgroup as part of the base-case analysis by the provision of estimates of clinical and cost effectiveness. The characteristics of participants in each subgroup should be clearly defined and, ideally, should be identified on the basis of an a priori expectation of differential clinical or cost effectiveness as a result of biologically plausible known mechanisms, social characteristics or other clearly justified factors.

Answer 'yes' if the study population is fully in line with that in the guideline question(s) and if the study differentiates appropriately between important subgroups.

Answer 'partly' if the study population is similar to that in the guideline question(s) but: (i) it differs in some important respects; or (ii) the study fails to differentiate between important subgroups. Answer 'no' if the study population is substantively different from that in the guideline question(s).

## 1.2    ARE THE INTERVENTIONS APPROPRIATE FOR THE GUIDELINE?

All relevant alternatives should be included, as specified in the guideline scope and any related review protocols. These should include routine and best practice in the NHS, existing NICE guidance and other feasible options. Answer 'yes' if the analysis includes all options considered relevant for the guideline, even if it also includes other options that are not relevant. Answer 'partly' if the analysis omits one or more relevant options but still contains comparisons likely to be useful for the guideline. Answer 'no' if the analysis does not contain any relevant comparisons.

## 1.3    IS THE HEALTHCARE SYSTEM IN WHICH THE STUDY WAS CONDUCTED SUFFICIENTLY SIMILAR TO THE CURRENT UK NHS CONTEXT?

This relates to the overall structure of the healthcare system within which the interventions were delivered. For example, an intervention might be delivered on an inpatient basis in one country whereas in the UK it would be provided in the community. This might significantly influence the use of healthcare resources and costs, thus limiting the applicability of the results to a UK setting. In addition, old UK studies may be severely limited in terms of their relevance to current NHS practice.

Answer 'yes' if the study was conducted within the UK and is sufficiently recent to reflect current NHS practice. For non-UK or older UK studies, answer 'partly' if differences in the healthcare setting are unlikely to substantively change the cost-effectiveness estimates. Answer 'no' if the healthcare setting is so different that the results are unlikely to be applicable in the current NHS.

## 1.4    ARE COSTS MEASURED FROM THE NATIONAL HEALTH SERVICE AND PERSONAL SOCIAL SERVICES PERSPECTIVE?

The decision-making perspective of an economic evaluation determines the range of costs that should be included in the analysis. NICE works in a specific context; in particular, it does not set the budget for the NHS. The objective of NICE is to offer guidance that represents an efficient use of available NHS and PSS resources. For these reasons, the perspective on costs used in the NICE reference case is that of the NHS and PSS. Productivity costs and costs borne by patients and carers that are not reimbursed by the NHS or PSS are not included in the reference case. The reference case also excludes costs to other government bodies, although these may sometimes be presented in additional analyses alongside the reference case.

Answer 'yes' if the study only includes costs for resource items that would be paid for by the NHS and PSS. Also answer 'yes' if other costs have been included in the study, but the results are presented in such a way that the cost effectiveness can be calculated from an NHS and PSS perspective. Answer 'partly' if the study has taken a wider perspective but the other non-NHS/PSS costs are small in relation to the total expected costs and are unlikely to change the cost-effectiveness results. Answer 'no' if non-NHS/PSS costs are significant and are likely to change the cost-effectiveness results. Some interventions may have a substantial impact on non-health outcomes or costs to other government bodies (for example, treatments to reduce illicit drug misuse may have the effect of reducing drug-related crime). In such situations, if the economic study includes non-health costs in such a way that they cannot be separated out from NHS/PSS costs, answer 'no' but consider retaining the study for critical appraisal. If studies containing non-reference-case costs are retained, use the comments column to note why.

### 1.5    ARE ALL DIRECT HEALTH EFFECTS ON INDIVIDUALS INCLUDED?

In the NICE reference case, the perspective on outcomes should be all direct health effects, whether for patients or, when relevant, other people (principally carers). This is consistent with an objective of maximising health gain from available healthcare resources. Some features of healthcare delivery that are often referred to as 'process characteristics' may ultimately have health consequences; for example, the mode of treatment delivery may have health consequences through its impact on concordance with treatment. Any significant characteristics of healthcare technologies that have a value to people that is independent of any direct effect on health should be noted. These characteristics include the convenience with which healthcare is provided and the level of information available for patients.

This question should be viewed in terms of what is **excluded** in relation to the NICE reference case; that is, non-health effects.

Answer 'yes' if the measure of health outcome used in the analysis excludes non-health effects (or if such effects can be excluded from the results). Answer 'partly' if the analysis includes some non-health effects but these are small and unlikely to change the cost-effectiveness results. Answer 'no' if the analysis includes significant non-health effects that are likely to change the cost-effectiveness results.

### 1.6    ARE BOTH COSTS AND HEALTH EFFECTS DISCOUNTED AT AN ANNUAL RATE OF 3.5%?

The need to discount to a present value is widely accepted in economic evaluation, although the specific rate varies across jurisdictions and over time. NICE considers it appropriate to discount costs and health effects at the same rate. The annual rate of 3.5%, based on the recommendations of the UK Treasury for the discounting of costs, applies to both costs and health effects.

Answer 'yes' if both costs and health effects (for example, quality-adjusted life years [QALYs]) are discounted at 3.5% per year. Answer 'partly' if costs and effects are discounted at a rate similar to 3.5% (for example, costs and effects are both discounted at 3% per year). Answer 'no' if costs and/or health effects are not discounted, or if they are discounted at a rate (or rates) different from 3.5% (for example, 5% for both costs and effects, or 6% for costs and 1.5% for effects). Note in the comments column what discount rates have been used. If all costs and health effects accrue within a short time (roughly a year), answer 'NA'.

## 1.7     IS THE VALUE OF HEALTH EFFECTS EXPRESSED IN TERMS OF QUALITY-ADJUSTED LIFE YEARS?

The QALY is a measure of a person's length of life weighted by a valuation of their health-related quality of life (HRQoL) over that period.

Given its widespread use, the QALY is considered by NICE to be the most appropriate generic measure of health benefit that reflects both mortality and effects on HRQoL. It is recognised that alternative measures exist (such as the healthy-year equivalent), but few economic evaluations have used these methods and their strengths and weaknesses are not fully established.

NICE's position is that an additional QALY should be given the same weight regardless of the other characteristics of the patients receiving the health benefit.

Answer 'yes' if the effectiveness of the intervention is measured using QALYs; answer 'no' if not. There may be circumstances when a QALY cannot be obtained or where the assumptions underlying QALYs are considered inappropriate. In such situations answer 'no', but consider retaining the study for appraisal. Similarly, answer 'no' but retain the study for appraisal if it does not include QALYs but it is still thought to be useful for GDG decision making: for example, if the clinical evidence indicates that an intervention might be dominant, and estimates of the relative costs of the interventions from a cost minimisation study are likely to be useful. When economic evaluations not using QALYs are retained for full critical appraisal, use the comments column to note why.

## 1.8     ARE CHANGES IN HEALTH-RELATED QUALITY OF LIFE REPORTED DIRECTLY FROM PATIENTS AND/OR CARERS?

In the NICE reference case, information on changes in HRQoL as a result of treatment should be reported directly by patients (and directly by carers when the impact of treatment on the carer's health is also important). When it is not possible to obtain information on changes in patients' HRQoL directly from them, data should be obtained from carers (not from healthcare professionals).

For consistency, the EQ-5D is NICE's preferred measure of HRQoL in adults. However, when EQ-5D data are not available or are inappropriate for the condition or the effects of treatment, other multi-attribute utility questionnaires (for example, SF6D, Quality of Well-being Scale or Health Utilities Index) or mapping methods from disease-specific questionnaires may be used to estimate QALYs. For studies not reporting QALYs, a variety of generic or disease-specific methods may be used to measure HRQoL.

Answer 'yes' if changes in patients' HRQoL are estimated by the patients themselves. Answer 'partly' if estimates of patients' HRQoL are provided by carers. Answer 'no' if estimates come from healthcare professionals or researchers. Note in the comments column how HRQoL was measured (EQ-5D, QWB, HUI and so on). Answer 'NA' if the cost-effectiveness study does not include estimates of HRQoL (for example, studies reporting 'cost per life year gained' or cost-minimisation studies).

## 1.9 IS THE VALUATION OF CHANGES IN HEALTH RELATED QUALITY OF LIFE (UTILITIES) OBTAINED FROM A REPRESENTATIVE SAMPLE OF THE GENERAL PUBLIC?

The NICE reference case specifies that the valuation of changes in HRQoL (utilities) reported by patients should be based on public preferences elicited using a choice-based method (such as the time trade-off or standard gamble) in a representative sample of the UK population.

Answer 'yes' if HRQoL valuations were obtained using the EQ-5D UK tariff. Answer 'partly' if the valuation methods were comparable to those used for the EQ-5D. Answer 'no' if other valuation methods were used. Answer 'NA' if the study does not apply valuations to HRQoL (for studies not reporting QALYs). In the comments column note the valuation method used (such as time trade-off or standard gamble) and the source of the preferences (such as patients or healthcare professionals).

## 1.10 OVERALL JUDGEMENT

Classify the applicability of the economic evaluation to the clinical guideline, the current NHS situation and the context for NICE guidance as one of the following:

- **Directly applicable** – the study meets all applicability criteria, or fails to meet one or more applicability criteria but this is unlikely to change the conclusions about cost effectiveness.
- **Partially applicable** – the study fails to meet one or more applicability criteria, and this could change the conclusions about cost effectiveness.
- **Not applicable** – the study fails to meet one or more applicability criteria, and this is likely to change the conclusions about cost effectiveness. Such studies would be excluded from further consideration and there is no need to continue with the rest of the checklist.

## SECTION 2: STUDY LIMITATIONS

### 2.1 DOES THE MODEL STRUCTURE ADEQUATELY REFLECT THE NATURE OF THE HEALTH CONDITION UNDER EVALUATION?

This relates to the choice of model and its structural elements (including cycle length in discrete time models, if appropriate). Model type and its structural aspects should be consistent with a coherent theory of the health condition under evaluation. The selection of treatment pathways, whether health states or branches in a decision tree, should be based on the underlying biological processes of the health issue under study and the potential impact (benefits and adverse consequences) of the intervention(s) of interest.

Answer 'yes' if the model design and assumptions appropriately reflect the health condition and intervention(s) of interest. Answer 'partly' if there are aspects of the model design or assumptions that do not fully reflect the health condition or intervention(s) but that are unlikely to change the cost-effectiveness results. Answer 'no' if the model omits some important aspect of the health condition or intervention(s) and this is likely to change the cost effectiveness results. Answer 'NA' for economic evaluations based on data from a clinical study which do not extrapolate treatment outcomes or costs beyond the study context or follow-up period.

### 2.2 IS THE TIME HORIZON SUFFICIENTLY LONG TO REFLECT ALL IMPORTANT DIFFERENCES IN COSTS AND OUTCOMES?

The time horizon is the period of analysis of the study: the length of follow-up for participants in a trial-based evaluation, or the period of time over which the costs and outcomes for a cohort are tracked in a modelling study. This time horizon should always be the same for costs and outcomes, and should be long enough to include all relevant costs and outcomes relating to the intervention. A time horizon shorter than lifetime could be justified if there is no differential mortality effect between options, and the differences in costs and

HRQoL relate to a relatively short period (for example, in the case of an acute infection).

Answer 'yes' if the time horizon is sufficient to include all relevant costs and outcomes. Answer 'partly' if the time horizon may omit some relevant costs and outcomes but these are unlikely to change the cost-effectiveness results. Answer 'no' if the time horizon omits important costs and outcomes and this is likely to change the cost-effectiveness results.

### 2.3 ARE ALL IMPORTANT AND RELEVANT HEALTH OUTCOMES INCLUDED?

All relevant health outcomes should include direct health effects relating to harms from the intervention (adverse effects) as well as any potential benefits.

Answer 'yes' if the analysis includes all relevant and important harms and bene-fits. Answer 'partly' if the analysis omits some harms or benefits but these would be unlikely to change the cost-effectiveness results. Answer 'no' if the analysis omits important harms and/or benefits that would be likely to change the cost-effectiveness results.

## 2.4      ARE THE ESTIMATES OF BASELINE HEALTH OUTCOMES FROM THE BEST AVAILABLE SOURCE?

The estimate of the overall net treatment effect of an intervention is determined by the baseline risk of a particular condition or event and/or the relative effects of the inter-vention compared with the relevant comparator treatment. The overall net treatment effect may also be determined by other features of the people comprising the popula-tion of interest.

The process of assembling evidence for economic evaluations should be system-atic – evidence must be identified, quality assessed and, when appropriate, pooled, using explicit criteria and justifiable and reproducible methods. These principles apply to all categories of evidence that are used to estimate clinical and cost effec-tiveness, evidence for which will typically be drawn from a number of different sources.

The sources and methods for eliciting baseline probabilities should be described clearly. These data can be based on 'natural history' (patient outcomes in the absence of treatment or with routine care), sourced from cohort studies. Baseline probabilities may also be derived from the control arms of experimental studies. Sometimes it may be necessary to rely on expert opinion for particular parameters.

Answer 'yes' if the estimates of baseline health outcomes reflect the best avail-able evidence as identified from a recent well-conducted systematic review of the literature. Answer 'partly' if the estimates are not derived from a systematic review but are likely to reflect outcomes for the relevant group of patients in routine NHS practice (for example, if they are derived from a large UK-relevant cohort study). Answer 'no' if the estimates are unlikely to reflect outcomes for the relevant group in routine NHS practice.

## 2.5      ARE THE ESTIMATES OF RELATIVE TREATMENT EFFECTS FROM THE BEST AVAILABLE SOURCE?

The objective of the analysis of clinical effectiveness is to produce an unbiased esti-mate of the mean clinical effectiveness of the interventions being compared.

The NICE reference case indicates that evidence on outcomes should be obtained from a systematic review, defined as the systematic location, inclusion, appraisal and synthesis of evidence to obtain a reliable and valid overview of the data relating to a clearly formulated question.

Synthesis of outcome data through meta-analysis is appropriate provided that there are sufficient relevant and valid data obtained using comparable measures of outcome.

Head-to-head RCTs provide the most valid evidence of relative treatment effect. However, such evidence may not always be available. Therefore, data from non-randomised studies may be required to supplement RCT data. Any potential bias arising from the design of the studies used in the assessment should be explored and documented.

Data from head-to-head RCTs should be presented in the base-case analysis, if available. When head-to-head RCTs exist, evidence from indirect or mixed treatment comparison analyses may be presented if it is considered to add information that is not available from the head-to-head comparison. This indirect or mixed treatment comparison must be fully described and presented as additional to the base-case analysis. (A 'mixed treatment comparison' estimates effect sizes using both head-to-head and indirect comparisons.)

If data from head-to-head RCTs are not available, indirect treatment comparison methods should be used. (An 'indirect comparison' is a synthesis of data from a network of trials that compare the interventions of interest with other comparators.)

When multiple interventions are being assessed that have not been compared within a single RCT, data from a series of pairwise head-to-head RCTs should be presented. Consideration should also be given to presenting a combined analysis using a mixed treatment comparison framework if it is considered to add information that is not available from the head-to-head comparison.

Only indirect or mixed treatment comparison methods that preserve randomisation should be used. The principles of good practice for standard meta-analyses should also be followed in mixed and indirect treatment comparisons.

The methods and assumptions that are used to extrapolate short-term results to final outcomes should be clearly presented and there should be documentation of the reasoning underpinning the choice of survival function.

Evidence for the evaluation of diagnostic technologies should normally incorporate evidence on diagnostic accuracy. It is also important to incorporate the predicted changes in health outcomes and costs resulting from treatment decisions based on the test result. The general principles guiding the assessment of the clinical and cost effectiveness of diagnostic interventions should be the same as for other technologies. However, particular consideration of the methods of analysis may be required, particularly in relation to evidence synthesis. Evidence for the effectiveness of diagnostic technologies should include the costs and outcomes for people whose test results lead to an incorrect diagnosis, as well as for those who are diagnosed correctly.

As for other technologies, RCTs have the potential to capture the pathway of care involving diagnostic technologies, but their feasibility and availability may be limited. Other study designs should be assessed on the basis of their fitness for purpose, taking into consideration the aim of the study (for example, to evaluate outcomes, or to evaluate sensitivity and specificity) and the purpose of the diagnostic technology.

Answer 'yes' if the estimates of treatment effect appropriately reflect all relevant studies of the best available quality, as identified through a recent well-conducted systematic review of the literature. Answer 'partly' if the estimates of treatment effect are not derived from a systematic review but are similar in magnitude to the best available estimates (for example, if the economic evaluation is based on a single large study with treatment effects similar to pooled estimates from all relevant studies). Answer 'no' if the estimates of treatment effect are likely to differ substantively from the best available estimates.

## 2.6      ARE ALL IMPORTANT AND RELEVANT COSTS INCLUDED?

Costs related to the condition of interest and incurred in additional years of life gained as a result of treatment should be included in the base-case analysis. This should include the costs of handling non-adherence to treatment and treating side effects. Costs that are considered to be unrelated to the condition or intervention of interest should be excluded. If introduction of the intervention requires additional infrastructure to be put in place, consideration should be given to including such costs in the analysis.

Answer 'yes' if all important and relevant resource use and costs are included given the perspective and the research question under consideration. Answer 'partly' if some relevant resource items are omitted but these are unlikely to affect the cost-effectiveness results. Answer 'no' if important resource items are omitted and these are likely to affect the cost-effectiveness results.

## 2.7      ARE THE ESTIMATES OF RESOURCE USE FROM THE BEST AVAILABLE SOURCE?

It is important to quantify the effect of the interventions on resource use in terms of physical units (for example, days in hospital or visits to a GP) and valuing those effects in monetary terms using appropriate prices and unit costs. Evidence on resource use should be identified systematically. When expert opinion is used as a source of information, any formal methods used to elicit these data should be clearly reported.

Answer 'yes' if the estimates of resource use appropriately reflect all relevant evidence sources of the best available quality, as identified through a recent well-conducted systematic review of the literature. Answer 'partly' if the estimates of resource use are not derived from a systematic review but are similar in magnitude to the best available estimates. Answer 'no' if the estimates of resource use are likely to differ substantively from the best available estimates.

## 2.8      ARE THE UNIT COSTS OF RESOURCES FROM THE BEST AVAILABLE SOURCE?

Resources should be valued using the prices relevant to the NHS and PSS. Given the perspective of the NICE reference case, it is appropriate for the financial costs relevant to the NHS/PSS to be used as the basis of costing, although these may not always reflect the full social opportunity cost of a given resource. A first point of reference in identifying costs and prices should be any current official listing published by the Department of Health and/or the Welsh Assembly Government.

When the acquisition price paid for a resource differs from the public list price (for example, pharmaceuticals and medical devices sold at reduced prices to NHS institutions), the public list price should be used in the base-case analysis. Sensitivity analysis should assess the implications of variations from this price. Analyses based on price reductions for the NHS will only be considered when the reduced prices are transparent and can be consistently available across the NHS, and if the period for which the specified price is available is guaranteed.

National data based on healthcare resource groups (HRGs) such as the Payment by Results tariff can be used when they are appropriate and available. However, data based on HRGs may not be appropriate in all circumstances (for example, when the definition of the HRG is broad, or the mean cost probably does not reflect resource use in relation to the intervention(s) under consideration). In such cases, other sources of evidence, such as micro-costing studies, may be more appropriate. When cost data are taken from the literature, the methods used to identify the sources should be defined. When several alternative sources are available, a justification for the costs chosen should be provided and discrepancies between the sources explained. When appropriate, sensitivity analysis should have been undertaken to assess the implications for results of using alternative data sources.

Answer 'yes' if resources are valued using up-to-date prices relevant to the NHS and PSS. Answer 'partly' if the valuations of some resource items differ from current NHS/PSS unit costs but this is unlikely to change the cost-effectiveness results. Answer 'no' if the valuations of some resource items differ substantively from current NHS/PSS unit costs and this is likely to change the cost-effectiveness results.

## 2.9   IS AN APPROPRIATE INCREMENTAL ANALYSIS PRESENTED OR CAN IT BE CALCULATED FROM THE DATA?

An appropriate incremental analysis is one that compares the expected costs and health outcomes of one intervention with the expected costs and health outcomes of the next-best non-dominated alternative.

Standard decision rules should be followed when combining costs and effects, and should reflect any situation where there is dominance or extended dominance. When there is a trade-off between costs and effects, the results should be presented as an ICER: the ratio of the difference in mean costs to the difference in mean outcomes of a technology compared with the next best alternative. In addition to ICERs, expected net monetary or health benefits can be presented using values placed on a QALY gained of £20,000 and £30,000.

For cost-consequence analyses, appropriate incremental analysis can only be done by selecting one of the consequences as the primary measure of effectiveness.

Answer 'yes' if appropriate incremental results are presented, or if data are presented that allow the reader to calculate the incremental results. Answer 'no' if: (i) simple ratios of costs to effects are presented for each alternative compared with a standard intervention; or (ii) if options subject to simple or extended dominance are not excluded from the incremental analyses.

## 2.10 ARE ALL IMPORTANT PARAMETERS WHOSE VALUES ARE UNCERTAIN SUBJECTED TO APPROPRIATE SENSITIVITY ANALYSIS?

There are a number of potential selection biases and uncertainties in any evaluation (trial- or model-based) and these should be identified and quantified where possible. There are three types of bias or uncertainty to consider:

- Structural uncertainty – for example in relation to the categorisation of different states of health and the representation of different pathways of care. These structural assumptions should be clearly documented and the evidence and rationale to support them provided. The impact of structural uncertainty on estimates of cost effectiveness should be explored by separate analyses of a representative range of plausible scenarios.
- Source of values to inform parameter estimates – the implications of different estimates of key parameters (such as estimates of relative effectiveness) must be reflected in sensitivity analyses (for example, through the inclusion of alternative scenarios). Inputs must be fully justified, and uncertainty explored by sensitivity analysis using alternative input values.
- Parameter precision – uncertainty around the mean health and cost inputs in the model. Distributions should be assigned to characterise the uncertainty associated with the (precision of) mean parameter values. Probabilistic sensitivity analysis is preferred, as this enables the uncertainty associated with parameters to be simultaneously reflected in the results of the model. In non-linear decision models – when there is not a straight-line relationship between inputs and outputs of a model (such as Markov models) – probabilistic methods provide the best estimates of mean costs and outcomes. Simple decision trees are usually linear.

The mean value, distribution around the mean, and the source and rationale for the supporting evidence should be clearly described for each parameter included in the model.

Evidence about the extent of correlation between individual parameters should be considered carefully and reflected in the probabilistic analysis. Assumptions made about the correlations should be clearly presented.

Answer 'yes' if an extensive sensitivity analysis was undertaken that explored all key uncertainties in the economic evaluation. Answer 'partly' if the sensitivity analysis failed to explore some important uncertainties in the economic evaluation. Answer 'no' if the sensitivity analysis was very limited and omitted consideration of a number of important uncertainties, or if the range of values or distributions around parameters considered in the sensitivity analysis were not reported.

## 2.11    IS THERE NO POTENTIAL CONFLICT OF INTEREST?

The *British Medical Journal* (BMJ) defines competing interests for its authors as follows: 'A competing interest exists when professional judgment concerning a primary interest (such as patients' welfare or the validity of research) may be influenced by a secondary interest (such as financial gain or personal rivalry). It may arise for the authors of a BMJ article when they have a financial interest that may influence, probably without their knowing, their interpretation of their results or those of others.' Whenever a potential financial conflict of interest is possible, this should be declared.

Answer 'yes' if the authors declare that they have no financial conflicts of interest. Answer 'no' if clear financial conflicts of interest are declared or apparent (for example, from the stated affiliation of the authors). Answer 'unclear' if the article does not indicate whether or not there are financial conflicts of interest.

## 2.12    OVERALL ASSESSMENT

The overall methodological study quality of the economic evaluation should be classified as one of the following:

- **Minor limitations** – the study meets all quality criteria, or the study fails to meet one or more quality criteria but this is unlikely to change the conclusions about cost effectiveness.
- **Potentially serious limitations** – the study fails to meet one or more quality criteria and this could change the conclusions about cost effectiveness.
- **Very serious limitations** – the study fails to meet one or more quality criteria and this is highly likely to change the conclusions about cost effectiveness. Such studies should usually be excluded from further consideration.

# APPENDIX 10: EVIDENCE TABLES FOR ECONOMIC STUDIES

## CASE IDENTIFICATION

| Study Country Study type | Intervention details | Study population Study design Data sources | Costs: description and values Outcomes: description and values | Results: cost-effectiveness | Comments |
|---|---|---|---|---|---|
| Hewitt *et al.*, 2009 UK Cost-utility analysis | Interventions: 14 identification strategies for postnatal depression: EPDS (cut points 7–16); Beck Depression Inventory (BDI) (cut-off point 10); and routine care (that is, routine case identification without the formal use of a diagnostic instrument) | Women in their 6th postnatal week Decision-analytic modelling Source of clinical effectiveness data: systematic literature review and meta-analysis and further assumptions Source of resource use estimates: *Antenatal and Postnatal Mental Health* NICE guideline (NCCMH, 2007), expert opinion Source of unit costs: national sources | Costs: Visits to clinical psychologist, health visitor, GP, community psychiatric nurse; structured psychological therapy, additional care Mean cost per person: EPDS: ranging between £73.49 and £187.32 BDI: £121.51 Routine care: £49.29 Outcome: Mean QALYs per person: EPDS: ranging between 0.846 and 0.847 BDI: 0.847 Routine care: 0.846 | ICER of the EPDS at a cut point of 16 versus routine care: £41,103 per QALY ICER of EPDS at a cut point of 14 versus EPDS at a cut point 16 was £49,928 per QALY Probability of routine care being cost effective at £20,000, £30,000 and £40,000 per QALY: 0.88, 0.59, and 0.39 respectively | Perspective: NHS and PSS Currency: UK£ Cost year: 2006/07 Time horizon: 12 months Discounting: not needed Applicability: directly applicable Quality: potentially serious limitations |

| Hakkaart *et al.*, 2006 Netherlands Cost-utility analysis | Interventions: Brief therapy: a formalised stepped-care approach<br><br>CBT: maximum number of sessions 15<br><br>Care as usual, not formalised. A multidisciplinary team can choose the suitable therapy from a variety of treatment options. The number of sessions depends on the therapy chosen | People with DSM-IV diagnoses of MDD, dysthymic disorder, panic disorder, social phobia and GAD<br><br>Source of clinical effectiveness data: multicentre randomised trial<br><br>Source of resource use: actual data using the TiC-P<br><br>Source of unit costs: published sources | Costs:<br>Contacts with healthcare providers (GPs, psychiatrists, medical specialist, physiotherapist, alternative health practitioner), day care and hospitalisation and medications. Productivity losses due to absenteeism from work<br><br>Total costs per person:<br>Direct medical costs:<br>Care as usual 3,360€<br>CBT: 3,127€<br>Brief therapy: 3,679€<br>Indirect costs:<br>Care as usual 6,151€<br>CBT: 6,621€<br>Brief therapy: 6,537€<br><br><u>Primary outcome</u>: number of QALYs<br><br>Care as usual: 0.91 QALYs<br>Brief therapy: 0.94 QALYs<br>CBT: 0.94 QALYs | Usual care is dominated by CBT as it is more expensive and less effective<br><br>ICER of brief therapy versus CBT: €222 956 per QALY gained<br><br>Sensitivity analysis – of the missing data using linear extrapolation and complete case analysis: No significant changes | Perspective: societal<br>Currency: Euros (€)<br>Cost year: 2002<br>Time horizon: 18 months<br>Discounting: not needed<br>Applicability: non-applicable |

# APPENDIX 11:

# HIGH PRIORITY RESEARCH RECOMMENDATIONS

*1. GAD-2 for people with suspected anxiety disorders*
In people with suspected anxiety disorders: What is the clinical utility of using the GAD-2 compared with routine case identification to accurately identify different anxiety disorders? Should an avoidance question be added to improve case identification?

**Why this is important**
There is good evidence of poor detection and under-recognition in primary care of anxiety disorders. Case identification questions for anxiety disorders are not well developed. There is reasonable evidence that the GAD-2 may have clinical utility as a case identification tool for anxiety disorders, in particular GAD, but there is greater uncertainly about its utility for other anxiety disorders, in particular those with an element of phobic avoidance. Understanding whether the GAD-2 plus or minus an additional phobia question would improve case identification for different anxiety disorders would be an important contribution to their identification.

These questions should be answered by a well-designed cohort study in which the GAD-2 is compared with a diagnostic gold-standard for a range of anxiety disorders. The cost-effectiveness of this approach should also be assessed.

*2. Comprehensive assessment versus a brief assessment*
For people with a suspected common mental health disorder, what is the clinical and cost effectiveness of using a comprehensive assessment (conducted by a mental health professional) versus a brief assessment (conducted by a paraprofessional)?

**Why this is important**
Uncertainty remains about the accuracy and consequent identification of appropriate treatment by paraprofessionals in primary care. An assessment by a mental health professional is likely to result in more accurate identification of problems and appropriate treatment, but is likely to entail greater cost and potentially significant longer wait times for interventions, both of which can have deleterious effects on care.

This question should be answered using a randomised controlled design that reports short- and medium-term outcomes (including cost-effectiveness outcomes) of at least 12 months' duration.

*3. 'Walking across' from one assessment instrument to another*
What methodology should be used to allow 'walking across' from one assessment instrument for common mental health disorders to another?

**Why this is important**

A number of different ratings scales for depression and anxiety disorders are in current use, both in research studies and clinical practice. This makes obtaining comparative estimates of clinical outcomes at the individual level difficult when moving between research and clinical settings, and also between clinical settings. A method that allows for prompt and easy 'walking across' between assessment instruments would have a potentially significant clinical benefit in routine care.

This question should be answered by developing a new method and subsequent data analysis of existing datasets to facilitate comparison between commonly used measures.

*4. Routine outcome measurement*

In people with a common mental health disorder, what is the clinical utility of ROM and is it cost effective compared with standard care?

**Why this is important**

ROM is increasingly a part of the delivery of psychological interventions, particular in the IAPT programme. There is evidence from this programme and from other studies that ROM may bring real benefits. However, there is much less evidence for pharmacological interventions on the cost-effectiveness of ROM. If ROM were shown to be cost effective across the range of common mental health disorders it could be associated with improved treatment outcomes because of its impact on healthcare professionals' behaviour and the prompter availability of appropriate treatment interventions in light of feedback from the measurement.

This should be tested in an RCT in which different frequencies of ROM are compared, for example at beginning and end of treatment at regular intervals and at every appointment.

*5. Use of a simple algorithm compared with a standard clinical assessment*

For people with a common mental health disorder is the use of a simple algorithm (based on factors associated with treatment response) when compared with a standard clinical assessment more clinically and cost effective?

**Why this is important**

There are well-established systems for the assessment of mental states, in primary and secondary care services, for common mental disorders. One key function of such assessment is to identify both appropriate treatments and to obtain an indication of likely response to such treatments, thereby informing patient choice and leading to clinically and cost-effective interventions. Although the reliability of diagnostic systems is much improved, data on appropriate treatment response indicators remain poor, with factors such as chronicity and severity emerging as some of the most reliable indicators. Other factors may also be identified, which, if they could be developed into a simple algorithms, could inform treatment choice decisions at many levels in the healthcare system. Treatment choice can include complex assessment and discussion of options but the validity of such assessments appears to be low. Would the use of a number of simple indicators (for example, chronicity, severity, comorbidity) provide a better indication of likely treatment response? Using existing individual patient data, could a simple algorithm be developed for testing in a prospective study?

This should be tested in a two-stage programme of research: first, a review of existing trial datasets to identify potential predictors and then to develop an algorithm; second, an RCT in which the algorithm is tested against expert clinical prediction.

*6. Priority of treatment for people with anxiety and depression*
For people with both anxiety and depression, which disorder should be treated first to improve their outcomes?

**Why this is important**
Comorbidity between depression and anxiety disorders is common. At present there is little empirical evidence to guide practitioners or patients in choosing which disorder should be treated first. Given that for many disorders the treatment strategies, particularly for psychological approaches, can be significantly different, guidance for healthcare professionals and patients on the appropriate sequencing of psychological treatment intervention would be likely to significantly improve interventions.

This should be tested in a randomised trial in which patients who have a dual diagnosis of an anxiety disorder and depression, and where there is uncertainty about the appropriate sequencing of treatment, should be randomised to different sequencing of treatment. The clinical and cost effectiveness of the interventions should be tested at end of treatment and at 12 months' follow-up.

# APPENDIX 12:
# COMPLETED METHODOLOGY CHECKLISTS FOR ECONOMIC STUDIES

The completed forms can be found on the CD accompanying this guideline.

# APPENDIX 13:

# GENERALIZED ANXIETY DISORDER SCALE

# (2 ITEMS) QUESTIONNAIRE

The GAD-2 short screening tool consists of the first two questions of the GAD-7 scale.

| GAD-7 | | | | |
|---|---|---|---|---|
| Over the <u>last 2 weeks</u>, how often have you been bothered by the following problems?<br><br>*(Use "✔" to indicate your answer)* | Not at all | Several days | More than half the days | Nearly every day |
| 1. Feeling nervous, anxious or on edge | 0 | 1 | 2 | 3 |
| 2. Not being able to stop or control worrying | 0 | 1 | 2 | 3 |
| 3. Worrying too much about different things | 0 | 1 | 2 | 3 |
| 4. Trouble relaxing | 0 | 1 | 2 | 3 |
| 5. Being so restless that it is hard to sit still | 0 | 1 | 2 | 3 |
| 6. Becoming easily annoyed or irritable | 0 | 1 | 2 | 3 |
| 7. Feeling afraid as if something awful might happen | 0 | 1 | 2 | 3 |

*(For office coding: Total Score T____ = ____ + ____ + ____ )*

Developed by Drs. Robert L. Spitzer, Janet B.W. Williams, Kurt Kroenke and colleagues, with an educational grant from Pfizer Inc. No permission required to reproduce, translate, display or distribute.

# 10    REFERENCES

Abramowitz, J. S. (2004) Treatment of obsessive-compulsive disorder in patients who have comorbid major depression. *Journal of Clinical Psychology, 60,* 1133–1141.

Abramowitz, J. S., Schwartz, S. A., Moore, K. M., *et al.* (2003) Obsessive-compulsive symptoms in pregnancy and the puerperium: a review of the literature. *Journal of Anxiety Disorders, 17,* 461–478.

Adler, R., Vasiliadis, A. & Bickell, N. (2010) The relationship between continuity and patient satisfaction: a systematic review. *Family Practice, 27,* 171–178.

Adli, M., Bauer, M. & Rush, A. J. (2006) Algorithms and collaborative-care systems for depression: are they effective and why? A systematic review. *Biological Psychiatry, 59,* 1029–1038.

Aertgeerts, B., Buntinx, F. & Kester, A. (2004) The value of the CAGE in screening for alcohol abuse and alcohol dependence in general clinical populations: a diagnostic meta-analysis. *Journal Clinical Epidemiology, 57,* 30–39.

Agarwal, G. & Crooks, V. A. (2008) The nature of informational continuity of care in general practice. *British Journal of General Practice, 58,* e17–e24.

AGREE Collaboration (2003) Development and validation of an international appraisal instrument for assessing the quality of clinical practice guidelines: the AGREE project. *Quality and Safety in Health Care, 12,* 18–23.

Akesson, K. M., Saveman, B. I. & Nilsson, G. (2007) Health care consumers' experiences of information communication technology: a summary of literature. *International Journal of Medical Informatics, 76,* 633–645.

Akiskal, H. S. (1986) A developmental perspective on recurrent mood disorders: a review of studies in man. *Psychopharmacology Bulletin, 22,* 579–586.

Allgulander, C., Jørgensen, T., Wade, A., *et al.* (2007) Health-related quality of life (HRQoL) among patients with generalised anxiety disorder: evaluation conducted alongside an escitalopram prevention trial. *Current Medical Research and Opinion, 23,* 2543–2549.

Almond, S. & Healey, A. (2003) Mental health and absence from work. *Work, Employment and Society, 17,* 731–742.

Altman, D. & Bland, M. (1994a) Statistics notes: diagnostic tests 2: predictive values. *British Medical Journal, 309,* 102.

Altman, D. & Bland, M. (1994b) Statistics notes: diagnostic tests 1: sensitivity and specificity. *British Medical Journal, 308,* 1552.

Anderson, C., Blenkinsopp, A. & Armstrong, M. (2001) Feedback from community pharmacy users on the contribution of community pharmacy to improving the public's health: a systematic review of the peer reviewed and non-peer reviewed literature 1990–2002. *Health Expectations, 7,* 191–202.

Anderson, L. M., Scrimshaw, S. C., Fullilove, M. T., *et al.* (2003) Culturally competent healthcare systems: a systematic review. *American Journal of Preventative Medicine, 24,* 68–79.

## References

Andlin-Sobocki, P., Jönsson, B., Wittchen, H. U., *et al.* (2005) Cost of disorders of the brain in Europe. *European Journal of Neurology*, *12*, 1–27.

Andrews, G. & Jenkins, R. (eds) (1999) *Management of Mental Disorders* (1st edn). Sydney: WHO Collaborating Centre for Mental Health and Substance Misuse.

Andrews, G. & Slade, T. (2001) Interpreting scores on the Kessler psychological distress scale (K10). *Australian and New Zealand Journal of Public Health*, *25*, 494–497.

Andrews, G., Slade, T. & Peters, L. (1999) Classification in psychiatry: ICD–10 versus DSM-IV. *British Journal of Psychiatry*, *174*, 3–5.

Andrews, G., Sanderson, K., Corry, J., *et al.* (2004) Utilising survey data to inform public policy: comparison of the cost-effectiveness of treatment of ten mental disorders. *The British Journal of Psychiatry*, *184*, 526–533.

Angst, J., Gamma, A. & Endrass, J. (2003) Risk factors for the bipolar and depression spectra. *Acta Psychiatrica Scandinavica*, *108*, 15–19.

Antony, M. M., Roth, D., Swinson, R. P., *et al.* (1998) Illness intrusiveness in individuals with panic disorder, obsessive-compulsive disorder, or social phobia. *Journal of Nervous and Mental Disease*, *186*, 311–315.

APA (2000) *Diagnostic and Statistical Manual of Mental Disorders* (4th edn). Washington DC: APA.

Apter, A., Horesh, N., Gothelf, D., *et al.* (2003) Depression and suicidal behavior in adolescent inpatients with obsessive compulsive disorder. *Journal of Affective Disorders*, *75*, 181–189.

Arnau, R., Meagher, M. W., Norris, M. P., *et al.* (2001) Psychometric evaluation of the Beck Depression Inventory-II with primary care medical patients. *Health Psychology*, *20*, 112–119.

Azarmina, P. & Wallace, P. (2005) Remote interpretation in medical encounters: a systematic review. *Journal of Telemedicine and Telecare*, *11*, 140–145.

Badamgarav, E., Weingarten, S. R., Henning, J. M., *et al.* (2003) Effectiveness of disease management programs in depression: a systematic review. *American Journal of Psychiatry*, *160*, 2080–2090.

Bajaj, P., Borreani, E., Ghosh, P., *et al.* (2008) Screening for suicidal thoughts in primary care: the views of patients and general practitioners. *Mental Health in Family Medicine*, 5, 229–235.

Balas, E. A., Jaffrey, F., Kuperman, G. J., *et al.* (1997) Electronic communication with patients: evaluation of distance medicine technology. *Journal of the American Medical Association*, *278*, 152–159.

Baldwin, D. S., Anderson, I. M., Nutt, D. J., *et al.* (2005) Evidence-based guidelines for the pharmacological treatment of anxiety disorders: recommendations from the British Association for Psychopharmacology. *Journal of Psychopharmacology*, *19*, 567–596.

Barbui, C. & Tansella, M. (2006) Identification and management of depression in primary care settings: a meta-review of evidence. *Epidemiologia e Psichiatria Sociale*, *15*, 276–283.

Barlow, D. H. (2000) Cognitive-behavioral therapy, imipramine, or their combination for panic disorder: a randomized controlled trial. *Journal of the American Medical Association*, *283*, 2529–2536.

Beach, M. C., Gary, T. L., Price, E. G., *et al.* (2006) Improving health care quality for racial/ethnic minorities: a systematic review of the best evidence regarding provider and organization interventions. *BMC Public Health, 6*, 104.

Bebbington, P. E., Dean, C., Der, G., *et al.* (1991) Gender, parity and the prevalence of minor affective disorder. *The British Journal of Psychiatry, 158*, 40–45.

Beck, A. T. (1996) *BDI-II: Beck Depression Inventory Manual* (2nd edn). Boston, MA: Harcourt Brace.

Bee, P. E., Bower, P., Lovell, K., *et al.* (2008) Psychotherapy mediated by remote communication technologies: a meta-analytic review. *BMC Psychiatry, 8*, 60.

Beney, J., Bero, L. A. & Bond, C. (2000) Expanding the roles of outpatient pharmacists: effects on health services utilisation, costs, and patient outcomes. *Cochrane Database of Systematic Reviews*, Issue 3. CD000336.

Berlin, J. A. (on behalf of University of Pennsylvania Meta-analysis Blinding Study Group) (1997) Does blinding of readers affect the results of meta-analysis? *Lancet, 350*, 185–186.

Bernal, G. (2006) Intervention development and cultural adaptation research with diverse families. *Family Process, 45*, 143–151.

Bernal, G. & Domenech Rodriguez, M. M. (2009) Advances in Latino family research: cultural adaptations of evidence-based interventions. *Family Process, 48*, 169–178.

Bhui, K., Stansfeld, S., Hull, S., *et al.* (2003) Ethnic variations in pathways to and use of specialist mental health services in the UK. *British Journal of Psychiatry, 182*, 105–116.

Biederman, J., Petty, C., Faraone, S. V., *et al.* (2004) Moderating effects of major depression on patterns of comorbidity in patients with panic disorder. *Psychiatry Research, 126*, 143–149.

Blake, D. D., Weathers, F. W., Nagy, L. M., *et al.* (1995) The development of a clinician-administered PTSD scale. *Journal of Traumatic Stress, 8*, 75–90.

Blashki, G., Judd, F. & Piterman, L. (2007) *General Practice Psychiatry*. NSW, Australia: McGraw-Hill.

Bobes, J., Gonzalez, M. P., Bascaran, M. T., *et al.* (2001) Quality of life and disability in patients with obsessive-compulsive disorder. *European Psychiatry, 16*, 239–245.

Bostwick, J. M. & Pankratz, V. S. (2000) Affective disorders and suicide risk: a reexamination. *American Journal of Psychiatry, 157*, 1925–1932.

Bouman, A., van Rossum, E., Nelemans, P., *et al.* (2008) Effects of intensive home visiting programs for older people with poor health status: a systematic review. *BMC Health Services Research, 8*, 74.

Bower, P. & Gilbody, S. (2005) Stepped care in psychological therapies: access, effectiveness and efficiency: narrative literature review. *British Journal of Psychiatry, 186*, 11–17.

Bower, P. & Sibbald, B. (2000) Systematic review of the effect of on-site mental health professionals on the clinical behaviour of general practitioners. *British Medical Journal, 320*, 614–617.

## References

Bower, P., Gilbody, S., Richards, D., *et al.* (2006) Collaborative care for depression in primary care: making sense of a complex intervention: systematic review and meta-regression. *British Journal of Psychiatry*, *189*, 484–493.

Breier, A., Charney, D. S. & Heninger, G. R. (1986) Agoraphobia with panic attacks: development, diagnostic stability, and course of illness. *Archives of General Psychiatry*, *43*, 1029–1036.

Breslau, N., Davis, G. C., Andreski, P., *et al.* (1991) Traumatic events and posttraumatic stress disorder in an urban population of young adults. *Archives of General Psychiatry*, *48*, 216–222.

Brewin, C. R., Andrews, B. & Valentine, J. D. (2000) Meta-analysis of risk factors for posttraumatic stress disorder in trauma-exposed adults. *Journal of Consulting and Clinical Psychology*, *68*, 748–766.

Bridges, K. W. & Goldberg, D. P. (1987) Somatic presentations of depressive illness in primary care. In *The Presentation of Depression: Current Approaches* (eds P. Freeling, L. J. Downey & J. C. Malkin), pp. 9–11. London: Royal College of General Practitioners.

British Medical Association & NHS Employers (2006) *Revisions to the GMS Contract 2006/07: Delivering Investment in General Practice.* London: NHS Employers & General Practitioners Committee. Available at: http://www.bma.org.uk/employmentandcontracts/independent_contractors/general_medical_services_contract/NewDEs0706.jsp

British Medical Association & NHS Employers (2008) *Quality and Outcomes Framework Guidance for GMS Contract* 2009/10: *Delivering Investment in General Practice.* London: NHS Employers & General Practitioners Committee. Available at: http://www.bma.org.uk/images/QoF%20Guidance%20-%20April%202008_tcm41-182872.pdf

British Medical Association & the Royal Pharmaceutical Society of Great Britain (2010) *British National Formulary (BNF 59).* London: British Medical Association and the Royal Pharmaceutical Society of Great Britain.

Brown, C., Schulberg, H. C., Madonia, M. J., *et al.* (1996) Treatment outcomes for primary care patients with major depression and lifetime anxiety disorders. *American Journal of Psychiatry*, *153*, 1293–1300.

Brown, G. & Harris, T. (1978) *The Social Origins of Depression: a Study of Psychiatric Disorder in Women.* London: Tavistock Publications.

Brown, T. A., O'Leary, T. A. & Barlow, D. H. (2001) Generalised anxiety disorder. In *Clinical Handbook of Psychological Disorders: a Step-by-Step Treatment Manual* (3rd edn) (ed. D. H. Barlow), pp. 154–208. New York: Guilford Press.

Bruce, M. L. & Hoff, R. A. (1994) Social and physical health risk factors for first-onset major depressive disorder in a community sample. *Social Psychiatry and Psychiatric Epidemiology*, *29*, 165–171.

Bunn, F., Byrne, G. & Kendall, S. (2005) The effects of telephone consultation and triage on healthcare use and patient satisfaction: a systematic review. *British Journal of General Practice*, *55*, 956–961.

Bushnell, J., McLeod, D., Dowell, A., *et al.* (2005) Do patients want to disclose psychological problems to GPs? *Family Practice*, *22*, 631–637.

Butler, R., Hatcher, S., Price, J., *et al.* (2007) Depression in adults: psychological treatments and care pathways. *BMJ Clinical Evidence*, *8*, 1016.

Byrne, G. J. & Pachana, N. A. (2011) Development and validation of a short form of the Geriatric Anxiety Inventory: the GAI-SF. *International Psychogeriatrics*, *23*, 125–131.

Callaghan, P., Eales, S., Coates, T., *et al.* (2003) A review of research on the structure, process and outcome of liaison mental health services. *Journal of Psychiatric and Mental Health Nursing*, *10*, 155–165.

Campbell, S., Roland, M. O. & Buetow, S. A. (2000) Defining quality of care. *Social Science and Medicine*, *51*, 1611–1625.

Campbell-Sills, L., Norman, S. B., Craske, M. G., *et al.* (2009) Validation of a brief measure of anxiety-related severity and impairment: the Overall Anxiety Severity and Impairment Scale (OASIS). *Journal of Affective Disorders*, *112*, 92–101.

Cassano, P. & Fava, M. (2002) Depression and public health: an overview. *Journal of Psychosomatic Research*, *53*, 849–857.

Centre for Reviews and Dissemination (2007) *NHS Economic Evaluation Database Handbook*. York: University of York. Available at http://www.york.ac.uk/inst/crd/pdf/nhseed-handb07.pdf

Chaix, B., Merlo, J. & Chauvin, P. (2005) Comparison of a spatial approach with the multilevel approach for investigating place effects on health: the example of healthcare utilisation in France. *Journal of Epidemiology and Community Health*, *59*, 517–526.

Chang-Quan, H., Bi-Rong, D., Zhen-Chan, L., *et al.* (2009) Collaborative care interventions for depression in the elderly: a systematic review of randomised controlled trials. *Journal of Investigative Medicine*, *57*, 446–455.

Chapman, J. L., Zechel, A., Carter, Y. H., *et al.* (2004) Systematic review of recent innovations in service provision to improve access to primary care. *British Journal of General Practice*, *54*, 374–381.

Christensen, H., Griffiths, K., Gulliver, A., *et al.* (2008) Models in the delivery of depression care: a systematic review of randomised and controlled intervention trials. *BMC Family Practice*, *9*, 25.

Christensen, K. S., Fink, P., Toft, T., *et al.* (2005) A brief case-finding questionnaire for common mental disorders: the CMDQ. *Family Practice*, *22*, 448–457.

Clark, D. A. (2004) *Cognitive-Behavioral Therapy for OCD*. New York: Guilford Press.

Clark, D. M., Layard, R., Smithies, R., *et al.* (2009) Improving Access to Psychological Therapy: initial evaluation of two UK demonstration sites. *Behaviour Research and Therapy*, *47*, 910–920.

Cochrane, L. J., Olson, C. A., Murray, S., *et al.* (2007) Gaps between knowing and doing: understanding and assessing the barriers to optimal health care. *Journal of Continuing Education in the Health Professions*, *27*, 94–102.

Cochrane Collaboration (2008) Review Manager (RevMan) Version 5.0. Copenhagen: The Nordic Cochrane Centre, The Cochrane Collaboration. [Computer programme].

Collacott, R. A. (1999) People with Down syndrome and mental health needs. In *Psychiatric and Behavioural Disorders in Developmental Disabilities and Mental Retardation* (ed. N. Barnes). Cambridge: Cambridge University Press.

Cooper, S., Smiley, E., Morrison, J., *et al.* (2007) Mental ill-health in adults with intellectual disabilities: prevalence and associated factors. *The British Journal of Psychiatry*, *190*, 27–35.

Cooper, S. A. (1997) Epidemiology of psychiatric disorders in elderly compared with younger adults with learning disabilities. *British Journal of Health Psychology*, *170*, 375–380.

Cougle, J. R., Keough, M. E., Riccardi, C. J., *et al.* (2009) Anxiety disorders and suicidality in the National Comorbidity Survey-replication. *Journal of Psychiatric Research*, *43*, 825–829.

Craven, M. A. & Bland, R. (2006) Better practices in collaborative mental health care: an analysis of the evidence base. *The Canadian Journal of Psychiatry*, *51* (Suppl. 1), 7S–72S.

Creamer, M., Burgess, P. & McFarlane, A. C. (2001) Post-traumatic stress disorder: findings from the Australian National Survey of Mental Health and Well-being. *Psychological Medicine*, *31*, 1237–1247.

CSIP Choice and Access Team (2007) *Improving Access to Psychological Therapies: Positive Practice Guide.* London: Department of Health.

Cuijpers, P. (1998) Psychological outreach programmes for the depressed elderly: a meta-analysis of effects and dropout. *International Journal of Geriatric Psychiatry*, *13*, 41–48.

Curtis, L. (2009) *Unit Costs of Health and Social Care.* Canterbury: PSSRU, University of Kent.

Das, A. K., Olfson, M., McCurtis, H. L., *et al.* (2006) Depression in African Americans: breaking barriers to detection and treatment. *Applied Evidence*, *55*, 30–39.

Das-Munshi, J., Goldberg, D., Bebbington, P. E., *et al.* (2008) Public health significance of mixed anxiety and depression: beyond current classification. *British Journal of Psychiatry*, *192*, 171–177.

Davidson, J. R., Zhang, W., Connor, K. M., *et al.* (2010) A psychopharmacological treatment algorithm for generalised anxiety disorder (GAD). *Journal of Psychopharmacology*, *24*, 3–26.

Davidson, J. R. T., Book, S. W., Colket, J. T., *et al.* (1997) Assessment of a new self-rating scale for post-traumatic stress disorder. *Psychological Medicine*, *27*, 153–160.

Dennis, C. & Chung-Lee, L. (2006) Postpartum depression help-seeking barriers and maternal treatment preferences: a qualitative systematic review. *Birth*, *33*, 323–331.

Dennis, R. E., Boddington, S. J. & Funnell N. J. (2007) Self-report measures of anxiety: are they suitable for older adults? *Aging & Mental Health*, *11*, 668–677.

Department of Health (1999) *National Service Framework for Mental Health: Modern Standards and Service Models.* London: Department of Health. Available at: http://www.dh.gov.uk/en/Publicationsandstatistics/Publications/PublicationsPolicy AndGuidance/DH_4009598

Department of Health (2001) National Service Framework for Older People. London: Department of Health. Available at: http://www.dh.gov.uk/ en/Publicationsandstatistics/Publications/PublicationsPolicyAndGuidance/DH_ 4003066

Department of Health (2006) *Models of Care for Alcohol Misusers.* London: Department of Health. Available at: http://www.dh.gov.uk/en/Publicationsandstatistics/Publications/PublicationsPolicyAndGuidance/DH_4136806

Department of Health (2009) *Delivering Race Equality in Mental Health Care: A Review.* London: Department of Health. Available at: http://www.dh.gov.uk/en/Publicationsandstatistics/Publications/PublicationsPolicyAndGuidance/DH_4139351

Dixon-Woods, M., Kirk, D. & Agarwal, S., *et al.* (2005) *Vulnerable Groups and Access to Health Care: a Critical Interpretive Review.* Report for the National Co-ordinating Centre for NHS Service Delivery and Organisation R & D (NCCSDO). London: National Co-ordinating Centre for NHS Service Delivery and Organisation. Available at: http://www.sdo.nihr.ac.uk/files/project/SDO_ES_08-1210-025_V01.pdf (accessed 10 August 2011).

Dodd, S. & Berk, M. (2004) Predictors of antidepressant response: a selective review. *International Journal of Psychiatry in Clinical Practice*, 8, 91–100.

Dowrick, C. (1995) Case or continuum? Analysing general practitioners' ability to detect depression. *Primary Care Psychiatry*, 1, 255–257.

Dowrick, C., Gask, L., Edwards, S., *et al.* (2009a) Researching the mental health needs of hard-to-reach groups: managing multiple sources of evidence. *BMC Health Services Research*, 9, 226.

Dowrick, C., Leydon, G. M., McBride, A., *et al.* (2009b) Patients' and doctors' views on depression severity questionnaires incentivised in UK quality and outcomes framework: qualitative study. *British Medical Journal*, 338, 663.

Dowrick, C., Gask, L. & Edwards, S. (2010) Programme to increase equity of access to high quality mental health services in primary care. *Journal of Affective Disorders*, 122, 18–19.

DuPont, R. L., Rice, D. P., Shiraki, S., *et al.* (1995) Economic costs of obsessive-compulsive disorder. *Medical Interface*, 8, 102–109.

DuPont, R. L., Rice, D. P., Miller, L. S., *et al.* (1998) Economic costs of anxiety disorders. *Anxiety*, 2, 167–172.

Dwamena, B. (2009) *MIDAS: Stata Module for Meta-Analytical Integration of Diagnostic Test Accuracy Studies.* Statistical Software Components S456880. Boston, MA: Boston College Department of Economics.

Dy, S. M., Garg, P., Nyberg, D., *et al.* (2005) Critical pathway effectiveness: assessing the impact of patient, hospital care, and pathway characteristics using qualitative comparative analysis. *Health Services Research*, 40, 499–516.

Eack, S. M., Greeno, C. G. & Lee, B. (2006) Limitations of the Patient Health Questionnaire in identifying anxiety and depression in community mental health: many cases are undetected. *Research on Social Work Practice*, 16, 625–631.

Eccles, M., Freemantle, N. & Mason, J. (1998) North of England evidence based guideline development project: methods of developing guidelines for efficient drug use in primary care. *British Medical Journal*, 316, 1232–1235.

Edlund, M. J. & Swann, A. C. (1987) The economic and social costs of panic disorder. *Hospital & Community Psychiatry*, 38, 1277–1288.

*References*

Ehlers A., Gene-Cos N. & Perrin M. (2009) Low recognition of post-traumatic stress disorder in primary care. *London Journal of Primary Care*, *2*, 36–42.

Emmerson, B., Frost, A., Fawcett, L., *et al.* (2006) Do clinical pathways really improve clinical performance in mental health settings? *Australasian Psychiatry*, *14*, 395–398.

European Agency for Safety and Health at Work (2000) *Research on Work-Related Stress*. Luxembourg: Office for Official Publication of the European Communities. Available at http://osha.europa.eu/en/publications/reports/203/view

Evans-Lacko, S. E., Jarrett, M., McCrone, P., *et al.* (2008) Clinical pathways in psychiatry. *The British Journal of Psychiatry*, *193*, 4–5.

Fava, M. & Kendler, K. (2000) Major depressive disorder. *Neuron*, *28*, 335–341.

Fechner-Bates, S., Coyne J. C. & Schwenk, T. L. (1994) The relationship of self-reported distress to depressive disorders and other psychopathology. *Journal of Consulting and Clinical Psychology*, *62*, 550–559.

Fekadu, A., Wooderson, S. C., Markoloulo, K., *et al.* (2009) What happens to patients with treatment resistant depression? A systematic review of medium to long term outcome studies. *Journal of Affective Disorders*, *116*, 4–11.

Fiellin, D. A., Reid, M. C. & O'Connor, P. G. (2000) Screening for alcohol problems in primary care: a systematic review. *Archives of Internal Medicine*, *160*, 1977–1989.

Fineberg, N. A. & Roberts, A. (2001) Obsessive compulsive disorder: a twenty-first century perspective. In *Obsessive Compulsive Disorder: a Practical Guide* (eds N. A. Fineberg, D. Marazziti & D. Stein), pp. 1–13. London: Martin Dunitz.

Fineberg, N. A., O'Doherty, C. & Rajagopal, S. (2003) How common is obsessive-compulsive disorder in a dermatology outpatient clinic? *The Journal of Clinical Psychology*, *64*, 152–155.

First, M. B., Spitzer, R. L., Gibbon, M., *et al.* (1997) *Structured Clinical Interview for DSM-IV Axis I Disorders: Clinician Version* (SCID-CV). Washington DC: American Psychiatric Press.

Fischer, J. E., Bachmann, L. M. & Jaeschke, R. (2003) A readers' guide to the interpretation of diagnostic test properties: clinical example of sepsis. *Intensive Care Medicine*, *29*, 1043–1051.

Fisher, T. L., Burnet, D. L., Huang, E. S., *et al.* (2007) Cultural leverage: interventions using culture to narrow racial disparities in health care. *Medical Care Research Review*, *64*, 243–282.

Flores, G. (2005) The impact of medical interpreter services on the quality of health care: a systematic review. *Medical Care Research Review*, *62*, 255–299.

Foa, E. B. & Kozak, M. J. (1996) Psychological treatment for obsessive-compulsive disorder. In *Long-Term Treatments of Anxiety Disorders* (eds M. R. Mavissakalian & R. F. Freeman), pp. 285–308. Washington DC: American Psychiatric Press.

Foa, E. B., Riggs, D. S., Dancu, C. V., *et al.* (1993) Reliability and validity of a brief instrument for assessing post-traumatic stress disorder. *Journal of Traumatic Stress*, *6*, 459–473.

Foa, E. B., Kozak, M. J., Goodman, W. K., *et al.* (1995) DSM-IV field trial: obsessive compulsive disorder. *American Journal of Psychiatry*, *152*, 90–96.

Foa, E. B., Cashman, L., Jaycox, L., *et al.* (1997) The validation of a self-report measure of posttraumatic stress disorder: the Posttraumatic Diagnostic Scale. *Psychological Assessment*, *9*, 445–451.

Foa, E. B., Keane, T. M. & Friedman, M. J. (2008) *Effective Treatments for PTSD: Practice Guidelines from the International Society for Traumatic Stress Studies.* New York: The Guilford Press.

Foy, R., Hempel, S., Rubenstein, L., *et al.* (2010) Meta-analysis: effect of interactive communication between collaborating primary care physicians and specialists. *Annals of Internal Medicine*, *152*, 247–258.

Francis, J. L., Weisberg, R. B., Dyck, I. R., *et al.* (2007) Characteristics and course of panic disorder and panic disorder with agoraphobia in primary care patients. *Primary Care Companion to The Journal of Clinical Psychiatry*, *9*, 173–179.

Frederick, J. T., Steinman, L. E., Prochaska, T., *et al.* (2007) Community-based treatment of late life depression: an expert panel-informed literature review. *American Journal of Preventive Medicine*, *33*, 222–249.

Freeston, M., Rheaume, J. & Ladouceur, R. (1996) Correcting faulty appraisals of obsessive thoughts. *Behaviour Research and Therapy*, *34*, 446.

Frost, R. & Steketee, G. (1999) Issues in the treatment of compulsive hoarding. *Cognitive and Behavioral Practice*, *6*, 397–407.

Gask, L., Dowrick, C., Dixon, C., *et al.* (2004) A pragmatic cluster randomised controlled trial of an educational intervention for GPs in the assessment and management of depression. *Psychological Medicine*, *34*, 63–72.

Gask, L., Lever-Green, G. & Hays, R. (2008) Dissemination and implementation of suicide prevention training in one Scottish region. *BMC Health Services*, *8*, 246.

Gensichen, J., Beyer, M., Muth, C., *et al.* (2005) Case management to improve major depression in primary health care: a systematic review. *Psychological Medicine*, *36*, 7–14.

Gerber, P. D., Barrett, J. E., Barrett, J. A., *et al.* (1992) The relationship of presenting physical complaints to depressive symptoms in primary care patients. *Journal of General Internal Medicine*, *7*, 170–173.

Gilbody, S., Whitty, P., Grimshaw, J., *et al.* (2003) Educational and organizational interventions to improve the management of depression in primary care: a systematic review. *Journal of the American Medical Association*, *289*, 3145–3152.

Gilbody, S., Bower, P., Fletcher, J., *et al.* (2006) Collaborative care for depression: a cumulative meta-analysis and review of longer term outcomes. *Archives of Internal Medicine*, *166*, 2314–2321.

Gilbody, S., Richards, D., Brealey S., *et al.* (2007) Screening for depression in medical settings with the Patient Health Questionnaire (PHQ): a diagnostic meta-analysis. *Journal of General Internal Medicine*, *22*, 1596–1602.

Gilbody, S. M., House, A. O. & Sheldon T. A. (2002) Psychiatrists in the UK do not use outcomes measures: national survey. *British Journal of Psychiatry*, *180*, 101–103.

## References

Giles, D. E., Jarrett, R. B., Biggs, M. M., *et al.* (1989) Clinical predictors of recurrence in depression. *American Journal of Psychiatry*, *146*, 764–767.

Gill, S. C., Butterworth, P., Rodgers, B., *et al.* (2007) Validity of the mental health component scale of the 12-item Short-Form Health Survey (MCS-12) as measure of common mental disorders in the general population. *Psychiatry Research*, *152*, 63–71.

Glover, G., Webb, M. & Evison, F. (2010) *Improving Access to Psychological Therapies: a Review of the Progress Made by Sites in the First Roll-out Year.* Stockton-on-Tees: North East Public Health Observatory.

Goldberg, D., Privett, M., Ustun, B., *et al.* (1998) The effects of detection and treatment on the outcome of major depression in primary care: a naturalistic study in 15 cities. *The British Journal of General Practice*, *48*, 1840–1844.

Goldberg, D. P. & Bridges, K. (1988) Somatic presentations of psychiatric illness in primary care settings. *Journal of Psychosomatic Research*, *32*, 137–144.

Goldberg, D. P. & Huxley, P. J. (1992) *Common Mental Disorders: a Bio-Social Model.* London: Tavistock/Routledge.

Goldberg, D. P., Steele, J. J. & Smith, C. (1980a) Teaching psychiatric interview techniques to family doctors epidemiological research as basis for the organization of extramural psychiatry: proceedings of the 'Second European Symposium on Social Psychiatry', Psychiatric Hospital in Aarhus 26–28 September, 1979. *Acta Psychiatrica Scandinavia*, *62*, 41–47.

Goldberg, D. P., Steele, J. J., Smith, C., *et al.* (1980b) Training family doctors to recognise psychiatric illness with increased accuracy. *Lancet*, *2*, 521–523.

Goldberg, D. P., Jenkins, L., Millar, T., *et al.* (1993) The ability of trainee general practitioners to identify psychological distress among their patients. *Psychological Medicine*, *23*, 185–193.

Goodwin, G. (2000) Neurobiological aetiology of mood disorders. In *New Oxford Textbook of Psychiatry* (eds M. G. Gelder, J. J. Lopez-Ibor & N. Andreasen), pp. 711–719. Oxford: Oxford University Press.

Gothelf, D., Aharonovsky, O., Horesh, N., *et al.* (2004) Life events and personality factors in children and adolescents with obsessive-compulsive disorder and other anxiety disorders. *Comprehensive Psychiatry*, *45*, 192–198.

Greenberg, P. E., Sisitsky, T., Kessler, R. C., *et al.* (1999) The economic burden of anxiety disorders in the 1990s. *Journal of Clinical Psychiatry*, *60*, 427–435.

Griffiths, K. M., & Christensen, H. (2008) Depression in primary health care: from evidence to policy. *Medical Journal of Australia*, *188*, 81–83.

Grilli, R., Ramsay, C. & Minozzi, S. (2002) Mass media interventions: effects on health service utilisation. *Cochrane Database of Systematic Reviews*, Issue 1. CD000389. DOI: 10.1002/14651858.CD000389

Griner, D. & Smith, T. (2006) Culturally adapted mental health intervention: a meta-analytic review. *Psychotherapy*, *43*, 531–548.

Gruen, R. L., Weeramanthri, T. S., Knight S. S., *et al.* (2003) Specialist outreach clinics in primary care and rural hospital settings. *Cochrane Database of Systematic Reviews*, Issue 1. CD003798.

Gulliford, M., Figueroa-Munoz, J., Morgan, M., *et al.* (2007) What does 'access to health care' mean? *Journal of Health Services Research & Policy*, *7*, 186–188.

Gunn, J., Diggens, J., Hegarty, K., *et al.* (2006) A systematic review of complex system interventions designed to increase recovery from depression in primary care. *BMC Health Services Research*, *6*, 88.

Hakkaart-van Roijen, L., van Straten, A., Al, M., *et al.* (2006) Cost-utility of brief psychological treatment for depression and anxiety. *British Journal of Psychiatry*, *188*, 323–329.

Hall, A., A'Hern, R. & Fallowfield, L. (1999) Are we using appropriate self-report questionnaires for detecting anxiety and depression in women with early breast cancer? *European Journal of Cancer*, *35*, 79–85.

Hansard (2004) *House of Commons: Written Answers from Mary Eagle, 27 May 2004, col. 1790W*. London: Stationery Office.

Hardeveld, F., Spijker, J., De Graaf, R., *et al.* (2010) Prevalence and predictors of recurrence of major depressive disorder in the adult population. *Acta Psychiatrica Scandinavica*, *122*, 184–191.

Harkness, E. F. & Bower, P. J. (2009) On-site mental health workers delivering psychological therapy and psychosocial interventions to patients in primary care: effects on the professional practice of primary care providers. *Cochrane Database of Systematic Reviews*, Issue 1. CD000532.

Harris, T. (2000) Introduction to the work of George Brown. In *Where Inner and Outer Worlds Meet: Psychosocial Research in the Tradition of George W. Brown*, (ed. T. Harris), pp. 1–52. London & New York: Routledge.

Haworth, J. E., Moniz-Cook, E., Clark, A. L., *et al.* (2007) An evaluation of two self-report screening measures for mood in an out-patient chronic heart failure population. *International Journal of Geriatric Psychiatry*, *22*, 1147–1153.

Heideman, J., van Rijswijk, E., van Lin, N, *et al.* (2005) Interventions to improve management of anxiety disorders in general practice. *British Journal of General Practice*, *55*, 867–873.

Heim, C. & Nemeroff, C. B. (2001) The role of childhood trauma in the neurobiology of mood and anxiety disorders: preclinical and clinical studies. *Biological Psychiatry*, *49*, 1023–1039.

Henkel, V., Mergl, R., Kohnen, R., *et al.* (2003) Identifying depression in primary care: a comparison of different methods in a prospective cohort study. *British Medical Journal*, *326*, 200–201.

Hettema, J. M., Neale, M. C. & Kendler, K. S. (2001) A review and meta-analysis of the genetic epidemiology of anxiety disorders. *American Journal of Psychiatry*, *158*, 1568–1578.

Hettema, J. M., Prescott, C. A. & Kendler, K. S. (2004) Genetic and environmental sources of covariation between generalized anxiety disorder and neuroticism. *American Journal of Psychiatry*, *161*, 1581–1587.

Hettema, J. M., Prescott, C. A., Myers, J. M., *et al.* (2005) The structure of genetic and environmental risk factors for anxiety disorders in men and women. *Archives of General Psychiatry*, *62*, 182–189.

Hewitt, C. E., Gilbody, S. M., Brealey, S., *et al.* (2009) Methods to identify postnatal depression in primary care: an integrated evidence synthesis and value of information analysis. *Health Technology Assessment*, *13*, 36.

## References

Horowitz, M. J., Wilner, N. & Alvarez, W. (1979) Impact of Event Scale: a measure of subjective stress. *Psychosomatic Medicine*, *41*, 209–218.

Huffman, J. C. & Pollack, M. H. (2003) Predicting panic disorder among patients with chest pain: an analysis of the literature. *Psychosomatics*, *44*, 222–236.

Humphris, G. M., Morrison, T. & Lindsay, S. J. (1995) The Modified Dental Anxiety Scale: validation and United Kingdom norms. *Community Dental Health*, *12*, 143–150.

IAPT (2010) *The IAPT Data Handbook: Guidance on Recording and Monitoring Outcomes to Support Local Evidence-Based Practice. Version 1.0.* See http://www.iapt.nhs.uk

Jadad, A. R., Moore, R. A. & Carroll, D. (1996) Assessing the quality of reports of randomised clinical trials: is blinding necessary? *Controlled Clinical Trials*, *17*, 1–12.

Jeffries, D. (2006) Ever been HAD? *British Journal of General Practice*, *56*, 885–886.

Jimison, H., Gorman, P., Woods, S., *et al.* (2008) Barriers and drivers of health information technology use for the elderly, chronically ill, and underserved. *Evidence Report/Technology Assessment*, *175*, 1–1422.

Jung, H. P., Baerveldt, C., Olesen, F., *et al.* (2003) Patient characteristics as predictors of primary health care preferences: a systematic literature analysis. *Health Expectations*, *6*, 160–181.

Kairy, D., Lehoux, P., Vincent, CF., *et al.* (2009) A systematic review of clinical outcomes, clinical process, healthcare utilization and costs associated with telerehabilitation. *Disability & Rehabilitation*, *31*, 1–21.

Katona, C. (2000) Managing depression and anxiety in the elderly patient. *European Neuropsychopharmacology*, *10*, 427–432.

Kendler, K. S. (1996) Major depression and generalised anxiety disorder same genes, (partly) different environments – revisited. *British Journal of Psychiatry*, *30*, 68–75.

Kendler, K. S., Gardner, C. O., Neale, M. C., *et al.* (2001) Genetic risk factors for major depression in men and women: similar or different heritabilities and same or partly distinct genes? *Psychological Medicine*, *31*, 605–616.

Kendler, L. & Prescott, C. (1999) A population-based twin study of lifetime major depression in men and women. *Archives of General Psychiatry*, *56*, 39–44.

Kendrick, T., Dowrick, C., McBride, A., *et al.* (2009) Management of depression in UK general practice in relation to scores on depression severity questionnaires: analysis of medical record data. *British Medical Journal*, *339*, b750.

Kendrick, T., King, F., Albertella, L., *et al.* (2005) GP treatment decisions for depression: an observational study. *British Journal of General Practice*, *55*, 280–286.

Kendrick, T., Stevens, L., Bryant, A., *et al.* (2001) Hampshire Depression Project: changes in the process of care and cost consequences. *British Journal of General Practice*, *51*, 911–913.

Kennedy, B. L. & Schwab, J. J. (1997) Utilization of medical specialists by anxiety disorder patients. *Psychosomatics*, *38*, 109–112.

Kessing, L. V. (2007) Epidemiology of subtypes of depression. *Acta Psychiatrica Scandinavica*, *433*, 85–89.

Kessler, D., Bennewith, O., Lewis, G., *et al.* (2002b) Detection of depression and anxiety in primary care: follow up study. *British Medical Journal*, *325*, 1016–1017.

Kessler, R. C., Sonnega, A., Bromet. E., *et al.* (1995) Posttraumatic stress disorder in the National Comorbidity Survey. *Archives of General Psychiatry*, *52*, 1048–1060.

Kessler, R. C., Stang, P., Wittchen, H. U., *et al.* (1999) Lifetime co-morbidities between social phobia and mood disorders in the US National Comorbidity Survey. *Psychological Medicine*, *29*, 555–567.

Kessler, R. C., Greenberg, P. E., Mickelson, K. D., *et al.* (2001) The effects of chronic mental health conditions on work loss and work cut back. *Journal of Occupational and Environmental Medicine*, *43*, 218–225.

Kessler, R. C., Berglund, P. A., Dewit, D. J., *et al.* (2002a) Distinguishing generalized anxiety disorder from major depression: prevalence and impairment from current pure and comorbid disorders in the US and Ontario. *International Journal of Methods in Psychiatric Research*, *11*, 99–111.

Kessler, R. C., Berglund, P., Demler, O., *et al.* (2003) The epidemiology of major depressive disorder: results from the National Comorbidity Survey Replication (NCS-R). *Journal of the American Medical Association*, *289*, 3095–3105.

Kessler, R. C., Berglund, P., Demler, O., *et al.* (2005a) Lifetime prevalence and age of onset distributions of DSM-IV disorders in the National Comorbidity Survey replication. *Archives of General Psychiatry*, *62*, 593–602.

Kessler, R. C., Chiu, W. T., Demler, O., *et al.* (2005b) Prevalence, severity and comorbidity of 12-month DSM-IV disorders in the National Comorbidity Survey Replication. *Archives of General Psychiatry*, *62*, 617–627.

Khan, A., Leventhala, R. M., Khan, S., *et al.* (2002) Suicide risk in patients with anxiety disorders: a meta-analysis of the FDA database. *Journal of Affective Disorders*, *68*, 183–190.

Khanna, S., Rajendra, P. N. & Channabasavanna, S. M. (1988) Life events and onset of obsessive compulsive disorder. *International Journal of Social Psychiatry*, *34*, 305–309.

King, M., Walker, C., Levy, G., *et al.* (2008) Development and validation of an international risk prediction algorithm for episodes of major depression in general practice attendees: the PredictD study. *Archives of General Psychiatry*, *65*, 1368–1376.

Kinnersley, P., Edwards, A., Hood, K., *et al.* (2008) Interventions before consultations to help patients address their information needs by encouraging question asking: systematic review. *British Medical Journal*, *337*, 485–494.

Kisely, S., Gater, R. & Goldberg, D. P. (1995) Results from the Manchester Centre. In *Mental Illness in General Health Care: an International Study* (eds T. B. Üstün & N. Sartorius), pp. 175–191. Chichester: Wiley.

Knapp, M. (2003) Hidden costs of mental illness. *British Journal of Psychiatry*, *183*, 477–478.

## References

Knapp, M. & Ilson, S. (2002) Economic aspects of depression and its treatment. *Current Opinion in Psychiatry*, *15*, 69–75.

Knaup, C., Koesters, M., Schoefer, D., *et al.* (2009) Effect of feedback of treatment outcome in specialist mental healthcare: a meta-analysis. *The British Journal of Psychiatry*, *195*, 15–22.

Kobak, K. A., Taylor, L. H., Dottl, S. L., *et al.* (1997) A computer-administered telephone interview to identify mental disorders. *Journal of the American Medical Association*, *278*, 905–910.

Kobak, K. A., Schaettle, S. C., Greist, J. H., *et al.* (1998) Computer-administered rating scales for social anxiety in a clinical drug trial. *Depression and Anxiety*, *7*, 97–145.

Koran, L. M., Ringold, A. L. & Elliott, M. A. (2000) Olanzapine augmentation for treatment-resistant obsessive-compulsive disorder. *Journal of Clinical Psychiatry*, *61*, 514–517.

Krasucki, C., Ryan, P., Ertan, T., *et al.* (1999) The FEAR: A rapid screening instrument for generalized anxiety in elderly primary care attenders. *International Journal of Geriatric Psychiatry*, *14*, 60–68.

Krefetz, D. G., Steer, R. A., Jermyn, R. T., *et al.* (2004) Screening HIV-infected patients with chronic pain for anxiety and mood disorders with the Beck Anxiety and Depression Inventory-Fast Screens for medical settings. *Journal of Clinical Psychology in Medical Settings*, *11*, 283–289.

Krochmalik, A., Jones, M. K., & Menzies, R. G. (2001) Danger ideation reduction therapy (DIRT) for treatment-resistant compulsive washing. *Behaviour Research and Therapy*, *39*, 897–912.

Kroenke, K., Jackson, J. L. & Chamberlin, J. (1997) Depressive and anxiety disorders in patients presenting with physical complaints: clinical predictors and outcome. *The American Journal of Medicine*, *103*, 339–347.

Kroenke, K., Spitzer, R. L. & Williams, J. B. (2001) The PHQ-9: validity of a brief depression severity measure. *Journal of General Internal Medicine*, *16*, 606–613.

Kroenke, K., Spitzer, R. L., Williams, J. B., *et al.* (2007) Anxiety disorders in primary care: prevalence, impairment, comorbidity and detection. *Annals of Internal Medicine*, *146*, 317–325.

Kupfer, D. J. (1991) Long-term treatment of depression. *Journal of Clinical Psychiatry*, *52*, 28–34.

Lambert, M. J., Whipple, J. L. & Hawkins, E. J. (2003) Is it time for clinicians to routinely track patient outcome? A meta-analysis. *Clinical Psychology: Science and Practice*, *10*, 288–301.

Lambert, M. J., Gregersen, A. T. & Burlingame, G. M. (2004) The Outcome Questionnaire-45. In *Use of Psychological Testing for Treatment Planning and Outcome Assessment* (3rd edn) (ed. M. E. Murish), vol. 3, pp. 191–234. New Jersey: Erlbaum.

Lang, A., Norman, S., Means-Christensen, A., *et al.* (2009) Abbreviated Brief Symptom Inventory for use as an anxiety and depression screening instrument in primary care. *Depression and Anxiety*, *26*, 537–543.

LaSalle, V. H., Cromer, K. R., Nelson, K. N., *et al.* (2004) Diagnostic interview assessed neuropsychiatric disorder comorbidity in 334 individuals with obsessive compulsive disorder. *Depression and Anxiety*, *19*, 163–173.

Layard, R. (2006) *The Depression Report: a New Deal for Depression and Anxiety Disorders*. London: Centre for Economic Performance. Available at: http://cep.lse.ac.uk/pubs/download/special/depressionreport.pdf

Lecrubier, Y., Sheehan, D., Weiller, E., *et al.* (1997) The MINI International Neuropsychiatric Interview (M.I.N.I.): a short diagnostic structured interview: reliability and validity according to the CIDI. *European Psychiatry*, *12*, 224–231.

Leon, A. C., Portera, L. & Weissman, M. M. (1995) The social costs of anxiety disorders. *British Journal of Psychiatry*, *166*, 19–22.

Lewinsohn, P. M., Solomon, A., Seeley, J. R., *et al.* (2000) Clinical implications of 'subthreshold' depressive symptoms. *Journal of Abnormal Psychology*, *109*, 345–351.

Liebowitz, M. R., Gorman, J. M., Fyer, A. J., *et al.* (1985) Social phobia: review of a neglected anxiety disorder. *Archives of General Psychiatry*, *42*, 729–736.

Lindesay, J., Jagger, C., Hibbett, M., *et al.* (1997) Knowledge, uptake and availability of health and social services among Asian Gujarati and white elderly persons. *Ethnicity and Health*, *2*, 59–69.

Lochner, C. & Stein, D. J. (2003) Heterogeneity of obsessive-compulsive disorder: a literature review. *Harvard Review of Psychiatry*, *11*, 113–132.

Love, A. W., Kissane, D. W., Bloch, S., *et al.* (2002) Diagnostic efficiency of the Hospital Anxiety and Depression Scale in women with early stage breast cancer. *Australian and New Zealand Journal of Psychiatry*, *36*, 246–250.

Lowe, B., Spitzer, R. L., Grafe, K., *et al.* (2004) Comparative validity of three screening questionnaires for DSM-IV depressive disorders and physicians' diagnoses. *Journal of Affective Disorders*, *78*, 131–140.

Malhi, G. S., Parker, G. B. & Greenwood, J. (2005) Structural and functional models of depression: from sub-types to substrates. *Acta Psychiatrica Scandinavica*, *111*, 94–105.

Mann, J. J., Apter, A., Bertolote, J., *et al.* (2005) Suicide prevention strategies: a systematic review. *Journal of the American Medical Association*, *294*, 2064–2074.

Mann, T. (1996) *Clinical Guidelines: Using Clinical Guidelines to Improve Patient Care within the NHS*. London: Department of Health.

Marciniak, M., Lage, M. J., Landbloom, R. P., *et al.* (2004) Medical and productivity costs of anxiety disorders: case control study. *Depression and Anxiety*, *19*, 112–120.

Marciniak, M. D., Lage, M. J., Dunayevich, E., *et al.* (2005) The cost of treating anxiety: the medical and demographic correlates that impact total medical costs. *Depression and Anxiety*, *21*, 178–184.

Marks, I. (1997) Behaviour therapy for obsessive-compulsive disorder: a decade of progress. *Canadian Journal of Psychiatry*, *42*, 1021–1027.

Marks, J., Goldberg, D. P. & Hillier, V. F. (1979) Determinants of the ability of general practitioners to detect psychiatric illness. *Psychological Medicine*, *9*, 337–353.

Marshall, M., Crowther, R., Almaraz-Serrano, A. M., *et al.* (2001) Systematic reviews of the effectiveness of day care for people with severe mental disorders: (1) acute day hospital versus admission; (2) vocational rehabilitation; (3) day hospital versus outpatient care. *Health Technology Assessment*, *5*, 1–75.

McCrone, P., Dhanasiri, S., Patel, A., *et al.* (2008) *Paying the Price: the Cost of Mental Health Care in England to 2026*. London: King's Fund. Available at: http://www.kingsfund.org.uk/publications/paying_the_price.html

McManus, S., Meltzer, H., Brugha, T., *et al.* (2009) *Adult Psychiatric Morbidity in England, 2007: Results of a Household Survey*. Leicester: Department of Health Sciences, University of Leicester.

McMillan, D., Gilbody, S., Beresford, E., *et al.* (2007) Can we predict suicide and non-fatal self-harm with the Beck Hopelessness Scale? A meta-analysis. *Psychological Medicine*, *37*, 769–778.

McNally, R. J. (2003) *Remembering Trauma*. Cambridge, MA: Harvard University Press.

Means-Christensen, A. J., Sherbourne, C. D., Roy-Byrne, P. P., *et al.* (2006) Using five questions to screen for five common mental disorders in primary care: diagnostic accuracy of the Anxiety and Depression Detector. *General Hospital Psychiatry*, *28*, 108–118.

Meghani, S. H., Brooks, J. M., Gipson-Jones, T., *et al.* (2009) Patient-provider race-concordance: does it matter in improving minority patients' health outcomes? *Ethnicity & Health*, *14*, 107–130.

Meltzer, H., Bebbington, P., Brugha, T., *et al.* (2000) The reluctance to seek treatment for neurotic disorders. *Journal of Mental Health*, *9*, 319–327.

Microsoft (2007) Microsoft Word and Excel [computer software]. Redmond, Washington: Microsoft.

Mitchell, A., Vaze, A. & Sanjay Rao, S. (2009) Clinical diagnosis of depression in primary care: a meta-analysis. *Lancet*, *374*, 609–619.

Mitchell, A. J. & Subramaniam, H. (2005) Prognosis of depression in old age compared to middle age: a systematic review of comparative studies. *American Journal of Psychiatry*, *162*, 1588–1601.

Moffat, J., Sass, B., McKenzie, K., *et al.* (2009) Improving pathways into mental health care for black and ethnic minority groups: a systematic review of the grey literature. *International Review of Psychiatry*, *21*, 439–449.

Montgomery, S. A., Kasper, S., Stein, D. J., *et al.* (2001) Citalopram 20 mg, 40 mg and 60 mg are all effective and well tolerated compared with placebo in obsessive compulsive disorder. *International Clinical Psychopharmacology*, *16*, 75–86.

Moscicki, E. K. (2001) Epidemiology of completed and attempted suicide: toward a framework for prevention. *Clinical Neuroscience Research*, *1*, 310–323.

Moussavi, S., Chatterji, S., Verdes, E., *et al.* (2007) Depression, chronic diseases, and decrements in health: results from the World Health Surveys. *Lancet*, *370*, 851–858.

Murray, C. & Lopez, A. D. (1997) Alternative projections of mortality and disability by cause 1990–2020: Global Burden of Disease Study. *Lancet*, *349*, 1498–1504.

Murray, C. J. L., Lopez, A. D. & Jamison, D. T. (1994) The global burden of disease in 1990: summary results, sensitivity analysis and future directions. *Bulletin of the World Health Organization*, *72*, 495–509.

Narrow, W. E., Rae, D. S., Robins, L. N., *et al.* (2002) Revised prevalence estimates of mental disorders in the United States: using a clinical significance criterion to reconcile 2 surveys' estimates. *Archives of General Psychiatry*, *59*, 115–123.

National Patient Safety Agency (2009) *Preventing Suicide: a Toolkit for Mental Health Services*. London: NHS NPSA.

NCCMH (2004a) *Depression: Management of Depression in Primary and Secondary Care*. Leicester & London: The British Psychological Society & the Royal College of Psychiatrists. [Full guideline]

NCCMH (2004b) *Self-harm: the Short-term Physical and Psychological Management and Secondary Prevention of Self-harm in Primary and Secondary Care*. Leicester & London: The British Psychological Society & the Royal College of Psychiatrists. [Full guideline]

NCCMH (2005) *Post-traumatic Stress Disorder (PTSD): the Management of PTSD in Adults and Children in Primary and Secondary Care*. Leicester & London: The British Psychological Society & the Royal College of Psychiatrists. [Full guideline]

NCCMH (2006) *Obsessive-compulsive Disorder: Core Interventions in the Treatment of Obsessive-compulsive Disorder and Body Dysmorphic Disorder*. Leicester & London: The British Psychological Society & the Royal College of Psychiatrists. [Full guideline]

NCCMH (2007) *Antenatal and Postnatal Mental Health: Clinical Management and Service Guidance*. Leicester & London: The British Psychological Society & the Royal College of Psychiatrists. [Full guideline]

NCCMH (2008a) *Drug Misuse: Psychosocial Interventions*. Leicester & London: The British Psychological Society & the Royal College of Psychiatrists. [Full guideline]

NCCMH (2008b) *Drug Misuse: Opioid Detoxification*. Leicester & London: The British Psychological Society & the Royal College of Psychiatrists. [Full guideline]

NCCMH (2010a) *Depression in Adults with a Chronic Physical Health Problem: Treatment and Management*. Leicester & London: The British Psychological Society & the Royal College of Psychiatrists. [Full guideline]

NCCMH (2010b) *Depression: the Treatment and Management of Depression in Adults*. (Updated edn.) Leicester & London: The British Psychological Society & the Royal College of Psychiatrists. [Full guideline]

NCCMH (2011a) *Generalised Anxiety Disorder in Adults: Management in Primary, Secondary and Community Care*. Leicester & London: The British Psychological Society & the Royal College of Psychiatrists. [Full guideline]

NCCMH (2011b) *Alcohol-use Disorders: Diagnosis, Assessment and Management of Harmful Drinking and Alcohol Dependence*. Leicester & London: The British Psychological Society & the Royal College of Psychiatrists. [Full guideline]

NCCMH (forthcoming) *Self-harm: Longer-term Management.* Leicester & London: The British Psychological Society & the Royal College of Psychiatrists.

Nelson, J. C., Delucchi, K. & Schneider, L. S. (2009) Anxiety does not predict response to antidepressant treatment in late life depression: results of a meta-analysis. *International Journal of Geriatric Psychiatry, 24*, 539–544.

Nestadt, G., Addington, A., Samuels, J., *et al.* (2003) The identification of OCD: related subgroups based on comorbidity. *Biological Psychiatry, 53*, 914–920.

Neumeyer-Gromen, A., Dipl-Soz, T. L., Stark, K., *et al.* (2004) Disease management programs for depression: a systematic review and meta-analysis of randomized controlled trials. *Medical Care, 42*, 1211–1221.

New Zealand Guidelines Group (2008) *Identification of Common Mental Disorders and Management of Depression in Primary Care: an Evidence-Based Best Practice Guideline.* Wellington: New Zealand Guidelines Group.

Newman, M. G., Zuellig, A. R., Kachin, K. E., *et al.* (2002) Preliminary reliability and validity of the Generalized Anxiety Disorder Questionnaire-IV: a revised self-report diagnostic measure of generalized anxiety disorder. *Behaviour Therapy, 33*, 215–233.

Newth, S. & Rachman, S. (2001) The concealment of obsessions. *Behaviour Research and Therapy, 39*, 457–464.

NHS Information Centre (2008) Quality and Outcomes Framework Database [website]. Available at: www.ic.nhs.uk/qof

NICE (2004a) *Anxiety: Management of Anxiety (Panic Disorder, With Or Without Agoraphobia, and Generalised Anxiety Disorder) in Adults in Primary, Secondary and Community Care.* NICE Clinical Guideline 22. Available at: www.nice.org.uk/CG22 [NICE guideline]

NICE (2004b) *Depression: Management of Depression in Primary and Secondary Care.* NICE Clinical Guideline 23. Available at: www.nice.org.uk/CG23 [NICE guideline]

NICE (2004c) *Self-harm: the Short-term Physical and Psychological Management and Secondary Prevention of Self-harm in Primary and Secondary Care.* NICE Clinical Guideline 16. Available at: www.nice.org.uk/CG16 [NICE guideline]

NICE (2005a) *Obsessive-compulsive Disorder: Core Interventions in the Treatment of Obsessive-compulsive Disorder and Body Dysmorphic Disorder.* NICE Clinical Guideline 31. Available at: www.nice.org.uk/CG31 [NICE guideline]

NICE (2005b) *Post-traumatic Stress Disorder (PTSD): the Management of PTSD in Adults and Children in Primary and Secondary Care.* NICE Clinical Guideline 26. Available at: www.nice.org.uk/CG26 [NICE guideline]

NICE (2006) *Bipolar Disorder: the Management of Bipolar Disorder in Adults, Children and Adolescents, in Primary and Secondary Care.* NICE Clinical Guideline 38. Available at: www.nice.org.uk/CG38 [NICE guideline]

NICE (2007a) *Antenatal and Postnatal Mental Health: Clinical Management and Service Guidance.* NICE Clinical Guideline 45. Available at: www.nice.org.uk/CG45 [NICE guideline]

NICE (2007b) *Drug Misuse: Psychosocial Interventions.* NICE Clinical Guideline 51. Available at: www.nice.org.uk/CG51www.nice.org.uk/CG51 [NICE guideline]

NICE (2007c) *Drug Misuse: Opioid Detoxification.* NICE Clinical Guideline 52. Available at: www.nice.org.uk/CG52 [NICE guideline]

NICE (2009a) *Depression: the Treatment and Management of Depression in Adults.* NICE Clinical Guideline 90. Available at: www.nice.org.uk/CG90 [NICE guideline]

NICE (2009b) *Depression in Adults with a Chronic Physical Health Problem: Treatment and Management.* NICE Clinical Guideline 91. Available at: www.nice.org.uk/CG91 [NICE guideline]

NICE (2009c) *Medicines Adherence: Involving Patients in Decisions about Prescribed Medicines and Supporting Adherence.* NICE Clinical Guideline 76. Available at: www.nice.org.uk/CG76

NICE (2009d) *The Guidelines Manual.* London: NICE.

NICE (2011a) *Generalised Anxiety Disorder and Panic Disorder (With or Without Agoraphobia) in Adults: Management in Primary, Secondary and Community Care.* NICE Clinical Guideline 113. Available at: www.nice.org.uk/CG113 [NICE guideline]

NICE (2011b) *Alcohol-use Disorders: Diagnosis, Assessment and Management of Harmful Drinking and Alcohol Dependence.* NICE Clinical Guideline 115. Available at: www.nice.org.uk/CG115. [NICE guideline]

NICE (2011c) *Self-harm: Longer-term Management.* NICE Clinical Guideline 133. Available at: www.nice.org.uk/CG133. [NICE guideline]

Nicholson, A., Kuper, H. & Hemingway, H. (2006) Depression as an aetiologic and prognostic factor in coronary heart disease: a meta-analysis of 6362 events among 146,538 participants in 54 observational studies. *European Heart Journal, 27,* 2763–2774.

Noyes, J., Clarkson, C., Crowe, R. R., *et al.* (1987) A family study of generalized anxiety disorder. *American Journal of Psychiatry, 144,* 1019–1024.

Nuechterlein, K. H. & Dawson, M. E. (1984) A heuristic vulnerability/stress model of schizophrenic episodes. *Schizophrenia Bulletin, 10,* 300–312.

Oakley Browne, M. A., Wells, J. E., Scott, K. M., *et al.* (2006) Lifetime prevalence and projected lifetime risk of DSM-IV disorders in Te Rau Hinengaro: the New Zealand Mental Health Survey. *Australian and New Zealand Journal of Psychiatry, 40,* 865–874.

O'Dwyer, L. A., Baum, F., Kavanagh, A., *et al.* (2007) Do area-based interventions to reduce health inequalities work? A systematic review of evidence. *Critical Public Health, 17,* 317–335.

Olfson, M. & Gameroff, M. J. (2007) Generalized anxiety disorder, somatic pain and health care costs. *General Hospital Psychiatry, 29,* 310–316.

Ostler, K., Thompson, C., Kinmonth, A. L. K., *et al.* (2001) The influence of socio-economic deprivation on the prevalence and outcome of depression in primary care: the Hampshire Depression Project. *British Journal of Psychiatry, 178,* 12–17.

Ouimette, P., Cronkite, R., Prins, A., *et al.* (2004) Posttraumatic stress disorder, anger and hostility, and physical health status. *The Journal of Nervous and Mental Disease, 192,* 566.

*References*

Ozer, E. J., Best, S. R., Lipsey, T. L., *et al.* (2003) Predictors of post-traumatic stress disorder and symptoms in adults: a meta-analysis. *Psychological Bulletin, 129,* 52–73.

Panella, M., Demarchi, M. L., Carnevale, L., *et al.* (2006) The management of schizophrenia through clinical pathways. *Value Health, 9,* 318.

Parkerson, G. R. J. & Broadhead, W. E. (1997) Screening for anxiety and depression in primary care with the Duke Anxiety-Depression Scale. *Family Medicine, 29,* 177–181.

Patel, V., Araya, R., de Lima, M., *et al.* (1999) Women, poverty and common mental disorders in four restructuring societies. *Social Science & Medicine, 49,* 1461–1471.

Patel, V., Kirkwood B. R., Pednekar, S., *et al.* (2006) Gender disadvantage and reproductive health risk factors for common mental disorders in women. *Archives of General Psychiatry, 63,* 404–413.

Patten, S. B. (1991) Are the Brown and Harris 'vulnerability factors' risk factors for depression? *Journal of Psychiatry and Neuroscience, 16,* 267–271.

Paulden, M., Palmer, S., Hewitt, C., *et al.* (2010) Screening for postnatal depression in primary care: cost effectiveness analysis. *British Medical Journal, 339,* b5203.

Petersen, T., Andreotti, C. F., Chelminski, I., *et al.* (2009) Do comorbid anxiety disorders impact treatment planning for outpatients with major depressive disorder? *Psychiatry Research, 169,* 7–11.

Piccinelli, M. & Wilkinson, G. (2000) Gender differences in depression: critical review. *British Journal of Psychiatry, 177,* 486–492.

Pies, R. (2009) Should psychiatrists use atypical antipsychotics to treat nonpsychotic anxiety. *Psychiatry, 6,* 29–37.

Pignone, M., DeWalt, D. A., Sheridan, S., *et al.* (2005) Interventions to improve health outcomes for patients with low literacy: a systematic review. *Journal of General Internal Medicine, 20,* 185–192.

Pignone, M. P., Gaynes, B. N., Rushton, J. L., *et al.* (2002) Screening for depression in adults: a summary of the evidence for the US Preventive Services Task Force. *Annals of Internal Medicine, 136,* 765–776.

Pilling, S. & Mavranezouli, I. (2010) Economic model misrepresents NICE guidance. [Letter]. *British Medical Journal,* 20 February 2010.

Ploeg, J., Feightner, J., Hutchison, B., *et al.* (2005) Effectiveness of preventive primary care outreach interventions aimed at older people: meta-analysis of randomized controlled trials. *Canadian Family Physician, 51,* 1244–1245.

Pompili, M., Serfini, G., Del Casale, A., *et al.* (2009) Improving assessment in mood disorders: the struggle against relapse, reoccurrence and suicide risk. *Expert Review of Neurotherapeutics, 9,* 985–1004.

Poole, N. A. & Morgan, J. F. (2006) Validity and reliability of the Hospital Anxiety and Depression Scale in a hypertrophic cardiomyopathy clinic: the HADS in a cardiomyopathy population. *General Hospital Psychiatry, 28,* 5–58.

Popay, J., Roberts, H., Sowden, A., *et al.* (2006) *Guidance on the Conduct of Narrative Synthesis in Systematic Reviews: a Product from the ESRC Methods Programme* (Version I). Lancaster: Institute of Health Research, 2006.

Powell, J. (2002) Systematic review of outreach clinics in primary care in the UK. *Journal of Health Services Research and Policy*, *7*, 177–178.

Priest, R. G., Vize, C., Roberts, A., *et al.* (1996) Lay people's attitudes to treatment of depression: results of opinion poll for Defeat Depression Campaign just before its launch. *British Medical Journal*, *313*, 858–859.

Prins, M. A., Verhaak, P. F. M., Bensing, J. M., *et al.* (2008) Health beliefs and perceived need for mental health care of anxiety and depression: the patients' perspective explored. *Clinical Psychology Review*, *28*, 1038–1058.

Rachman, S. (1998) A cognitive theory of obsessions: elaborations. *Behaviour Research and Therapy*, *36*, 385–401.

Rachman, S. (2002) A cognitive theory of compulsive checking. *Behaviour Research and Therapy*, *40*, 625–639.

Rachman, S. (2004) Fear of contamination. *Behaviour Research and Therapy*, *42*, 1227–1255.

Ramachandani, P. & Stein, A. (2003) The impact of parental psychiatric disorder on children. *British Medical Journal*, *327*, 242–243.

Richards, M., Maughan, B., Hardy, R., *et al.* (2001) Long-term affective disorder in people with mild intellectual disability. *British Journal of Psychiatry*, *179*, 523–527.

Rodriguez, M., Valentine, J. M., Son, J. B., *et al.* (2009) Intimate partner violence and barriers to mental health care for ethnically diverse populations of women. *Trauma Violence Abuse*, *10*, 358–374.

Rogers A., Hassell, K. & Nicolaas, G. (1999) *Demanding Patients? Analysing the Use of Primary Care*. Milton Keynes: Open University Press.

Rosenfeld, R., Dar, R., Anderson, D., *et al.* (1992) A computer-administered version of the Yale-Brown Obsessive Compulsive Scale. *Psychological Assessment*, *4*, 329–332.

Roth, A. & Fonagy, P. (2004) *What Works For Whom? A Critical Review of Psychotherapy Research*. New York: Guilford Publications.

Rowe, S. K. & Rapaport, M. H. (2006) Classification and treatment of sub-threshold depression. *Current Opinion in Psychiatry*, *19*, 9–13.

Rush, J. A., Trivedia, M. T., Carmodya, T. J., *et al.* (2004) One-year clinical outcomes of depressed public sector outpatients: a benchmark for subsequent studies. *Biological Psychiatry*, *56*, 46–53.

Salkovskis, P. M., Shafran, R., Rachman, S., *et al.* (1999) Multiple pathways to inflated responsibility beliefs in obsessional problems: possible origins and implications for therapy and research, *Behaviour Research and Therapy*, *37*, 1055–1072.

Salokangas, R. K. R. & Poutanen, O. (1998) Risk factors for depression in primary care: findings of the TADEP project. *Journal of Affective Disorders*, *48*, 171–180.

Sareen, J., Jacobi, F., Cox, B. J., *et al.* (2006) Disability and poor quality of life associated with comorbid anxiety disorders and physical conditions. *Archives of Internal Medicine*, *166*, 2109–2116.

Sartorius, N. (2001) The economic and social burden of depression. *Journal of Clinical Psychiatry*, *62*, 8–11.

Sartorius, N. (2002) Eines der letzen Hindernisse einer verbesserten psychiatrischen Versorgung: das Stigma psychisher Erkrankung [One of the last obstacles to better mental health care: the stigma of mental illness]. *Neuropsychiatrie, 16*, 5–10.

Scheppers, E., van Dongen, E., Dekker, J., *et al.* (2006) Potential barriers to the use of health services among ethnic minorities: a review. *Family Practice, 23*, 325–348.

Schmitz, N., Kruse, J., Heckrath, C., *et al.* (1999) Diagnosing mental disorders in primary care: the General Health Questionnaire (GHQ) and the Symptom Check List (SCL-90-R) as screening instruments. *Social Psychiatry and Psychiatric Epidemiology, 34*, 360–366.

Schnurr, P. P. & Green, B. L. (eds) (2003) *Trauma and Health: Physical Consequences of Exposure to Extreme Stress.* Washington, DC: American Psychological Association

Schünemann, H. J., Best, D., Vist, G., *et al.* (2003) Letters, numbers, symbols and words: how to communicate grades of evidence and recommendations. *Canadian Medical Association Journal, 169*, 677–680.

Scogin, F., Hanson, A. & Welsh, D. (2003) Self-administered treatment in stepped-care models of depression treatment. *Journal of Clinical Psychology, 59*, 341–349.

Shah, R., McNiece, R. & Majeed, A. (2001) General practice consultation rates for psychiatric disorders in patients aged 65 and over: prospective cohort study. *International Journal of Geriatric Psychiatry, 16*, 57–63.

Sherbourne, C. D., Wells, K. B. & Judd, L. L. (1996) Functioning and well-being of patients with panic disorder. *American Journal of Psychiatry, 153*, 213–218.

Shimokawa, K., Lambert, M. J., Smart, D. W. (2010) Enhancing treatment outcome of patients at risk of treatment failure: meta-analytic and mega-analytic review of a psychotherapy quality assurance system. *Journal of Consulting and Clinical Psychology, 78*, 298–311.

Simon, G., Ormel, J., VonKorff, M., *et al.* (1995) Health care costs associated with depressive and anxiety disorders in primary care. *American Journal of Psychiatry, 152*, 352–357.

Simon, G. E., Goldberg, D. P., von Korff, M., *et al.* (2002) Understanding crossnational differences in depression prevalence. *Psychological Medicine, 32*, 585–594.

Simpson, S. M., Krishnan, L. L., Kunik, M. E., *et al.* (2007) Racial disparities in diagnosis and treatment of depression: a literature review. *Psychiatric Quarterly, 78*, 3–14.

Singleton, N., Bumpstead, R., O'Brien, M., *et al.* (2001) *Psychiatric Morbidity Among Adults Living in Private Households.* London: The Stationery Office.

Skoog, G. & Skoog, I. (1999) A 40-year follow-up of patients with obsessive compulsive disorder. *Archives of General Psychiatry, 56*, 121–127.

Skultety, K. M. & Zeiss, A. (2006) The treatment of depression in older adults in the primary care setting: an evidence-based review. *Health Psychology, 25*, 665–674.

Slattery, M. J., Dubbert, B. K., Allan, A. J., *et al.* (2004) Prevalence of obsessive compulsive-disorder in patients with systemic lupus erythematosis. *Journal of Clinical Psychiatry*, *65*, 301–306.

Smiley, E. (2005) Epidemiology of mental health problems in adults with learning disabilities: an update. *Advances in Psychiatric Treatment*, *11*, 214–222.

Smith, A. B., Wright, E. P., Rush, R., *et al.* (2006) Rasch analysis of the dimensional structure of the Hospital Anxiety and Depression Scale. *Psycho-Oncology*, *15*, 817–827.

Smolders, M., Laurant, M., Roberge, P., *et al.* (2008) Knowledge transfer and improvement of primary and ambulatory care for patients with anxiety. *Canadian Journal of Psychiatry*, *53*, 277–293.

Solomon, S. D. & Davidson, J. R. T. (1997) Trauma: prevalence, impairment, service use and cost. *Journal of Clinical Psychiatry*, *58*, 5–11.

Souêtre, E., Lozet, H., Cimarosti, I., *et al.* (1994) Cost of anxiety disorders: impact of comorbidity. *Journal of Psychosomatic Research*, *38*, 151–160.

Spitzer, R. L., Kroenke, K., Williams, J. B., *et al.* (1999) Validation and utility of a self-report version of the PRIME-MD: the PHQ primary care study. *Journal of the American Medical Association*, *282*, 1737–1744.

Spitzer, R. L., Kroenke, K., Williams, J. B. W., *et al.* (2006) A brief measure for assessing generalized anxiety disorder: the GAD-7. *Archives of Internal Medicine*, *166*, 1092–1097.

Stansfeld, S. A., Fuhrer, R., Shipley, M. J., *et al.* (1999) Work characteristics predict psychiatric disorder: prospective results from the Whitehall II study. *Occupational and Environmental Medicine*, *56*, 302–307.

Stark, D., Kiely, M., Smith, A., *et al.* (2002) Anxiety disorders in cancer patients: their nature, associations, and relation to quality of life. *Journal of Clinical Oncology*, *14*, 3137–3148.

StataCorp (2007) *Stata Statistical Software: Release 10*. College Station, TX: StataCorp LP.

Steketee, G., Frost, R. & Bogart, K. (1996) The Yale-Brown Obsessive Compulsive Scale: interview versus self-report. *Behaviour Research and Therapy*, *34*, 675–684.

Taylor, S. (1995) Assessment of obsessions and compulsions: reliability, validity, and sensitivity to treatment effects. *Clinical Psychology Reviews*, *15*, 261–296.

Taylor, S., Thordarson, D. S. & Sachting, I. (2002) Obsessive-compulsive disorder. In *Handbook of Assessment and Treatment Planning for Psychological Disorders* (eds M. M. Anthony & D. H. Barlow), pp. 182–214. New York: Guilford Press.

Thomas, C. M. & Morris, S. (2003) Cost of depression among adults in England in 2000. *British Journal of Psychiatry*, *183*, 514–519.

Thompson, C., Kinmonth, A. L., Steven, L., *et al.* (2000) Effects of a clinical-practice guideline and practice-based education on detection and outcome of depression in primary care: Hampshire Depression Project randomized controlled trial. *Lancet*, *355*, 50–57.

Thompson, C., Ostler, K., Peveler, R. C., *et al.* (2001) Dimensional perspective on the recognition of depressive symptoms in primary care. *British Journal of Psychiatry*, *179*, 317–323.

Tiemens, B. G., Ormel, J., Jenner, J. A., *et al.* (1999) Training primary-care physicians to recognize, diagnose and manage depression: does it improve patient outcomes? *Psychological Medicine, 29,* 833–845.

Titov, N., Andrews, G., Robinson, E., *et al.* (2009) Clinician-assisted internet-based treatment is effective for generalized anxiety disorder: randomized controlled trial. *Australian and New Zealand Journal of Psychiatry, 43,* 905–912.

Tylee A. & Walters P. (2007) Underrecognition of anxiety and mood disorders in primary care: why does the problem exist and what can be done? *Journal of Clinical Psychiatry, 68,* 27–30.

Tyrer, P. & Baldwin, D. (2006) Generalised anxiety disorder. *The Lancet, 368,* 2156–2166.

Tyrer, P., Seivewright, H. & Johnson, T. (2004) The Nottingham study of neurotic disorder: predictors of 12-year outcome of dysthymia, panic disorder and generalized anxiety disorder. *Psychological Medicine, 34,* 1385–1394.

Üstün, T. B. & Sartorius, N. (eds) (1995) *Mental Illness in General Health Care: an International Study.* Chichester: Wiley.

Van Citters, A. D. & Bartels, S. J. (2004) A systematic review of the effect of community-based mental health outreach services for older adults. *Psychiatric Services, 55,* 1237–1249.

van Oppen, P. & Arntz, A. (1994) Cognitive therapy for obsessive-compulsive disorder. *Behaviour Research and Therapy, 32,* 79–87.

Van Voorhees, B. W., Walters, A. E., Prochaska, M., *et al.* (2007) Reducing health disparities in depressive disorders outcomes between non-Hispanic whites and ethnic minorities: a call for pragmatic strategies over the life course. *Medical Care Research and Review, 64,* 157–194.

Vanhaecht, K., Bollmann, M., Bower, K., *et al.* (2007) Prevalence and use of clinical pathways in 23 countries: an international survey by the European Pathway Association. *Journal of Integrated Care Pathways, 10,* 28–34.

Vanherck, P., Vanhaecht, K. & Sermeus, W. (2004) Effects of clinical pathways: do they work? *Journal of Integrated Pathways, 8,* 95.

Von Korff, M., Shapiro, S., Burke, J. D., *et al.* (1987) Anxiety and depression in a primary care clinic: comparison of Diagnostic Interview Schedule, General Health Questionnaire, and practitioner assessments. *Archives of General Psychiatry, 44,* 152–156.

Waraich, P., Goldner, E. M., Somers, J. M. *et al.* (2004) Prevalence and incidence studies of mood disorders: a systematic review of the literature. *Canadian Journal of Psychiatry, 49,* 124–138.

Warrilow, A. E. & Beech, B. (2009) Self-help CBT for depression: opportunities for primary care mental health nurses? *Journal of Psychiatric and Mental Health Nursing, 16,* 792–803.

Weathers, F. W. & Ford, J. (1996) Psychometric properties of the PTSD Checklist (PCL–C, PCL–S, PCL–M, PCL–PR). In *Measurement of Stress, Trauma and Adaptation* (ed. B. H. Stamm). Lutherville, MD: Sidran Press.

Webb, S. A., Diefenbach, G., Wagener, P., *et al.* (2008) Comparison of self-report measures for identifying late-life generalized anxiety in primary care. *Journal of Geriatric Psychiatry and Neurology, 21,* 223–231.

Weich, S. & Lewis, G. (1998a) Poverty, unemployment and common mental disorders: population based study. *British Medical Journal, 317,* 115–119.

Weich, S. & Lewis, G. (1998b) Material standard of living, social class, and the prevalence of the common mental disorders in Great Britain. *Journal of Epidemiology & Community Health, 52,* 8–14.

Weiss, D. S. & Marmar, C. R. (1997) The Impact of Event Scale – Revised. In *Assessing Psychological Trauma and PTSD* (eds J. P. Wilson & T. Keane), pp. 399–411. New York: Guilford Press.

Weissman, M. M. & Merikangas, K. R. (1986) The epidemiology of anxiety and panic disorders: an update. *Journal of Clinical Psychiatry, 47,* 11–17.

Weissman, M. M., Broadhead, W. M., Olfson, M., *et al.* (1998) A diagnostic aid for detecting (DSM-IV) mental disorders in primary care. *General Hospital Psychiatry, 20,* 1–11.

Welkowitz, L. A., Struening, E. L., Pittman, J., *et al.* (2000) Obsessive-compulsive disorder and comorbid anxiety problems in a national anxiety screening sample. *Journal of Anxiety Disorders, 14,* 471–482.

Wells, A. (2000) *Emotional Disorders and Metacognition: Innovative Cognitive Therapy.* New York: John Wiley & Sons.

Westen, K. & Morrison, A. (2001) A multidimensional meta-analysis of treatments for depression, panic, and generalized anxiety disorder: an empirical examination of the status of empirically supported treatments. *Journal of Consulting and Clinical Psychology, 69,* 875–899.

Wetherell, J. L., Kim, D. S., Lindamer, L. A., *et al.* (2007) Anxiety disorders in a public mental health system: clinical characteristics and service use patterns. *Journal of Affective Disorders, 104,* 179–183.

Whelan-Goodinson, R., Ponsford, J. & Schonberger, M. (2009) Validity of the Hospital Anxiety and Depression Scale to assess depression and anxiety following traumatic brain injury as compared with the Structured Clinical Interview for DSM-IV. *Journal of Affective Disorders, 114,* 94–102.

Whitaker, S. & Read, S. (2006) The prevalence of psychiatric disorders among people with intellectual disabilities: an analysis of the literature. *Journal of Applied Research in Intellectual Disabilities, 19,* 330–345.

Whittle, C. & Hewison, A. (2007) Integrated care pathways: pathways to change in health care? *Journal of Health Organization and Management, 21,* 297–306.

WHO (1992) *The ICD–10 Classification of Mental and Behavioural Disorders: Clinical Descriptions and Diagnostic Guidelines.* Geneva, Switzerland: WHO.

WHO (2002) *The World Health Report 2002: Reducing Risks, Promoting Healthy Life.* Geneva, Switzerland: WHO.

Whooley, M. A., Avins, A. L., Miranda, J., *et al.* (1997) Case-finding instruments for depression: two questions are as good as many. *Journal of General Internal Medicine, 12,* 439–445.

Wilkinson, M. J. B. & Barczak, P. (1988) Psychiatric screening in general practice: comparison of the general health questionnaire and the hospital anxiety depression scale. *The Journal of Royal College of General Practitioners*, *38*, 311–313.

Williams, J. W., Noel, P. H., Cordes, J. A., *et al.* (2002) Is this patient clinically depressed? *Journal of the American Medical Association*, *287*, 1160–1170.

Williamson, R. J., Neale, B. M., Sterne, A., *et al.* (2005) The value of four mental health self-report scales in predicting interview-based mood and anxiety disorder diagnoses in sibling pairs. *Twin Research and Human Genetics*, *8*, 101–107.

Wilson, A., Tobin, M., Ponzio, V., *et al.* (1997) Developing a clinical pathway in depression: sharing our experience. *Australasian Psychiatry*, *7*, 17–9.

Wittchen, H. U. & Jacobi, F. (2005) Size and burden of mental disorders in Europe-a critical review and appraisal of 27 studies. *European Neuropsychopharmacology*, *15*, 357–376.

Wittchen, H. U., Carter, R., Pfister, H., *et al.* (2000) Disabilities and quality of life in pure and comorbid generalized anxiety disorder and major depression in a national survey. *International Clinical Psychopharmacology*, *15*, 319–328.

Wittchen, H. U., Kessler, R. C., Beesdo, K., *et al.* (2002) Generalised anxiety and depression in primary care: prevalence, recognition, and management. *Journal of Clinical Psychiatry*, *63*, 24–34.

World Bank (1993) *World Development Report: Investing in Health Research Development.* Geneva, Switzerland: World Bank.

Yonkers, K. A., Warshaw, M. G., Massion, A. O., *et al.* (1996) Phenomenology and course of generalised anxiety disorder. *The British Journal of Psychiatry*, *168*, 308–313.

Zatzick, D. F., Marmar, C. R., Weiss, D. S., *et al.* (1997) Posttraumatic stress disorder and functioning and quality of life outcomes in a nationally representative sample of male Vietnam veterans. *American Journal of Psychiatry*, *154*, 1690–1695.

Zhu, B., Zhao, Z., Ye, W., *et al.* (2009) The cost of comorbid depression and pain for individuals diagnosed with generalized anxiety disorder. *Journal of Nervous & Mental Disease*, *197*, 136–139.

Zigmond, A. S. & Snaith, R. P. (1983) The Hospital Anxiety and Depression Rating Scale. *Acta Psychiatrica Scandinavica*, *67*, 361–370.

Zimmerman, M., McDermut, W. & Mattia, J. I. (2000) Frequency of anxiety disorders in psychiatric outpatients with major depressive disorder. *American Journal of Psychiatry*, *157*, 1337–1340.

Zohar, J. & Judge, R. (1996) Paroxetine versus clomipramine in the treatment of obsessive-compulsive disorder. OCD Paroxetine Study Investigators. *British Journal of Psychiatry*, *169*, 468–474.

# 11    GLOSSARY

This provides definitions of a number of terms, based on definitions from related NICE guidelines. The list aims to cover the most commonly used terms and is not intended to be exhaustive.

**Active monitoring**: an active process of assessment, monitoring symptoms and functioning, advice and support for people with mild common mental health disorders that may spontaneously remit. It involves discussing the presenting problem(s) and any concerns that the person may have about them, providing information about the nature and course of the disorder, arranging a further assessment, normally within 2 weeks, and making contact if the person does not attend follow-up appointments. Also known as 'watchful waiting'.

**Applied relaxation**: a psychological intervention that focuses on applying muscular relaxation in situations and occasions where the person is or might be anxious. The intervention usually consists of 12 to 15 weekly sessions (fewer if the person recovers sooner, more if clinically required), each lasting 1 hour.

**Alcohol dependence**: characterised by craving, tolerance, a preoccupation with alcohol and continued drinking in spite of harmful consequences.

**Befriending**: meeting and talking with someone with a mental health problem usually once a week; this would be provided as an adjunct to any psychological or pharmacological intervention. The befriender may accompany the befriendee on trips to broaden their range of activities and offer practical support with ongoing difficulties.

**Behavioural activation**: a psychological intervention for depression that aims to identify the effects of behaviour on current symptoms, mood and problem areas. It seeks to reduce symptoms and problematic behaviours through behavioural tasks related to reducing avoidance, activity scheduling, and enhancing positively reinforced behaviours. The intervention usually consists of 16 to 20 sessions over 3 to 4 months.

**Behavioural couples therapy**: a psychological intervention that aims to help people understand the effects of their interactions on each other as factors in the development and maintenance of symptoms and problems, and to change the nature of the interactions so that the person's mental health problems improve. The intervention should be based on behavioural principles and usually consists of 15 to 20 sessions over 5 to 6 months.

**Cognitive behavioural therapy (CBT)**: a psychological intervention where the person works collaboratively with the therapist to identify the effects of thoughts, beliefs and interpretations on current symptoms, feelings states and problems areas. They learn the skills to identity, monitor and then counteract problematic thoughts, beliefs and interpretations related to the target symptoms or problems, and appropriate coping skills. Duration of treatment varies depending on the disorder and its severity but for people with depression it should be in the range of 16 to 20 sessions over 3 to 4 months; for people with GAD it should usually consist of 12 to 15 weekly sessions (fewer if the person recovers sooner, more if clinically required), each lasting 1 hour.

**Collaborative care**: in the context of this guideline, a coordinated approach to mental and physical healthcare involving the following elements: case management which is supervised and has support from a senior mental health professional; close collaboration between primary and secondary physical health services and specialist mental health services; a range of interventions consistent with those recommended in this guideline, including patient education, psychological and pharmacological interventions, and medication management; and long-term coordination of care and follow-up.

**Computerised cognitive behavioural therapy (CCBT)**: a form of cognitive behavioural therapy that is provided via a stand-alone computer-based or web-based programme. It should include an explanation of the CBT model, encourage tasks between sessions, and use thought-challenging and active monitoring of behaviour, thought patterns and outcomes. It should be supported by a trained practitioner who typically provides limited facilitation of the programme and reviews progress and outcome. The intervention typically takes place over 9 to 12 weeks, including follow-up.

**Counselling**: a short-term supportive approach that aims to help people explore their feelings and problems, and make dynamic changes in their lives and relationships. The intervention usually consists of six to ten sessions over 8 to 12 weeks.

**Eye movement desensitisation and reprocessing (EMDR)**: a psychological intervention for PTSD. During EMDR, the person is asked to concentrate on an image connected to the traumatic event and the related negative emotions, sensations and thoughts, while paying attention to something else, usually the therapist's fingers moving from side to side in front of the person's eyes. After each set of eye movements (about 20 seconds), the person is encouraged to discuss the images and emotions they felt during the eye movements. The process is repeated with a focus on any difficult, persisting memories. Once the person feels less distressed about the image, they are asked to concentrate on it while having a positive thought relating to it. The treatment should normally be 8 to 12 sessions when the PTSD results from a single event. When the trauma is discussed in the treatment session, longer sessions than usual are generally necessary (for example 90 minutes). Treatment should be regular and continuous (usually at least once a week).

**Exposure and response prevention (ERP)**: a psychological intervention used for people with OCD that aims to help people to overcome their need to engage in obsessional and compulsive behaviours. With the support of a practitioner, the person is exposed to whatever makes them anxious, distressed or fearful. Rather than avoiding the situation, or repeating a compulsion, the person is trained in other ways of coping with anxiety, distress or fear. The process is repeated until the person no longer feels this way.

**Facilitated self-help**: in the context of this guideline, facilitated self-help (also known as guided self-help or bibliotherapy) is defined as a self-administered intervention, which makes use of a range of books or other self-help manuals, and electronic materials based on the principles of CBT and of an appropriate reading age. A trained practitioner typically facilitates the use of this material by introducing it, and reviewing progress and outcomes. The intervention consists of up to six to eight sessions (face-to-face and via telephone) normally taking place over 9 to 12 weeks, including follow up.

**Group-based peer support (self-help) programme**: in the context of this guideline, a support (self-help) programme delivered to groups of patients with depression and a shared chronic physical health problem. The focus is on sharing experiences and feelings associated with having a chronic physical health problem. The programme is supported by practitioners who facilitate attendance at the meetings, have knowledge of the patients' chronic physical health problem and its relationship to depression, and review the outcomes of the intervention with the individual patients. The intervention consists typically of one session per week over a period of 8 to 12 weeks.

**Harmful drinking**: a pattern of alcohol consumption causing health problems directly related to alcohol. This could include psychological problems such as depression, alcohol-related accidents or physical illness such as acute pancreatitis.

**Interpersonal therapy (IPT)**: a psychological intervention that focuses on interpersonal issues. The person works with the therapist to identify the effects of problematic areas related to interpersonal conflicts, role transitions, grief and loss, and social skills, and their effects on current symptoms, feelings states and problems. They seek to reduce symptoms by learning to cope with or resolve such problems or conflicts. The intervention usually consists of 16 to 20 sessions over 3 to 4 months.

**Low-intensity interventions**: brief psychological interventions with reduced contact with a trained practitioner, where the focus is on a shared definition of the presenting problem, and the practitioner facilitates and supports the use of a range of self-help materials. The role adopted by the practitioner is one of coach or facilitator. Examples include: facilitated and non-facilitated self-help, CCBT, physical activity programmes, group-based peer support (self-help) programmes, and psychoeducational groups.

**Mindfulness-based cognitive therapy**: a group-based skills training programme using techniques drawn from meditation and cognitive therapy designed specifically to prevent depressive relapse or recurrence of depression. Its aim is to enable people to learn to become more aware of bodily sensations, and thoughts and feelings associated with depressive relapse. The intervention usually consists of eight weekly 2-hour sessions and four follow-up sessions in the 12 months after the end of treatment.

**Non-facilitated self-help**: in the context of this guideline, non-facilitated self-help (also known as pure self-help or bibliotherapy) is defined as a self-administered intervention, which makes use of written or electronic materials based on the principles of CBT and of an appropriate reading age. The intervention usually involves minimal contact with a practitioner (for example an occasional short telephone call of no more than 5 minutes) and includes instructions for the person to work systematically through the materials over a period of at least 6 weeks.

**Paraprofessional**: a staff member who is trained to deliver a range of specific healthcare interventions, but does not have NHS professional training, such as a psychological wellbeing practitioner.

**Physical activity programme**: in the context of this guideline, physical activity programmes are defined as structured and group-based (with support from a competent practitioner) and consist typically of three sessions per week of moderate duration (24 minutes to 1 hour) over 10 to 14 weeks (average 12 weeks).

**Psychoeducation**: the provision of information and advice about a disorder and its treatment. It usually involves an explanatory model of the symptoms and advice on how to cope with or overcome the difficulties a person may experience. It is usually of brief duration, instigated by a healthcare professional, and supported by the use of written materials.

**Psychoeducational groups**: a psychosocial group-based intervention based on the principles of CBT that has an interactive design and encourages observational learning. It may include presentations and self-help manuals. It is conducted by trained practitioners, with a ratio of one therapist to about 12 participants and usually consists of six weekly 2-hour sessions.

**Somatic symptoms**: physical symptoms of common mental health disorders, which form part of the cluster of symptoms that are necessary for achieving a diagnosis. They may include palpitations or muscular tension in an anxiety disorder or lethargy and sleep disturbance in depression. In some cases they may be the main symptom with which a person first presents; they do not constitute a separate diagnosis and should be distinguished from somatoform disorders and medically unexplained symptoms.

**Short-term psychodynamic psychotherapy**: a psychological intervention where the therapist and person explore and gain insight into conflicts and how these are represented in current situations and relationships including the therapeutic relationship. Therapy is non-directive and recipients are not taught specific skills (for example, thought monitoring, re-evaluating, and problem solving.) The intervention usually consists of 16 to 20 sessions over 4 to 6 months.

**Severity**: see the section on 'assessing severity of common mental health disorders' below.

**Trauma-focused CBT**: a type of CBT specifically developed for people with PTSD that focuses on memories of trauma and negative thoughts and behaviours associated with such memories. The structure and content of the intervention are based on CBT principles with an explicit focus on the traumatic event that led to the disorder. The intervention normally consists of 8 to 12 sessions when the PTSD results from a single event. When the trauma is discussed in the treatment session, longer sessions than usual are generally necessary (for example 90 minutes). Treatment should be regular and continuous (usually at least once a week).

*Assessing severity of common mental health disorders: definitions*
Assessing the severity of common mental health disorders is determined by three factors: symptom severity, duration of symptoms and associated functional impairment (for example, impairment of vocational, educational, social or other functioning).

**Mild** generally refers to relatively few core symptoms (although sufficient to achieve a diagnosis), a limited duration and little impact on day-to-day functioning.

**Moderate** refers to the presence of all core symptoms of the disorder plus several other related symptoms, duration beyond that required by minimum diagnostic criteria, and a clear impact on functioning.

**Severe** refers to the presence of most or all symptoms of the disorder, often of long duration and with very marked impact on functioning (for example, an inability to participate in work-related activities and withdrawal from interpersonal activities).

**Persistent subthreshold** refers to symptoms and associated functional impairment that do not meet full diagnostic criteria but have a substantial impact on a person's life, and which are present for a significant period of time (usually no less than 6 months and up to several years).

# 12   ABBREVIATIONS

| | |
|---|---|
| **ADD** | Anxiety and Depression Detector |
| **ADS-GA (-3)** | Anxiety Disorder Scale – Generalised Anxiety Subscale (three items) |
| **AGREE** | Appraisal of Guidelines for Research and Evaluation Instrument |
| **APA** | American Psychiatric Association |
| **ASSIA** | Applied Social Sciences Index and Abstracts |
| **AUC** | area under the curve |
| | |
| **BAI (-FS)** | Beck Anxiety Inventory (– Fast Screen) |
| **BDI (-II)** | Beck Depression Inventory (2nd edition) |
| **BHS** | Beck Hopelessness Scale |
| **BME** | black and minority ethnic |
| **BMJ** | *British Medical Journal* |
| **BSI** | Brief Symptom Inventory |
| | |
| **CBT** | cognitive behavioural therapy |
| **CCBT** | computerised cognitive behavioural therapy |
| **CDSR** | Cochrane Database of Systematic Reviews |
| **CENTRAL** | Cochrane Central Register of Controlled Trials |
| **CES-D** | Center for Epidemiological Studies Depression scale |
| **CI** | confidence interval |
| **CIDI (-Auto)** | Composite International Diagnostic Interview (– Computerized) |
| **CINAHL** | Cumulative Index to Nursing and Allied Health Literature |
| **CMDQ** | Common Mental Disorder Questionnaire |
| | |
| **DALY** | disability-adjusted life year |
| **DARE** | (Cochrane) Database of Abstracts of Reviews of Effects |
| **DSM (-III, -IV, -R, TR)** | *Diagnostic and Statistical Manual of Mental Disorders* of the American Psychiatric Association (3rd edition, 4th edition, Revised, Text Revision) |
| | |
| **EconLit** | The American Economic Association's electronic bibliography |
| **ECT** | electro-convulsive therapy |
| **EED** | Economic Evaluation Database |
| **EMBASE** | Excerpta Medical Database |
| **EMDR** | eye movement desensitisation and reprocessing |
| **EPDS** | Edinburgh Postnatal Depression scale |
| **EPQ-N** | Eysenck Personality Questionnaire – Neuroticism Scale |

| | |
|---|---|
| EQ-5D | European Quality of Life – 5 Dimensions |
| ERP | exposure and response prevention |
| FN | false negative |
| FP | false positive |
| | |
| G-I-N | Guidelines Internationalï Network |
| GAD | generalised anxiety disorder |
| GAD-2, -7) | Generalized Anxiety Disorder scale -2 items, -7 items |
| GAD-Q-IV | Generalized Anxiety Disorders Questionnaire 4th Edition |
| GAI-SF | Geriatric Anxiety Inventory – Short Form |
| GDG | Guideline Development Group |
| GHQ-12 | General Health Questionnaire – 12 item version |
| GP | general practitioner |
| GRADE | Grading of Recommendations: Assessment, Development and Evaluation |
| | |
| HADS (-A) | Hospital Anxiety and Depression Scale (–Anxiety subscale) |
| HE | health economic |
| HIV | human immunodeficiency virus |
| HoNOS-PbR | Health of the Nation Outcome Scales, Payment by Results |
| HRG | healthcare resource group |
| HRQoL | health-related quality of life |
| HTA | Health Technology Assessment |
| | |
| IAPT | Improving Access to Psychological Therapies programme |
| ICD-10 | *International Classification of Diseases* (10th revision) |
| ICER | incremental cost-effectiveness ratio |
| IPT | interpersonal therapy |
| | |
| k | number of studies |
| | |
| LR− | negative likelihood ratio |
| LR+ | positive likelihood ratio |
| | |
| MCS (-12) | Mental Health Component Summary scale (12 items) |
| MD | mean difference |
| MDD | major depressive disorder |
| MEDLINE | Medical Literature Analysis and Retrieval System Online |
| | |
| n | number of participants in a group |
| N | total number of participants |
| NA or N/A | not applicable |
| NCCMH | National Collaborating Centre for Mental Health |
| NHS | National Health Service |
| NICE | National Institute for Health and Clinical Excellence |
| NIMH | National Institute of Mental Health |

*Abbreviations*

| | |
|---|---|
| **OASIS** | Overall Anxiety Sensitivity and Impairment Scale |
| **OCD** | obsessive-compulsive disorder |
| **ONS** | Office for National Statistics |
| **OR** | odds ratio |
| | |
| **PHQ (-A, -9)** | Patient Health Questionnaire (– Anxiety module; – nine items) |
| **PICO** | patient/population, intervention, comparison and outcome |
| **PRIME-MD** | Primary Care Evaluation of Mental Disorders |
| **PSS** | personal social services |
| **PSWQ (-A)** | Penn State Worry Questionnaire (– Abbreviated) |
| **PsyINDEX** | |
| **PsycLIT** | |
| **PsycINFO** | Psychological Information Database |
| **PTSD** | post-traumatic stress disorder |
| **PubMed** | National Library of Medicine's collection database |
| | |
| **QALY** | quality-adjusted life year |
| **QI** | quality improvement |
| **QOF** | *Quality and Outcomes Framework Guidance for GMS Contract* |
| | |
| **RCT** | randomised controlled trial |
| **ROC** | receiver operator characteristic |
| **ROM** | routine outcome monitoring |
| **RR** | relative risk |
| **RSCL** | Rotterdam Symptom Checklist |
| | |
| **SCID-IV** | Structured Clinical Interview for DSM-IV Axis I Disorders |
| **SF (-12, 6D)** | Short Form Health Survey (12 items, six dimensions) |
| **SIGN** | Scottish Intercollegiate Guidelines Network |
| **SMD** | standardised mean difference |
| **SSRI** | selective serotonin reuptake inhibitor |
| | |
| **TiC-P** | Trimbos/iMTA Questionnaire on Costs Associated with Psychiatric Illness |
| **TN** | true negative |
| **TP** | true positive |
| | |
| **VAS** | Visual Analogue Scale |
| | |
| **WHO** | World Health Organization |
| **WHO-5** | World Health Organization Wellbeing Index |

310